C000272020

Everything is Washable*

And other life lessons

(Almost)

Sali Hughes

Also by Sali Hughes

Our Rainbow Queen

Pretty Iconic: A Personal Look at the Beauty Products that Changed the World

Pretty Honest: The Straight-Talking Beauty Companion

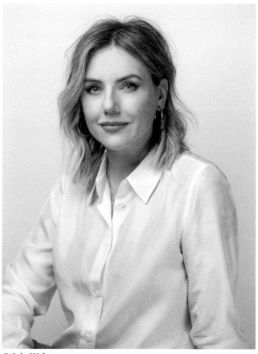

© Jake Walters

SALI HUGHES is a leading journalist, presenter and broadcaster with over 24 years' experience. A former magazine editor, she has written extensively for *Vogue, Elle, Grazia,* the *Telegraph,* the *Observer, Red* and *Radio Times.* She has been beauty editor on the *Guardian* since 2011, where she is known for her intelligent, straight-talking advice and honest product recommendations.

Sali is a very experienced radio broadcaster, appearing frequently on BBC Radio 4's *Woman's Hour,* and her own popular YouTube series of 'In the Bathroom With ...' interviews has won three industry awards.

In 2018 she co-founded Beauty Banks, a nationwide charity providing essential toiletries to people living in poverty, for which she and co-founder Jo Jones have won several major awards. In 2022 she was awarded an Honorary Fellowship from Cardiff University for services to journalism and charity.

Sali has a large social media presence and can be found on Twitter and Instagram @salihughes. She lives in Brighton.

Everything is Washable*

And other life lessons

(Almost)

Sali Hughes

4th Estate · London

4th Estate
An imprint of HarperCollins*Publishers*
1 London Bridge Street
London SE1 9GF
www.4thEstate.co.uk

HarperCollins*Publishers*
1st Floor, Watermarque Building, Ringsend Road, Dublin 4, Ireland

First published in Great Britain in 2022 by 4th Estate

1

Text copyright © Sali Hughes 2022

A catalogue record for this book is available from the British Library
ISBN 978-0-00-828417-6

This book has been written by Sali Hughes based on her own experiences and knowledge; the advice in it should be used to complement, and not as a substitute for, professional advice.

Always follow the manufacturer's instructions when using kitchen appliances and other electrical tools and equipment.

Designed by Jack Smyth
Typeset by GS Typesetting

Printed and bound by GPS Group

This book is produced from independently certified FSC™ paper to ensure responsible forest management.

For more information visit: www.harpercollins.co.uk/green

For Daniel Maier, with love

Acknowledgements

First and foremost, I must thank Georgia Garrett, who supports me, believes in me and frightens me, all at the optimal levels. Truly, I cannot believe my good fortune. And to Louise Haines and her team at 4th Estate. Their generosity, patience, kindness and continued enthusiasm during a very difficult time personally made all the difference professionally. I really can't thank them enough. Huge thanks to my brother, Wyn, who filled some of my memory gaps and remains the family's best lighter of fires (literally, not metaphorically). Thank you also to the indefatigable Jo Jones, Lauren Oakey and Leo Pemberton for generously allowing me to shirk some of my Beauty Banks responsibilities towards the end of the writing process, shouldering my workload as well as their own, to ensure our services weren't interrupted. Thanks also to Jimmy Bent and Marco Mini, who will be furious if Leo is mentioned without them. And to the brilliantly talented and decent Ed Griffiths and Megan Pidgeon at Insanity Group for moving around the other half of my life to accommodate the book.

Thank you to TT, for unfailingly being there, and always understanding me. This book couldn't exist without the quarterlies, dailies, hourlies. Your love and support means the world. For a long time, I stopped being able to write this book because my mind was so fogged by thoughts of those who I knew would hate it. In the end, the advice I gave myself is the same advice I'd now give any writer struggling to proceed: choose just one person who'd appreciate the piece, someone who'd find it helpful and valuable, and write it for them and them only. And so on that basis, a huge thanks must go to my dear friend Lucy Mangan, the person who asks me the most questions in life (many of them repeated verbatim in this book), who never left my mind, and for whom it remains a challenge and a pleasure to stay on my game.

Finally, thank you to my beloved husband, Daniel Maier, who forced me to get up while at my lowest ebb and pushed me forwards until it was done, and to Marvin and Arthur, the most interesting, funny, kind, supportive and understanding sons any mother could ask for. You three truly are the best, and you proved the book's title correct.

Contents

Home

'The most beautiful homes are not made with money, they are made with love, and no amount of cash alone can disguise an unhappy one.'

Several years ago, my boyfriend and I had to be at the Hay Literary Festival, and in an uncharacteristic fit of nostalgia, I suggested we drive to the village in which I grew up, some forty-five minutes away. We toured the landmarks – my grandparents' house, where I was born, the primary school I'd attended, the comprehensive I barely went to, the library where I sometimes hid until school had finished and I could return home – and, of course, my childhood homes, ending at where I had started: the small end-of-terrace I shared with my two big brothers and my father, following my mother's departure to a tiny flat a mile or so away. Dan and I had been stood outside for no more than a minute or two, peering as politely as we could at the house, when the door opened and a friendly older couple asked us if they could help. I told them I'd grown up in their house and they immediately invited us inside for tea. I feel tearful whenever I think of them, not only because their home – now bright, lovingly decorated and happy – holds so many unusual memories for me, but also because the owners were so generous and warm that I somehow felt more at home than I did when I could rightfully call that house my own.

As they showed us around, sharing with us all the work they'd done over the past thirty-plus years, the conversation turned to how they'd come to buy the place. They told us that some time after my family must have moved on, a man had moved in – an older Englishman whose wife had left him. He'd apparently become so depressed that he'd developed a drink problem and become what we'd now call a hoarder. There had been vermin, they told me. Litter throughout the house. Damp, mould. Every room was full of junk – old newspapers, broken furniture, filthy carpets and bags and bags of rubbish. The overgrown garden concealed broken glass, scrap and yet more rubbish bags. They were glad, they told me, that I'd never had to see my former home – the house we all loved – in such squalor. It had been a very sorry state of affairs. I nodded and smiled because I had too much pride, and felt too much shame, to tell them – and my new boyfriend – that the Englishman was my father and the house sounded much the same as when we'd left it.

I tell this story because, as sad as it made me in some ways, that day also showed me how a house's entire soul can be transplanted with proper cleaning, some organisational care and a few cherished, meaningful possessions. The most beautiful homes are not made with money, they are made with love, and no amount of cash alone can disguise an unhappy one. Because of the circumstances in which I grew up, and the unpredictable and precarious nature of my housing once I left home at nearly fifteen and came to London, I am undeniably obsessed with my home, which is the most important thing in my life after the people I love. I confess, I fetishise domesticity. Not in a frantic cushion-plumping, door-knocker-polishing, doorstep-scrubbing kind of way (though I am full of admiration and envy for the diligently house-proud), but insofar as there is nowhere in the world I'd rather be than on my own sofa or bed. I simply can't believe my good fortune in having a home that I love and I would do pretty much anything legal to hold on to it. It's where I feel safest, comfiest, happiest and most like myself.

You may be the same. Our homes give us so much, so I feel taking care of them is the least we can try to do in return. For me, that means keeping mine clean, of course. But more personally, it means owning things I truly treasure and not allowing the things I don't to obscure and overshadow them. It means keeping everything in good repair and proper working order, using the skills I learned from my maternal grandparents and great-godmother, who taught the very little me how to light a fire, sew on a button and operate a twin tub. It also means designing rooms, choosing colours, arranging photographs and decorations in a way that allows me to have the affectionate and intimate relationship with my home that, for a variety of reasons, my father was sadly unable to form. Here's how I've done it.

Old is usually better

I will not shop for a single item of furniture until I have first explored the second-hand options available. I estimate that at least half of my furniture is pre-owned and, in all honesty, I'd like that share to be higher. Vintage furniture is, in my unshakable view, unfailingly of a much higher quality than its modern-day equivalent, and often very much more beautiful, too.

Please don't feel I'm talking about precious antiques here – I own very few expensive pieces and even those were fairly cheap when I bought them. I'm mostly talking about the sort of stuff your parents or grandparents might have bought. Old, mass-produced, high-street furniture is at least as sturdy as luxury brands are now. My 1970s tan leather Chesterfield sofa (probably made by someone like MFI) cost £136 on eBay in 2003. It has been the birthplace of two babies, the climbing frame of two children, the bed of two dogs and the overcrowded host to countless party guests. It has seen two smart, new, infinitely more expensive sofas come and go, and I suspect it'll outlive the third. Its nearest neighbour, my 1960s G Plan cabinet, has also been in the family longer than my children and cost me less than a Deliveroo for four. My original Art Deco towel rail was a mere fiver and yet somehow elevates the look of the whole bathroom. My beautiful Edwardian dressing table and matching three-way mirror (no doubt unexceptional in the 1930s) was destined for the skip and cost me £45 for a delivery company to fetch it from London. I could go on and on, room to room, but suffice to say that every single one of these items is more solid, more soulful, attractive and meaningful than the – albeit lovely – new items I've bought to live alongside them. Vintage furniture gives me great joy and zero guilt over money and waste. Just one well-chosen piece will, in my view, make your room look and feel so much better.

I know people who want to buy old furniture but worry that it's impractical and intimidating. It's true that one can't get a mid-century modern dining table delivered by Amazon Prime, but a little effort will save you just as much money. There are furniture couriers all over the country whose surprisingly manageable fees (£50–60 for a table a hundred or so miles away is normal in 2022) when added to purchase price still make vintage pieces a steal. And they adapt beautifully to modern life. When furniture needs a purpose the past couldn't have anticipated, consider whether something old can be tweaked. Take AV units, for example. They are mostly enormous, soulless, revolting-looking things

3

'Vintage furniture gives me great joy and zero guilt over money and waste.'

that cost a fortune and gradually fall apart. It is almost always much nicer to buy a vintage sideboard and pay someone handy to reconfigure the interior shelves for a Sky box and PlayStation, and drill holes in the back for the cables. If a very old desk is looking too shabby to be chic, get it lacquered shiny, or stripped back and painted in a colour of your choice. I guarantee it will still outlive the new one bought on the high street. A sturdy chair frame can easily and cheaply be reupholstered to make it smart and comfy. My tall, glass-fronted bathroom cabinet was an optician's display unit – everything can undergo a career change. The point is that breathing new life into old things isn't just the more moral, sustainable and responsible choice. It is, with some practice, the infinitely more satisfying and rewarding one. Please do get involved.

Where I find my vintage furniture

eBay

My favourite for vintage finds, since the selection is vast and prices are mostly very reasonable. Just type in your search term ('Vintage Danish Dining Table', for example), and browse the results, taking a close look at the photographs and asking any questions not answered in the listing. The only problem with eBay is the risk of getting carried away, so stay focused on the items you actually need, and stick to your budget.

Etsy

There are some terrific finds on Etsy, where most vintage dealers and enthusiasts now gather globally. Here you're likely to find more professional sellers rather than individuals selling their possessions, and that can make for a higher-quality selection. Things typically cost a little more than on eBay as a result, but prices are, on the whole, fair. I've bought all sorts from Etsy, from my Art Deco diamond engagement ring to a rocking chair. Lots of items come from America, so check before buying anything hefty.

Vinterior

A really brilliant site for the vintage enthusiast seeking a special piece: high-quality furniture, barware, upholstery, textiles and more, costing more than the average eBay or Etsy offering, but usually much less than mid- to low-end reproduction. For example, an original, beautiful 1960s cocktail chair will cost around £200, while a high-street copy manufactured in China might set you back £350.

The Old Cinema

A discerning and eclectic marketplace in West London for everything from vintage clocks and film posters (of which I'm a collector), to office chairs and huge Italian sofas. The website is wonderful, but the physical store is a joy. I love buying from here and I visit in person whenever I'm near Chiswick. Usefully, they also restore whatever you already own (as will many a local professional. All major cities have plenty of upholsterers and restorers. You'd be surprised). There's doubtlessly a skew towards mid-century modern here, which suits me down to the ground, but try to get a feel for your own preferred eras – there are sites for every conceivable style.

Are posh candles a waste of money?

People are seemingly divided into those who love scented candles, and those with an almost principled objection to their very existence. I've seen people become furious at the suggestion of parting with cash for something that they then effectively set alight. While I disagree (I adore candles), I do want to set them – as well as those more naturally inclined towards home fragrance – straight on something crucial: candles are not meant to be burned for as long as you plan to enjoy them. What I mean by that is this: if you are spending a cosy evening in front of the fire, your candle only kicks off the proceedings. The light from a scented candle is the pleasing but secondary benefit of burning one. Its primary purpose is not as a light source, but as a room scent. If you want the soft, flattering flicker of candlelight, get cheap church pillars from IKEA. If you want to fragrance the whole house without wasting money, do this:

1. Wick-trimming is very important to keep your candle at its best. Take your solid, unlit candle and trim the wick to a quarter of an inch with scissors or, even better, an angled wick trimmer. The wick should never be trimmed when the wax is still warm.
2. Light the candle and stand it somewhere safe. It must be away from any draughts in order to burn evenly.
3. Keep a casual eye on it, to see when the entire top layer has melted and become clear. There's no exact science to this, since waxes and sizes vary, but as a general rule of thumb, a single-wicked, standard glass-jarred candle (a 190–200g, classic-sized Jo Malone or Diptyque, for example) will take around thirty to forty minutes to reach this

point. A travel-sized candle will take around half as much time, though remember the scent won't pervade as far into the house.

4. If your candle develops a central tunnel over time, it has one or more of the following problems:

    (i) Your wick is too short and burns down faster than it can heat the wax around it.

    (ii) Your candle doesn't have enough wicks – i.e. a very large one will need three or even five wicks to melt evenly – a single flame has too much ground to cover and can't cast its heat far or fast enough. Never buy a large candle with only one wick.

    (iii) Your candle has been placed in a draught, which is throwing the flame down on a slant, meaning one part of the candle is being exposed to more heat than the rest.

    (iv) You have relit the candle when it's still warm. Candles should be left to cool completely and solidify between burnings.

If your candle becomes black and sooty, your wick is too long. If it crackles and fizzes, it's a little dusty; be sure to replace its lid between burnings, or give it a blow or a dust before lighting.

How to clean out a votive candle or jar

7

I always reuse my prettier scented candle jars for pens and pencils, makeup brushes and the like. Jars from brands like Bella Freud, Cire Trudon and Fornasetti are decorative items in themselves, so I will typically put a cheap, squat pillar candle inside them when they're spent.

1. Place the nearly empty candle jar in a bowl of almost boiling water, to soften the wax.

2. Grab a butter knife or cereal spoon and dig out the wick and its metal base plate. Discard.

3. Place the candle and jar in the microwave and heat for twenty to thirty seconds, or until all the remaining wax has liquefied. Discard. (I tend to pour it into the central cavity of an unscented candle, but I'm obsessive about avoiding waste.)

4. Wash the jar in hot, soapy water or place in the dishwasher with your glasses. I have never known the label on a high-quality scented candle jar to peel off in the wash.

Tips on hiring a cleaner

I find middle-class British people utterly ridiculous on the subject of paying for help with cleaning. I have cleaned for money myself, in three very different London homes varying dramatically in family set-up and wealth. I cleaned bathrooms, did the ironing, mopped floors, polished wood, dusted surfaces and hoovered top to bottom four times a week, and much as I mostly didn't feel like doing it (it is undoubtedly hard graft), I never felt my job anything short of decent and satisfactorily transactional. Much later on, in a rented flatshare, I happily contributed towards paying a cleaner who earned more than my own hourly rate at a clothes shop. I then went without a cleaner for several years, either because I couldn't afford one, was rarely in to make any mess anyway, or later, because I was home all the time with small children. I re-employed one when I became a single parent and, in improved financial and marital circumstances, I still employ the same cleaner now. She has become a part of our family, we respect her utterly and pay her properly, whether she is able to work or not. I find it amusing that right-on types think nothing of getting a Deliveroo rider to pedal over a noodle soup, or giving an exploited immigrant god-knows-how-tiny a portion of £20 to clean their car, or getting a zero-hour-contracted courier to next-day deliver a single ream of printer paper, or, for that matter, leaving out the dishes for their girlfriend to clean up for free, but mention a woman with the audacity to outsource some housework in exchange for a fair wage, and it's all sneering judgement and social media class wars. Having been on both sides of the transaction, I find this response patronising, out of touch and completely disingenuous. So yes, I employ a cleaner and will continue to do so for as long as I can justify both the need and the cost. And yes, I would clean for cash again if I needed to.

I'm grateful for having only ever had reliable, skilled and honest cleaners in my home, but this may not be a coincidence, so here's how I manage it:

Consider using agencies
Agencies are useful insofar as they will usually be able to cover holidays and sickness with another cleaner, and they should also have an insurance policy in place to cover any accidents or breakages (find out – if they don't, walk away). But remember, agency cleaners will involve two payments: your monthly subscription premium to the agency, and your payment of

wages directly to the agency cleaner whenever they finish a shift. This can stack up and, personally, I'd rather pay the whole thing to a cleaner direct, but this very much depends on finding a good one yourself. If you go with an agency, take the time to ask the cleaner privately how they find working with them. Are they paid properly? Are they happy there? Are they being charged by the agency for the privilege of providing their services? Ask plenty of questions.

Tidy up

Cleaners come to clean, and it's impossible for them to do that when your house is in chaos and disarray. Unless you've previously agreed otherwise, it is polite and respectful to have your house in order prior to your cleaner's arrival, which means keeping on top of things and even having a good tidy up if necessary.

Get out of the way

It is hugely annoying for anyone to have to clean around you and unless you simply can't avoid it, it's unhelpful and discourteous to get in the cleaner's way. We work from home and make a point of making ourselves scarce on a Friday. Taking your laptop to the library or parking in a coffee shop gives the cleaner a chance to do his or her job properly and in peace. If I have to be in, I don't interrupt with chatter beyond offering the occasional cuppa. I know from personal experience that people who work alone generally just want to shove in their earbuds and crack on.

Provide refreshments

Make your tea and coffee facilities fully available and let anyone working in your home know where everything is, how to work the coffee machine and so on.

Supply products

It's unusual for a cleaner to bring their own products, though I have heard of this happening. The default is to provide them yourself. Ask for any specific brand preferences. We have a system where our cleaner leaves whatever's nearly empty next to the sink, to remind us to buy more before next week, and it works well. Machine-wash cloths so they're all clean and stacked for your cleaner's arrival.

Consult on equipment

I would not typically make a big purchase like a vacuum cleaner without first consulting our cleaner, since she also has to use it. For what it's worth, I've never employed a cleaner who didn't have a preference for Henry Hoovers, but I hear extremely enthusiastic reviews for Sharks. Similarly, if your cleaner irons (ours doesn't, and nor do we), ask them if there's a type of iron they favour.

Bleach loos

Cleaners aren't sewage workers. As much as cleaning loos is part of the job, I think it's respectful to always squirt a cursory coating of bleach or suitable eco substitute into the toilet bowl in advance of a cleaner's visit. It's just polite.

Pay properly

The single most important duty of any employer is to pay someone properly. If your plans change and you need your cleaner to skip a visit (as we did when we had builders everywhere), you still need to pay them. If you go on holiday, you still need to pay them. If you can't afford this, then have your cleaner visit but draw up a different to-do list of rarely done jobs, like cleaning the oven or inside the cupboards. Always have your cleaner's wages ready on the kitchen counter, so they never have to ask, or pay them in advance via direct debit.

Add a Christmas bonus

We pay our cleaner a bonus inside her Christmas card every year, and we increase this amount annually. What you pay is obviously down to what you can afford, but an extra two shifts' wages is a good place to start if it's doable.

Get insurance

If you're not with a cleaning agency, or don't have a very experienced cleaner with her own policy, you will need to either get insurance or take breakages on the chin. Human error and misadventure are inevitable, but most home and contents policies won't cover anything caused by someone working in your home, so you'll need to inform your provider and ask for an amendment. More importantly, think about what would happen if someone had an accident and hurt themselves. Many cleaners will have personal indemnity policies, but don't take this for granted – ask.

10

Don't be neurotic

Cleaners come to work. It's important to be friendly, kind and courteous, but don't start frantically attempting to force a bond of friendship, like David Brent telling jokes from the edge of a desk. It suggests an awkwardness and embarrassment at having someone work in your home, and while I can only speak for myself, I found it somewhat belittling. People want their employers to be pleasant and grateful. They don't want to be their best friends.

Be flexible

It's vital to be understanding about public holidays and celebrations, especially if your cleaner's family isn't in the UK and they are likely to want to travel home. I get completely that people want a clean house for Christmas, and this is where an agency can be very useful and can book you in a replacement. Lots of cleaners have colleagues in their network who swap around shifts in these situations, which is also great. If all else fails, set aside half a day for everyone in your family to muck in and get the job done.

Don't let your kids rely on a cleaner

This is utterly essential. Our job as parents is to prepare our children for adulthood, and being a grown-up means knowing how to look after your own home. A sense of entitlement makes for the least-charming children and the very worst adults, so don't indulge it for a second. I never wanted my children to think it was anyone's job or responsibility to clean up after them, or to think this is how everyone lives. They benefit amply from the cleanliness of the shared living space, so they are made to tidy their bedrooms in advance of our cleaner's weekly visit and never leave out anything on the assumption that she'll take care of it. No adult should be picking up the pants, socks and cereal bowls of a perfectly capable teenager they played no part in creating. Even I feel decidedly disinclined – and I pushed them both out.

Key management

Of course, you should give a spare set of keys to your most trustworthy and least-sociable neighbours. But if you're a serial misplacer of keys, consider investing in some Tile Bluetooth trackers – little keyrings, credit cards and stickers that inform your smartphone or Alexa of the location of your keys, wallet and just about anything else you can't be without. We kitted out the whole family for about £40.

How to decorate a Christmas tree

I'm obsessed with Christmas trees and would quite like one all year round. There's just something completely and brilliantly mad about plonking a large tree incongruously in your living room and effectively dressing it in drag. The way you decorate yours is very personal, of course. I have an almost allergic aversion to the kind of tasteful, colour-coordinated trees you might see behind a cordon in the middle of a shopping centre – all tartan bows and red baubles, or a vision in silver and lilac. My feeling is that Christmas is no time for good taste and restraint, and I opt always for a riot of clashing colour and too many decorations amassed over many years – bought anywhere, from supermarket to souvenir shop. I also keep a VIP box of decorations made at nursery and school by my children, like the clothes-peg angel, the loo-roll centre painted in glitter and the large twig wrapped in green and gold ribbon. They'd be among the first things I'd grab in a fire and I look forward all autumn to seeing them again.

I order my tree from a local business, which delivers it to my house at the end of November (much respect to you if you actively enjoy the ritual of choosing and dragging your tree home yourself. Completely understandable). I clear the area in advance, moving the record player out of the way, shoving the sofa over a few feet, sweeping the floor and assembling the stand. When the tree is in place, I always start with string lights – it is the only way. I walk 360 degrees around the tree, laying the string (about 50ft for a 6–7ft tree), climbing one level of branches with each full circle. I then lay another set more haphazardly at the base, so the lights peep through the presents when they finally appear. Then I decorate with a mixture of ornaments and baubles, spaced out fairly evenly to avoid duplication. Sets of identical baubles are split up, so there's a bit of everything from every point of view. With Christmas trees, I very much take the view that less is a bore, and so I keep going until not a single outward-facing branch remains unadorned. My one concession to restraint is tinsel – I don't use it on the tree because it obscures the baubles, but I do drape it lavishly from the staircase. For wall and ceiling decorations, I use brightly coloured tissue-paper pompoms, lanterns and garlands, which you never see in the shops but are available for not very much money at all on party supplies sites. I hang them from light fittings, mirrors, ceilings and anything else that stays still long enough. They are – to me – beautiful, and as I write this in spring, some remain cheerfully on display.

'With Christmas trees, I very much take the view that less is a bore.'

How to throw meaningful things away

I am hugely sentimental, and for many years I wouldn't throw away, donate or sell anything that had once belonged to someone who was no longer with us. I understand this is, to an extent, normal and human and I wouldn't want to change in any fundamental sense, but it can become a problem when the sheer volume of kept items detracts from the truly precious ones. It's easily done. The penny finally dropped for me when I was preparing to give away some of my own furniture and it occurred to me, rather morbidly, that if I were to die in that moment, those left behind might assume that a 2001 Habitat CD rack was an item of some significance to me. But it was simply somewhere to store my CDs at a price I could then afford; it fitted in the gap in a former flat and was the same colour as a neighbouring chair I didn't much care about either. My point is that our grandmothers, like anyone else at any time, bought things they needed, that they may not have loved, based purely on what was affordably available to them. The dressing table at which my late, beloved grandmother sat each morning to make up her face was from B&Q and falling apart. It wasn't special – she was, the memory is. I understand now that she probably looked at it with, at best, indifference. We assume that old objects are intrinsically more meaningful, but they're not. Some are, of course, and we should treasure them. As for the rest, we still own our memories without owning their props.

Wood or carpet?

It really depends where and how you live. My only fitted carpet is a stair runner and as someone with a moulting dog and multiple teenagers – my own and their friends – bounding enthusiastically around the house, I'd have it no other way. We would destroy carpet in weeks, if not minutes. My husband starts sneezing in dusty environments, which is another reason to choose hard flooring. But my bare wooden floors are a privilege that comes with living in a house with no neighbours beneath us to complain about the stampede, and which still has the original floorboards I could tart up with a sander, saving me a small fortune. Things become trickier in flats, where floorboards cause noise pollution – if they even exist at all. Laminate flooring is even noisier. Carpets are a better option here; they cushion the acoustics and, it must be said, create warmth in a chilly room. When choosing carpet, I would always opt for a neutral shade and plain design, though I'd avoid grey entirely, since it's the carpet that every property developer fits for their tenants and consequently feels cold and generic. Shades like beige go with everything, and while they're unexciting, carpet doesn't need to be exciting any more than a blank canvas needs to be – it's all about what goes on top. Whatever carpet you choose, never scrimp on proper fitting. A well-fitted, cheap carpet will look infinitely better than a badly fitted luxury one. If you'd like the characterful feel and low-effort maintenance of floorboards but your originals are irredeemably screwed, think about engineered boards. They share the same style as hardwood, are less noisy and nicer looking than laminate, and they cost somewhere between the two.

Whether your floors are wooden, laminated, carpeted, corked or tiled, it's a good idea to lay rugs. My preference is for a medium rug on which the furniture partially sits, since it makes the room appear larger but still cosy. But you can place a small rug in the centre – perhaps under a coffee table – or a huge rug to act simply as a shrunken floor carpet (great if you're renting and hate the landlord's floor). Natural matting – sisal, coir and jute (the latter is softest) – is durable and goes with everything, while a bold, colourful graphic mat can make a drab room look spectacular. Design is more important than quality, unless your rug is in a particularly high-traffic area. Next make terrific rugs, as do John Lewis and Habitat, and with all three, do check eBay first. I routinely see barely used rugs for a fraction of their retail price – even when you factor in carpet cleaner hire to freshen your purchase.

How to measure for new curtains

Measure the width of your window. If your curtains will be thick (velvet, wool or corduroy, for example), double the width. If your curtains are thin or sheer (muslin, poplin, linen), triple it. If the fabric is midweight, i.e. somewhere between the two extremes, then split the difference and order 2.5 times the width of the window. As for length, it's more a matter of personal preference. I only really like curtains that hit the floor and then some, falling into a shallow puddle (maybe an inch or two) on the floor – I find short curtains a bit Wendy house. But you may prefer them to stop beneath the window (sometimes necessary if there's a windowsill and the fabric is especially thick). In which case, measure from the top of the pole to the sill and add 1.5 inches to avoid draughts. While you wait for your curtains to arrive, if you need to, buy self-adhesive paper blinds from Amazon – they just stick to the top of the window frame, come down again without mess and go into your recycling when the curtains arrive. They're genius.

How to get rid of moths

I love all creatures except rats, flies and moths, and know only how to deal effectively with the last (if I spotted a rat, I fear I'd just have to burn down my house and never return in case something crawled from the embers). Moths offend me partly because they are creepy and flappy, but mainly because the babies of certain moths like to eat my clothes and I won't take it lying down. That said, it's only in the past three years, many moth treatments later and god knows how many jumpers down on the deal that I've really managed to rid the little sods from my life. Here are a few tips:

- As soon as you buy a precious item of clothing, whether a cashmere jumper, wool coat or silk dress, take it to the dry cleaners. The chemicals used really do seem to deter moths for several months at a time.
- Hang Rentokil FM41 Clothes Moth Killer Cassettes in your wardrobes. They're sold in packs of two or four, and a pair of cassettes will be effective in one cubic metre of hanging space, for up to six months. It is essential you keep track of how long they've been active, as the minute the effect wears off, the moths invade like fans on a pitch at the whistle blow. There's a little sliding date reminder on the cassette to help you.
- If you own special and rarely worn items (an evening gown, for example), it's best to store this in a suit carrier, but this will also mean it requires its own personal Rentokil cassette inside the hanging bag, so buy extra.
- Line drawers with Rentokil REN0125 Moth Killer Papers. They're sold in packs of ten and I use at least three per drawer. For under the bed, or infrequently accessed storage for things like blankets and bedding, I use all ten. I use a pencil to scribble the changeover date on the papers, as a reminder.
- Cedar balls certainly won't do any harm, smell nothing like traditional mothballs and are cheap enough for a punt, so you might as well put them in your pockets and in the base of suit carriers for good measure.

- Try not to leave items undisturbed for long. If you don't wear half your wardrobe in summer, pack the cold-weather clothing into plastic tubs lined with Rentokil papers and put away. Your garments are safer there than hanging untouched for the summer, when moths are most rife.

How to descale

If you live in a hard-water area, as I do, you'll know the effect it has on your kettle and shower head. If you want something fast and low maintenance, use Oust, but vinegar works just as well. For a kettle, pour 750ml white vinegar (the cheap stuff, not something you'd use in salad dressing) and 250ml water into your kettle. Bring it to the boil but stop just before it begins to bubble. Leave for at least an hour – a couple if you can stand to be without tea – or overnight. Take a toothbrush to any stubborn bits, throw away the solution, rinse twice, fill with water and boil. Discard and repeat if you can still smell chip shops.

For your shower, pour the same solution as above into a plastic bag containing a sponge or cloth. Raise the bag so the fixed shower head is pushed into the saturated sponge and tie the bag handles snugly around it to secure in place. Leave for a few hours and rinse. Removable shower heads are very easy. Just dangle them in a bowl of the vinegar solution until descaled.

How to fold a fitted sheet

I love sleeping on crispy flat sheets if I'm paying to stay in a hotel, but at home, it's fitted or bust. Life is short. While they're much easier and quicker to put on, and the act of stretching the elasticated corners taut reduces or eliminates the need for ironing, people seem to come a cropper when folding a fitted sheet. I concede that fresh from the line or dryer they seem unwieldy, but there is a knack to it.

- Fold the sheet in half, top to bottom.
- Tuck the bottom elastic corners inside-out, into the top corners, so they're nestled inside.
- Now lay the sheet down and fold the corners and flaps down the sides inwards, much as you'd fold in the sleeves on a T-shirt to get that square, stackable shape.
- Now the flaps and corners are folded over, you should have square edges. Fold the sheet as if it were a flat one and put away.

Should I get a gas, electric or induction cooker?

I think I've lived with every combination and I don't hesitate to say you should get a gas hob and an electric oven. Gas cookers give you the most instantly controllable heat, can be used with any pan, and are energy efficient. Electric ovens heat most accurately, cook most evenly and can best employ helpful features like delay timers and so on. Modern kitchens are certainly moving towards induction hobs, however, so if you are choosing a new cooker now, you'll want to consider it. I didn't take the plunge myself because I didn't want to buy new cookware and the on-off reflex whenever you lift a pan drives me mad. The rhythm of cooking is still too strange. I will get there when required.

The wild card in the pack is an AGA. These are brilliant but very much dependent on having a lot of space, very strong floorboards and joists, plenty of patience to learn a new way of cooking and a large budget to buy one (though no one in their right mind buys an AGA new, when there are so many reconditioned ones put up for adoption by people who buy them because they're pretty and don't think much beyond that). With a little practice, AGAs are actually very easy to use and produce fantastic food (you will never eat a better Yorkshire), economical to use, heat the whole house and, of course, are very beautiful. I just don't have the gigantic kitchen to house one.

How to hang pictures

Rooms look sad without artwork hanging on their walls. And when I say 'artwork', I really do use the term so very loosely – photographs of friends and relatives, collages made of snapshots, vintage wallpaper panels, especially pretty wrapping-paper scraps, playing cards or collectors' stickers, childhood memorabilia, pressed flowers, graphic-design posters, old vinyl records, even an item of clothing – all can be framed to add heaps of style and character to a room. My preference for most things is a white wooden frame with square edges. They're much less expensive than the fancier ones and, to me, look the nicest – there's good reason why most galleries use them. I do occasionally, where appropriate, go for a full-on, Mona Lisa-style gold decorative frame, because why not have some fun? A large portrait of my dear, departed dog Margot lives in one of these, and it makes me smile whenever I catch her grumpy face staring down from her gaudy, mock-baroque surround. The only styles I won't consider are clip frames. There was an argument for them when they were the only cheap option available (I had them everywhere), but that ship has long since sailed. I always hang my own pictures, because I invariably find fault when someone else does it. Here's my method for large and/or heavy pictures (for small or light pictures, see: 'How to build a gallery wall', page 34).

1. First, ensure your frame has an attached string, sturdy ledge or integrated hanging hole at the back, from which it can hang.
2. Measure between 1.45 and 1.55 metres up from the floor, depending on your ceiling height and the average height of your household members (if some are short and some are tall, as in my house, split the difference). That point will be where the centre of your artwork should sit. Mark it on the wall with a pencil.
3. Alternatively, if your artwork is being hung behind a sofa or table, then forget the height from the floor – it should be around 20-25cm above the top of the furniture. If you want to play around with placement, cut wrapping paper to the size of your artworks and experiment with them, anchoring the sheets into different positions with Blu Tack until you're happy.
4. If this is to be the only picture on the wall, it's usually ideal to place it at the centre point along the wall, with equal space on either side. If there are multiple pictures already on the same wall, measure to the midpoint of your chosen gap between artworks.
5. Stick some felt dots on the back corners of the artwork, to protect your wall's paintwork (these also hold the picture still if it gets knocked accidentally as you brush past). You can buy these very cheaply in hardware shops.
6. If your artwork is relatively light, you should at this point be able to hammer a nail into the wall, at your pencil mark. The vast majority of large pictures in my house are hung this way and remain very secure.
7. If your artwork is especially heavy, get a picture hook that's appropriate for its weight. I find hardware shop staff are very good at advising here. For a very heavy artwork, you'll need a drill, Rawlplug and a thicker nail – again, hardware shop staff will know which fixings go with the appropriate hook and weight. Drill your hole at your pencil mark, push in the Rawlplug so it's snug with the surface of the wall, then bang in the nail with a hammer.

'I do occasionally go for a full-on, Mona Lisa-style gold decorative frame, because why not have some fun?'

8. Hang your picture from the nail. If you can't see what you're doing behind the picture, then lower a dining fork onto the nail, facing outwards, the tines straddling the nail at the centre. Then lower the artwork string onto the fork handle, down onto the nail. Remove the fork.
9. Lie a spirit level across the top of your picture, adjusting the frame until it's level.

What to do if your freezer defrosts

I once made the mistake of allowing the useless boyfriend of a non-useless friend to look after my London flat and dog while away on my honeymoon. When I returned, the dog was insane from lack of exercise, there was a cigarette burn on my sofa, and the freezer, which had absent-mindedly been left open for what must have been several days, stood in a puddle on the floor. In these situations, you must not close the door and allow things to refreeze and therefore become unusable (essentially, only peas and other vegetables are safe to go again), but instead, get everything out and cook and eat what you can. Challenge yourself to use as many ingredients as possible and throw the mother of all eating parties. But before you do that, be sure the freezer really did defrost, by squeezing the foods behind those at the immediate front to see if they're soft. House removal companies are generally insured for the contents of an unplugged freezer for twenty-four hours after their removal, so if yours has been off for just a few hours, you'll be perfectly fine – the freezer will have kept everything sufficiently cold. (Reader, she dumped him and is now happily married to a good man.)

21

How to deliberately defrost a freezer
1. Cook and eat as much as you can in the preceding weeks. This is a good time to clear out anything that's hanging around unduly.
2. Replace what you eat with ice packs (the kinds you put in packed lunches and picnics) and if you don't already have one, buy a foil-lined freezer bag from the checkout display at the supermarket.
3. Take out any remaining frozen foods and put them, and the ice packs, into the freezer bag and zip it up. Throw away anything that's become crystallised or discoloured by freezer burn.
4. Unplug the freezer and remove all the drawers for cleaning (I throw mine in the dishwasher, but check what's safe for yours).

5. Place a washing-up bowl (if it fits) or a shallow rectangular casserole dish (if it doesn't) at the bottom of the freezer, where the bottom drawer sat. Pour boiling water into the bowl from the kettle, so that the steam rises up into the freezer. Use shallower dishes to do the same thing on the upper shelves. You'll need to swap out or top up the hot water a few times as ice drops into the bowl and it cools.

6. Place a black bin liner flat on the floor, around the freezer door (you may need to cut it with scissors to cover every inch of space), then place a beach towel that you don't much love on top, to absorb any overspill.

7. While the steam gets to work, grab your hairdryer and blow hot air into the solid ice. This accelerates the process quite dramatically.

8. When the freezer is fully defrosted, get a clean cloth and some hot soapy water and wipe it all over from top to bottom. Replace the now-pristine drawers and switch the freezer back on. Return the remainder of the food and the ice packs to the freezer, and close the door.

How to improve scruffy or limited outside space

I live in central Brighton, where few but the very rich own sizeable gardens. In my case, this is probably for the best, since my horticultural skills are non-existent. What I am good at is making the most of my outside space, and never has this been more useful than in a pandemic, where my few square metres were a godsend, and for which I was extremely grateful. I tart up the area twice a year, at the beginning of the main seasons, with my husband taking ownership of anything green and me in charge of everything else. The whole thing takes a weekend.

Firstly, if your outdoor space is paved, hire a power washer from your nearest tool hire shop or dry cleaners. They are the most satisfying piece of kit and will improve your surroundings more than anything else. Clean around drains, steps, slate, walls and stones, going easy at first in case anything is loose. The pressure of the water will do all the work for you, so don't use washing-up liquid or detergent, otherwise the blast of the water will transform your garden into an unmanageable foam party that takes ages to rinse away. Use the pressure washer to clean your garden furniture, too, since it gets dirty and mouldy, particularly at the end of winter, even if it's been stored in a shed.

'There's also something very convivial about sitting around on the floor and chatting, though I may of course outgrow it as my bones age.'

If you have no garden furniture and you need some, or if yours is nearing death, then you may need to buy new. I say this with a heavy heart because I loathe most garden furniture and don't wish to encourage its manufacturers, who cheerfully charge the earth for mostly ugly furniture that survives only in homes massive enough to afford them hibernation in a conservatory or watertight shed. There is a huge gap in the market for affordable outdoor items that are attractive in their own right, cost less than comfortable indoor furniture and last longer than your average house slippers. Funnily enough, by far my most lasting and agreeable garden furniture has been the cheapest – wirework sofas and chairs for £100–250 from John Lewis, and a bistro table and matching chair costing about £30 from Asda (who have a surprisingly good selection overall). Because I like throwing parties in summer but don't have masses of outdoor space, I supplement these with large outdoor floor cushions and squishy beanbags from Amazon and Homesense. The advantage of these, apart from being very comfortable, is that they're so close to the ground that you don't need to supply tables – your guests' glasses are always close to hand, the covers are stain- and water-resistant but machine washable, and they don't rust. There's also something very convivial about sitting around on the floor and chatting, though I may of course outgrow it as my bones age.

Lighting is of huge importance in creating an atmosphere that is conducive to outdoor living. Festoon lights (which look like fairground lightbulbs dangling from a line) strung in zigzags in trees or between opposing walls are the best option. For £200, you can light a small garden lavishly and easily to look utterly fabulous, and in winter you can redeploy your lighting indoors if you please. It's well worth the investment.

If you're useless with beds and lawns, buy pebbles, wood or slate chips to add texture to the ground space. If you have no lawn but do own a fussy pet who pees only on grass, get a boxed AstroTurf mat (available in larger pet shops) and hose regularly with Fairy Liquid and water.

How to clean jewellery

John Lewis sells cheap dippy pots (complete with integrated draining racks) of gold and silver jewellery cleaner and they are deeply satisfying, but warm soapy water works just as well and keeps jewellery in great nick. Just fill a bowl (not the sink – it's asking for trouble) with warm water and some unscented handwash and use an old, knackered toothbrush to clean gently around the settings, stones and any engraving. Dry on a fresh towel. You can give cheap silver jewellery an extra shine by rubbing in some toothpaste with your fingers and rinsing off with warm water. However diligent you are, it's still worth dropping your special pieces in to a jeweller once in a while for expert cleaning and attention.

How to remove stains from clothing

This is your essential household kit for accidents and stain removal, to be kept together and handy, but safely out of reach – such as in the under-sink, child-locked cupboard:

- Bicarbonate of soda
- Acetone nail polish remover
- A spare dishwasher liquid capsule
- Non-oily eye makeup remover (The Body Shop's Camomile is best. I am never without it under the sink)
- Cheap, generic aspirin
- Colourless, clear alcohol hand sanitiser spray or gel
- Magic Eraser sponge (the best stain remover for any hard surface, like pale walls and white trainers. You can buy one in Lakeland, John Lewis, Robert Dyas and large supermarkets)
- White vinegar
- Toothbrush (old is better than new, as it'll be softer)
- A stain-removing product for posh and super-delicate fabrics – I like The Laundress Stain Solution, which works brilliantly on new marks.

Common stains

Biro
Alcohol hand sanitiser spray or gel is brilliant here. I use The Sanctuary Spa sanitiser spray at home and it works like magic – but any clear, colourless sanitiser will do (as will hairspray, at a push). Place the item, stain uppermost, on a worktop (covered in a clean white tea towel, if you're worried), and spray or douse the stain liberally, saturating it in sanitiser. Leave well alone while it takes effect. Most stains, when caught early, will disappear entirely in a few minutes. Finish with a machine wash.

Lipstick

Use the same technique as with Biro stains, but this time use gel rather than spray, and after soaking for a few minutes, work the gel into the fabric with a clean white flannel. If the fabric is extremely delicate, use non-oily eye makeup remover (see: 'Makeup', overleaf).

Turmeric

The least movable of stains, so be exceptionally careful when handling it – especially if you have Corian, melamine or wood surfaces in your kitchen. I never unpack our weekly Indian takeaway until the white worktop is covered with a tea towel – it's a two-second job that saves tears. If any turmeric liquid or curry paste spills during cooking, cover it immediately in granulated sugar, then use a piece of kitchen paper to sweep and scoop it away. If you spill dry turmeric powder on the worktop or floor, do not attempt to wipe in the first instance. Immediately grab a vacuum and place the pipe vertically above the powder to suck it up directly. If any marks remain, make a paste of bicarbonate of soda and water, and apply to the stain for ten minutes.

Red wine (and coffee)

Do not under any circumstances pour over white wine. This does not work and is an unforgivable waste of wine. Instead, drape the garment, single ply, over an open bowl, like a mixing bowl or loo pan. Sprinkle the stain generously with table salt and pour boiling water through the salt and the fabric. Machine wash to finish. If the item is static – for example, a carpet – then pour fizzy soda water (all households should keep some safe – a soda machine is even better) over the stain. Press down a clean towel to absorb the soda water, then pour on more soda water and repeat. Continue this process many times, lifting the stain to the surface, then absorbing it, until it's faded significantly or gone. Use the same technique for coffee stains.

Sweat

If a precious garment becomes stained with sweat rings, you must move quickly. Crush a packet of aspirin into a bowl and add warm water, smooshing with a soup spoon to make a paste. Spoon this paste onto the stains, pressing in firmly. Leave for fifteen minutes. Finish with a machine wash containing a scoop of stain powder (I use Vanish Oxi Action).

'Do not under any circumstances pour over white wine. This does not work and is an unforgivable waste of wine.'

Makeup

Your course of action here depends very much on the fabric stained. A solution of water, vinegar and a tiny drop of acetone-based nail polish remover works extremely well, but can be used only on natural, sturdy fibres like cotton. Something manmade, like a pleather skirt or polythene raincoat, will melt and ruin. For delicate clothing, carpets and upholstery, I always use a non-oily makeup remover such as The Body Shop's Camomile Gentle Eye Makeup Remover, but anything oil-free works. Test a tiny and inconspicuous area first (like the underside of a shirt placket) to make sure the colour doesn't run. If the coast is clear, saturate the stain with the remover, using an unbleached cotton bud to gently rub the wet stain. Finish with a machine wash.

Ketchup

In the first instance, place the stained item outside in sunlight (it doesn't have to be a hot or very bright day) for a few hours. Sunlight is magic on tomato and many other stains. If that doesn't work, squeeze the contents of a dishwasher tablet into a dish and add some white vinegar. Mix together to a paste and use a clean toothbrush to work the solution into the stain until removed. Follow with a machine wash.

Chewing gum

Do not attempt to remove the gum. Fold the item with the gum uppermost and place immediately into the deep freeze. Leave for a couple of hours. Remove and rub a fresh ice cube around the gum to moisten the area. Lift off the gum with fingers and follow with a machine wash.

Sun cream

I'm sorry to say that there's nothing that works particularly well, which is why I mostly buy holiday clothes on the high street. It's less traumatic. Scrub neat Fairy liquid into the stain and rinse.

Other laundry issues

Underwired bras

The most maddening habit of underwires is when the wires themselves pierce out an escape route and stab the wearer in either the breastplate or underarm. This is almost always down to poor laundry care, as is the loss of elasticity in the straps and the shrinking of the cups. At the same time, lingerie care labels are absurd. Who on earth has time to handwash their scanties in a basin? The answer is a 'Delicates' machine cycle, adjusted down to 30°C if your machine allows, and a lingerie bag for each bra. These are small mesh zip-up pouches (get them cheaply from Lakeland, John Lewis, Robert Dyas or Amazon) for isolating bras and other delicates from the rest of the wash. You can get large, partitioned washbags for posh knickers (useful for stopping tangling and colour transfer) and different-sized bags for containing whole undies sets or several bras. I buy multipacks and use one small bag per bra and two pairs of matching knickers, but if you wash multiple items in one, always do up your bra on the outermost hooks before washing, partly to keep the shape intact, but mainly to stop stray hooks from damaging your other items.

Towels

The only way to keep towels bright white is to wash them only with other white towels, on a high heat, without fabric conditioner but with a scoop of Vanish Oxi Action. Tumble drying will keep them bouncy and soft, but not everyone has that luxury. If you are dryerless, do try to dry towels outside, never on a hot radiator, as that will send them crispy.

Cashmere

I don't subscribe at all to the notion that cashmere must only be dry-cleaned. I can understand why this was the case when cashmere cost fortunes, but in the time of Uniqlo and Autograph at M&S (both of whom make some of the best cashmere sweaters around), who can face forking out a tenner every time they need a clean? I wash all my cashmere – socks, sweaters, cardis – inside out (to prevent pilling) at 30°C, on the woollen cycle, then dry either in the shade outside, or in winter, over the bath. Tumble drying is disastrous unless you plan to donate your clothing to a Barbie doll. Placing cashmere (or wool) against any direct heat source like a radiator or heated rail causes shrinkage and a change in texture. Even this is a bit too much of a faff to do too often, so I always wear a thin T-shirt underneath my cashmere and wool jumpers, to cut down dramatically on the number of times they need washing. I de-bobble with a cashmere comb, or if the disease is particularly rife, a battery-powered clothes shaver (I have a posh £30 one that is no better than the cheap £5 one I had before it).

'Tumble drying
is disastrous
unless you plan
to donate your
clothing to a
Barbie doll.'

Quilted fabric

If washing sleeping bags, puffa coats, down gilets and other puffy items, add a couple of plastic laundry balls to the wash (and dry, where appropriate) – the softly spiked ones from Lakeland are ideal. Do not follow the YouTuber meme's top tip of using tennis balls to do the same job. They are almost always neon yellow and give your laundry a sort of nicotine-tinged sadness that you won't shift.

Washer-dryers

I always presume that all those people who declare washer-dryers 'a waste of time and money' have never lived in a flat without a garden and washing line, and have been spoiled for interior space their whole lives. Washer-dryers are a godsend when you don't have the space for separate appliances and would a) prefer garments to not become cardboard-stiff, and b) quite like to cook your dinner without tainting your fresh-smelling clothing hanging from every available chair and radiator. Washer-dryers actually just need more careful use to keep them in working order. First and foremost – and this is where practically everyone goes wrong – a washer-dryer can only dry HALF of its washing load. This is vital if you want to get your clothes dry and keep your machine operational. Frequently, those who own washer-dryers decide they know better than the manual and switch immediately from washing to drying without first half emptying the machine and setting aside the second drying batch. They are wrong. The clothes will stay damp and need hours of ironing. The machine will ultimately break. The landlord will blame and possibly charge them. People will erroneously lecture them on how washer-dryers never work. They will be left with what is now a washing machine and blouses that smell of Tuesday's sausage casserole.

Choosing a washing machine

If you have the immense luxury of space, a big budget or a home you can furnish to your specifications, do always look for a washing machine with the largest drum you can accommodate, a freshen-up cycle, and customisable programmes that allow you to select your own temperature with a separate dial or button, rather than one with those programme menus that wash cottons at 40, 60 or 90°C whether you like it or not. I wash sheets and towels on 60°C and cottons, woollens, cashmere and delicates on 30°C, but I also want the option of a 20°C wash for something super-fragile, or 40°C for particularly gross PE kits. Having been broke with a cheap, rented machine, well-off with a state-of-the-art bought one, and having lived at some time with practically everything in between, I can say with absolute conviction that if you can get German, do. Miele (my favourite), Bosch, Siemens and so on are the best of the pricier machines (ask a washing machine engineer – she or he usually has a Miele at home) and live for many years longer than machines costing £200 less. The best of the affordable machines are, in my view, by Beko.

Condenser dryer 101

I have been Team Condenser for many years and so cannot speak of the maintenance routine of a vented dryer. For the uninitiated, vented dryers are the ones with a white plastic hose taking steam through an exterior wall, while condenser dryers (and their newer relations, heat pump dryers) can theoretically be placed anywhere as they keep the water drawn from your laundry in a removable tank. Regarding the latter type, the price of this freedom is small, but the hint is there in the word 'removable'. You must remember to take out and empty the tank after every two or three drying cycles. Or one, in the case of a big load, especially of sopping towels. The other thing to be aware of in a condenser dryer, though, is – and forgive me if you saw this coming – the condenser. While level one maintenance involves emptying the tank as described and, just as regularly, cleaning lint from the filter usually located in the door opening (if you've left it too long and the filter resembles a comfort blanket, poking up around the channel either side of this filter may bring further fluffy rewards), level two involves the occasional de-linting of the condenser itself. This is generally located behind a panel at the lower front of the machine. The panel may be push-release or require a tool to open. Behind it, usually secured by plastic catches, is a metal and plastic block of tubes, smaller than a shoebox. This is your condenser. It has no electrical parts so can be safely cleaned with water – a shower head in the bath is one way, though you may wish to take precautions to stop all the fluff clogging your plughole. An outdoor hose with spray attachment is another option. Give the condenser a thorough spray both length- and widthways and leave to dry off a little before clipping back into the machine.

Never, ever leave a tumble dryer running when you're out or asleep. I know of two home fires that started this way.

Keeping clothes in shape

Before loading the machine, always button up blouses, zip up hoodies, hook up bras – clothes left undone flap, stretch, tangle and crease, lose their shape faster, and are more prone to becoming damaged. Never dry wet clothes on hangers unless they can withstand very hot ironing (shirts, for example) to remove shoulder protrusions. Knitwear should be dried flat.

The best laundry baskets

The proper hampers and wooden boxes may look nice, but I find the lidded ones make clothes smell fusty, sometimes even staining them with tiny mould spores if you've dropped in something damp like a flannel, and you can't move them. I use white, flexible tubs from hardware stores – they nest to save space; can be carried around the house easily; they bend to get into narrow spaces; and can be used to hold dirty clothes, washed wet clothes and dried folded clothes. Also, they're cheap, available in many colours and look fine.

Sluttish ironing

I understand that ironed clothes are vital to many, but not to me. I categorically refuse to iron large piles of clothing myself, nor will I pay to outsource the misery to another (unless getting things dry cleaned counts), chiefly because I have earned money this way myself, hated it, and now believe there is little need for most ironing unless one is a member of the armed forces. Shaking and carefully folding clothing while still warm keeps casual clothing smooth. If the occasional unruly pyjama placket or hemline offends, turn on your hair straighteners and smooth it back down in seconds. For anything bigger, like a silk shirt or dress, a hand-held steamer is your best friend. As an ironing hater who has worked on hundreds of photo shoots, I know that a garment can be steamed and smoothed to perfection, with none of the pressure marks, limescale deposits, stickiness and scalding of an iron, in a fraction of the time. Steamers are also brilliantly useful in freshening up delicates, silk dresses, cashmere and outerwear, reducing the need for expensive dry cleaning. If you're one of those unfathomable people who irons sheets, tea towels, pants and kids' tracksuits, you'll need a mains-powered one with a stand (around £150). I have a portable steamer unit by Philips, and I love it. If you de-crease even less frequently than me (I doff my crumpled cap), then just hang your item onto a shower pole, move the shower head away to avoid splashing, and turn on the water for a couple of minutes. As the room steams up, pull taut the sleeves and hemline to shape and smooth. Allow to cool before dressing.

Static

If your skirt or dress sticks unflatteringly to your tights, apply hand cream or body lotion to your hands and massage in as normal. Then use your moisturised hands to stroke briskly your stockinged legs, from top to bottom. The fabric should stop clinging. You can also spray your tights lightly with hair lacquer, which works just as well, but smells stronger in a way you might enjoy less.

Laddering

If your tights ladder in an inconspicuous place, nip it in the bud by painting clear nail polish thinly all around the top and bottom of the run and allow to dry hard. If the ladder is more visible, lose the tights altogether, or get changed as soon as convenient. Ladders are one of those infuriating mishaps that, whatever you tell yourself in the moment, are always noticed by others, like spinach caught in a tooth.

How to build a gallery wall

My gallery wall – eighty-odd assorted photo frames, containing photographs of our favourite people and family memories and arranged Tetris-style on the wall – stretches from the bottom of my ground-floor hallway to the top of the staircase. It is my pride and joy, mainly, I think, because I always assumed it would be so complex and hard to put together that I'd need to pay someone professional to do it. In reality, it took me around three weeks of planning and just five extremely happy hours to execute one Sunday morning. I can't stress enough that I am not a natural DIYer, and my method would almost certainly horrify an expert, but mine looks brilliant and I've become so good at them that several friends have asked me to make theirs. But you don't need me or anyone else to project-manage your gallery wall. It's just not hard. To delegate would be to deny yourself the purest pleasure and satisfaction of building the focal point to your home.

So, to create your own gallery wall, you'll need:

Frames

And lots of them. I was adamant that my frames would all be white and wood, but that their styles would be varied and mismatched, so I spent a few weeks buying different shapes, textures and sizes from all over

'I now believe there
is little need for most
ironing unless one
is a member of the
armed forces.'

– TK Maxx, M&S, Next, House of Fraser, Amazon, B&Q, Homesense, Zara and more. Mixing three colours also looks lovely – black, white and gold, for example (see: 'The three-colour rule', page 135). If you want all your frames to match in colour and size, then your task is extremely easy – just get a job lot in different sizes from the same range. It is worth also sourcing some square frames as well as rectangular, which are usually sold separately, and one or two multi-aperture frames for variety. Don't buy round or oval – they're a total pain in the arse. Regardless of your design preferences, what is of vital importance is that you buy 'picture frames' not 'photo frames', because the latter have a hinged stand on the back that stops your frame lying flush against the wall, thus stopping it from being hung. You can sometimes remove these with pliers, but it's a world of faff and only successful on some frames, so only buy one that's truly worth the hassle.

Photographs

Go through your phone, your Instagram, Facebook, old albums. Ask your friends to send you files of old favourites. Then upload them to a photo printing site. I used Photobox for all mine, but they all seem to be equally straightforward. Order single prints in assorted sizes to match the frames you have (not the other way around – having to find frames to match existing pictures is much harder).

A good mix would be:

- Eleven to twenty-one 6 × 4-inch prints
- Five to nine 7 × 5-inch prints
- Three 8 × 10-inch prints
- A handful of 5 × 5-inch square prints
- One to three 8 × 8-inch square prints

Remember that odd numbers always look better than even, and consider that the smaller the picture's digital file, the worse quality it will be when enlarged. I recommend ordering matte prints, as gloss looks cheaper and can cause glare. They're very inexpensive (pennies per print), so it's worth doubling up on a few to give yourself different-sized options when you come to build the wall.

Command Strips

I use only these for hanging small to medium pictures and replaceable items. They're a sort of adhesive strip that snaps in on itself to leave both sides sticky and the interiors locked together like Velcro. They allow you to stick frames directly to the wall and remove the need for nails, Rawlplugs, string or hooks. When instructions are followed correctly, they make for fast, secure hanging that doesn't damage plaster or paintwork. You'll need lots of them – at least two strips per little picture, four for larger frames. You can safely budget for around £2 in strips per picture. Don't use them on wallpaper (which can tear) or fresh paint – it needs to have had a good week to dry before you apply the strips.

Sharp, sturdy scissors

For snipping Command Strips and photos to size where needed.

Spirit level

This is vital, especially since my method is a mostly non-measuring one. A fairly thin, one-hand-held spirit level (as opposed to a massive builder's one) is perfect, as it also then acts as a spacer between frames. My method, with apologies to DIY experts everywhere:

1. Place all your photos in their frames. When complete, place the largest one flat on the floor.
2. Arrange the other frames around it on the floor. Spread out the subjects, so photographs of the same people or visual themes, similar crops (like portraits) and sizes aren't clustered together. Make sure the gaps between frames don't align, like tiling, but overlap, like brickwork. The goal here is for the placement to look varied and haphazard.
3. Keep moving your framed pictures around until you're happy with your overall design. Take a photograph with your smartphone so that you still have a complete visual record when you start removing frames.
4. Find your midpoint (see: 'How to hang pictures', page 18). Get your large middle frame and apply your Command Strips according to the instructions (they also have a good YouTube tutorial on best practice). Check it's straight with your spirit level – do not attempt to follow the lines of a wonky ceiling or floor. Ignore them and make your frame dead straight. Apply Command Strips to the next frame out, according to your design.

5. Turn the spirit level on its side, where it's usually narrower. This is generally an ideal width for your gaps between frames. Place it on top of the centre frame. Get your next frame – the one nearest to the centre frame according to your floor plan. Rest it on the spirit level, so the spirit level is sandwiched between the middle frame and its neighbour. Repeat the sticking process.

6. Keep going like this, referring back to the floor-plan photo on your phone. After each frame is stuck to the wall, use the spirit level to check it's straight and make any adjustments. Always use the spirit level as your gap guide, both over and under that centre frame. This will give you a neat and even finish.

The odd rule

When it comes to interiors, unless items naturally come in pairs to live on either side of something (bookends, for example), they will look better in odd numbers. When decorating a table, cluster three, five or seven tealights, not two, four or six. In a floral arrangement, uneven numbers of roses look better than a symmetrical assortment. Two or four cushions on a sofa looks formal and sparse. Three or five looks relaxing and inviting. Three photo frames look like a fun gathering; two look like an interview panel. Planting in gardens looks prettier grouped into threes. Almost every time, odd is the stylish way to go.

Are artificial flowers acceptable?

I used to be a snob about artificial flowers, but now think better of it because modern artificial flowers can be absolutely beautiful. I still somehow never think that I'm looking at real flowers, more that I'm looking at a clever and very lovely decorative accessory that looks really great in its own right. Artificial flowers are also excellent if you are away from home a lot, simply find fresh flowers a faff, or if you or a loved one are allergic to the real thing (more common than you'd think – I've somehow managed to marry not one, but two men with rhinitis. I daren't hazard a third). One thing good artificial flowers are not is cheap. The very low-cost arrangements (£10–20) are pretty awful and plasticky and you're wasting your cash. The best I've seen are by Diane James or John Richard at LuxDeco – but the prices are eye-wateringly high. A happy medium are those by UK-based Abigail Ahern, and also Amaranthine

'When it comes to interiors, unless items naturally come in pairs to live on either side of something (bookends, for example), they will look better in odd numbers.'

Blooms, who hand-paint each of their stems individually. Again, both are expensive – about the cost of four to six high-quality fresh bouquets, but should last for many years, especially if spruced up weekly with a feather duster, and should (depending on your fresh cut-flower habits) ultimately prove a more sustainable choice. No cloudy, stinky water, no having to wash vases constantly. I am dangerously close to buying my own.

A note on cheap fresh flowers

While I swoon over divine-smelling, velvety roses and big, fat, luxurious peonies, I simultaneously believe that there are few things lovelier than a jug of 99p daffodils. Cheap petrol station, supermarket or greengrocer daffs, tulips, daisies, gerbera, goldenrods, sweet Williams and carnations (yes, carnations) can be utterly gorgeous and an immediately uplifting purchase, and I'd sooner buy those if I'm feeling indulgent. That said, I believe almost all of these bright, cheap and cheerful blooms look better in their own company, rather than in a pre-arranged supermarket bouquet, which always seem a bit generic and sparse. Three bunches of daffs, costing £2.97 for the lot, are infinitely more elegant than a £9.99 bouquet containing three daffs, a handful of tulips and some baby's breath. There's just something particularly stylish, luxurious and appealing about a fat bunch of single floral species, packed lavishly into a jug or vase. Mixing colours doesn't seem to ruin the effect. Arrangements and mixed bouquets are done best by proper florists in flower shops, not factory production lines.

How to make fresh flowers last

Clean your vase properly
Florists sterilise their buckets to prolong the life of flowers, but the chances of me taking the time to sterilise my vases are nil. That said, a cursory rinse isn't enough either. Bacteria causes flowers to decay faster, so give them a really good go (see: 'How to clean a vase', opposite).

Remove leaves
Always remove any leaves at water level. Submerging leaves in the vase water will pollute it, and your flowers will be drinking dirty water, which will shorten their life and cause the vase to smell bad.

Remove the bottom inch of each stem

The tips of your flowers will be filled with air. You need to remove these to let them have a big drink. If you have rose cutters, use those, but I don't, so I use a bread knife (household scissors pinch the hard stems and crush them). Slice or cut through them on a slant, to increase the surface area of the drinking hole.

Use the flower food

That little sachet of powder stuck to the side of the cellophane isn't a con. Flower food isn't so much nourishment for flowers as it is a preventer of slime. Taking a moment to pour in the food will prolong your blooms' health by keeping their environment cleaner.

Change the water

Murky brown water smells gross, looks ugly and accelerates the ageing process of your arrangement. Swapping out your vase water every other day makes a big difference and adds on several days of enjoyment.

Give it a shot

Many people swear by a dash of bleach in the vase water, and it certainly does help, since it kills the bacteria. But mentally, I can't quite get past what feels to me, quite irrationally, to be 'a bit murdery'. I prefer a few drops of Milton Sterilising Fluid or a dash of neat vodka, both of which work well.

How to clean a vase

I hate cleaning vases and if you do too, I strongly recommend you invest a little over a fiver in some Magic Balls from Lakeland, John Lewis or your local hardware shop. Just pour them into the bottom of a dirty vase, add a little water, and swirl. They're brilliant at removing scummy stains quickly and painlessly. Add washing-up liquid to clean the stem of the vase, pour the whole thing through a sieve to catch the balls, rinse them off, then pour back into their pot for next time.

Flower alternatives

Flowers are very expensive, not to everyone's taste, environmentally unsound and, unless you're Sir Elton John, no one expects you to have fresh arrangements arriving as often as milk. What is necessary, at least for me, is that a room has some organic and natural elements, but there are lots of ways to do this. Pebbles, driftwood, cacti, feathers – all look great and don't need replacing. My own favourite affordable substitute for flowers is a single variety of fruit used as decoration. A large wooden or glass bowl of shiny Granny Smith apples or of bright, sunny lemons makes a striking and cheerful centrepiece in any room (a mixed fruit bowl is less stylish and attracts flies). A dozen pieces of fruit costs much less (and lasts much longer) than a floral arrangement that you can't chuck in a tart when it starts to lose its looks.

Don't be conned by Black Friday

I love to shop and am all for a bargain – particularly if it involves me not having to move further than my sofa. But it may be that now UK retailers have adopted the US Black Friday sales phenomenon we fail to realise that we are actually saving not very much money at all. According to *Forbes* business magazine, the average Black Friday discount is just 5 per cent. Frankly, I do better out of an average Monday morning's spam folder or overfamiliar postcard from Johnnie Boden. The week before Christmas, meanwhile, offers a much greater average discount of 17.5 per cent. Black Friday is demonstrably not worth it unless you're shopping for an item that would never normally go into an end-of-season sale – a Dyson vacuum, a Magimix processor, a favourite face cream or lipstick, perhaps – otherwise you're probably getting less of a discount than you would in any other upcoming sale. We've unwittingly swallowed the hype on a US marketeer's invention that simply doesn't deliver on its very noisy promise.

If Black Friday isn't saving us much money, then what is it for? To me, it seems to be yet another imported American phenomenon – like pulled pork, school proms, Halloween as religion – used by marketeers to part us from our cash. When checks and balances are calculated, the only people who gain significantly from Black Friday are the companies coining it in, and the superior, self-satisfied gits sneering at poor people fighting over a new telly in Tesco. Have you ever known this happen in real life? Truly, in the world of wholly improbable but reliably popular tabloid stories, this rarely witnessed scene is the new 'woke lefties banned my child's nativity'.

'When checks and balances are calculated, the only people who gain significantly from Black Friday are the companies coining it in.'

Washing glassware

Regardless of what the box tells me to do, I put all my nice glasses into the dishwasher except for the very tall-stemmed ones that don't fit. I put them through as normal, then every year, I soak them for a few minutes in cheap white vinegar, which rids them of all their streaks and cloudy stains. If glassware emerges from the dishwasher with dried-on food from neighbouring dishes, do not put it back in. The food will not shift. Instead, you must soak it in warm soapy water and finish off manually. For parties, I have the cheapest available (about a pound each) red wine, white wine and Martini glasses that live in the attic, descending for twenty-four-hour periods before being packed away again in their boxes. They're dishwashable, much kinder to the environment than disposables and within just a handful of parties, cheaper, too.

How to remove the smell of cigarettes

Whenever we throw a party, I always promise my husband I won't let anyone smoke inside and invariably, the evening reaches a point where my kitchen disco spirits are so high that I can't face throwing someone into the garden to spark up and before I know it, it's a free for all. I don't mind as long as the kids are away (which they usually choose to be to avoid the sight of middle-aged people vogueing), because I have my fumigation routine down pat.

First, open all doors and windows where it's safe to do so. Empty any ashtrays into an outside bin, clean their interiors with wet kitchen paper, then wash up as normal. If people have been smoking near sofas, or if you have carpets and rugs, sprinkle them all well with baking powder (it's worth keeping a flour shaker full of it – baking powder is useful for all sorts of household tasks and is usually available in large bags in the pound shop), and leave while you do the rest. Take a few small clean bowls, half-fill with water and add in some lemon juice (the squeezy supermarket kind is fine) or some slices of fresh lemon in the unlikely event that you have some left over from the gin. Place each of the bowls on top of a radiator. Next, you'll need to light a candle – again, only where it's safe and where you will be able to supervise (especially important when there are open windows). I find Price's inexpensive 'Anti-Tobacco' candles, available at most hardware shops and on Amazon, to be brilliantly effective, and the tin container makes things very simple for the hungover brain. You'll need a couple on the go, maybe even three, in the offending room. Take any fabrics lying around – tea towels, abandoned sweatshirts and the like – and throw them in the washing machine. Hoover up the baking powder on the carpets and soft furnishings. You'll be good as new in a couple of hours.

How to make a home cosy

Cosiness is my religion. I can't describe it as what is fashionably referred to as hygge, as that makes it sound a bit more 'aspirational Pinterest board' than it deserves. I am someone who very much likes to be at home. I really do love nature, and the outdoors, but engaging with both requires more persuasion and effort than will ever be needed for me to lie in an elasticated waistband to watch a Scorsese triple bill with a nap interval. My natural habitat is a sofa, my default eyeline about a third of a room's height from the floor. I like my rooms to be built for this lifestyle, but just as importantly, I want them to invite in my guests to relax, too. I once interviewed a well-known actress in her beautiful, very expensive apartment, and realised ten minutes into our conversation that despite her undeniable friendliness and warmth, I felt extremely uncomfortable because the room didn't want me there. White marble tabletops and immaculate arrangements of calla lilies interrupting the eyeline. Designer sofas with wooden arms that could never cushion a weary head. A pale carpet that looked as though it might wince if you were to carry in a mug or pizza slice. I wasn't in the least bit surprised when she told me she found it hard to unwind and do nothing. Cosiness is an essential component of inactivity. It is the difference between boredom and bliss. It's a state of mind encouraged by the comfort and warmth of our surroundings.

45

Fairy lights

It is an indisputable fact that any room is made instantly more cosy by warm, white fairy lights. Inexpensive and available everywhere, they require zero imagination or skill and make every room look better and more homely. Hang a set like curtains on windows, like artwork on walls, clustered in inactive fireplaces, trailing up staircases, gathered under sofas – wherever you feel like putting fairy lights, I promise they'll work. I have lots of sets, but my preferred option is a battery-operated, extra-long string, since they're mobile, the most versatile and you're not confined to areas near a plug socket.

'Cosiness is my religion ... It is the difference between boredom and bliss.'

Something old in every room

See: 'Old is usually better' (page 3). Something that has lived a life is almost always going to be more comfortable and more welcoming than something boxfresh. Even if your furniture is new, some vintage accessories, photo frames or textiles add depth and soul to any room and, importantly, stop everything from matching. Coordinating furniture 'sets', like a vanity dresser, bedside cabinets and wardrobe all in the same colour and style look extremely old-fashioned and boring. Throwing in a curveball like a vintage blanket box or dressing table gives a bedroom some quality, personality and depth. All rooms benefit from a past.

Blankets and textiles

I keep blankets everywhere (see: 'Make everything a bed', overleaf), but not only for lying under. Even if blankets live draped over the arm of a chair, or on the back of the sofa, their varied textures and relaxed feel make any room seem warmer and more inviting. I collect colourful vintage Welsh blankets, bought second-hand for a fraction of the cost of newly woven, and combine them with myriad other inexpensive, machine-washable styles – from Zara faux-fur bedspreads to knitted John Lewis blankets and shantung silk throws from Dusk (my favourite bargain bedding website). Cushions are another good way of introducing new fabrics. Matching them to your sofa is a missed opportunity for texture and comfort. Instead, contrast them – velvet cushions on a linen sofa, corduroy and fur on leather and so on. Mix them up in size, shape, fabric and placement. No one wants to cosy up with four identical squares lined up like soldiers.

47

Low-level lighting

Overhead lights (or the 'big light' as it was always known to me until I met posh people) are primarily for switching on when you'd like everyone to bugger off. For almost everything else post-daylight – reading, eating, listening to music, watching TV, chatting and general idling, side lamps are much nicer. Generally speaking, lamps with bulbs pointing upwards add mood and glow, and those with bulbs pointing downwards serve a purpose, such as easy reading or sewing. For the former, I find 60 watts is usually ideal. Reading lights are trickier – I can do no fewer than 60 watts, no more than 75, but an older person or someone with even weaker eyesight may need up to 100, depending on any other light in the room.

The exceptions are kitchen lights, which should be bright for safety when you're dealing with sharp knives and direct heat. I'd also use a high wattage in the hallway, since they are usually windowless and a place where one often has to get organised and look for things before leaving the house, and in the bathroom, on a dimmer switch, turned up for spot squeezing and leg shaving, and right down for bathing with the additional glow of a scented candle.

Books

Books add warmth, texture and colour to a room, as well as a welcoming feel that almost invites you to sit down and interact with the objects inside it. I'm not suggesting we surrender entire walls to bookshelves (I wish that I could), but a compact, freestanding bookshelf or even just a small pile of books, whether fancy coffee table photography or paperback novels, will always make a room feel much more human and homely. A shelf of well-thumbed cookery books is also a great way of giving a modern kitchen a more hospitable, personal feel.

Make everything a bed

A more active, outdoorsy sort of a reader need not bother, but it is extremely important to me, a slovenly homebody, that every soft seat in my house is a bed waiting to happen. If a sofa can't be lain on comfortably, then it's no good to me. An armchair that forces its occupier to sit upright like a Bond villain, rather than curled up like a cat, is a literal waste of space. I must know that I can snooze in everything, or put up a minibus load of visitors if I have to. So to that end, I have my Welsh wool blankets on every seat, and a hamper full of inexpensive but soft, machine-washable throws so that any of us can slope in and unthinkingly pull out something snuggly for watching telly or catching forty winks with the dog. I wouldn't have it any other way.

How to store pan lids

If you have the space, turn the lid upside down and place it convexly in its own pan, then stack a smaller pan on top of the upturned lid and repeat. If you don't have the cupboard height for a stack, buy a cheap plate rack from a hardware shop and line up the lids in slots, as though they are crockery. Depending on the design, it is often a more effective use of space to have the lids facing one another like bookends, rather than pointing in the same direction like spoons.

How to deal with mice

If you have only the occasional mouse scurry across the floor then fail to reappear for several months at a time, I'd personally be tempted to turn a blind eye. If you have a family, nest or colony and want to be the good guy, then know this: humane traps don't work. Trust me, I've been there and seen myself thwarted in my humanitarian endeavours. However far you drive from your home, your humane traps securely onboard, heaving with painlessly squeaking, freedom-seeking vermin, the mice will find their way back to you. It will go on for months, as they multiply, peeing and pooing germs and potential illness around your house and in your food packaging. They will chew through wires and cables in a way that will compromise your family members' and pets' safety. You will reach a point where you can take no more and you outsource the cruelty to traditional mousetraps or Rentokil, only now you'll be killing far, far more mice than if you'd grasped the nettle from the off. You will feel infinitely worse, spend much more money (£400 in my case, not including the various humane methods tried previously) and you'll have far more damage to repair. When you reach this point – and you will – you must fill or mesh every cavity in the house, to prevent a comeback tour.

How to catch a spider

I am a fan of spiders. They're clever, don't like to socialise, they make beautiful things and kill annoying, germ-carrying flies. I see them very much as life's good guys and generally leave them to their business. But I realise this is as pointless a statement to arachnophobes as when my friend Caitlin tries to convince me of the goodness of rats, who are the literal worst of all things. But it seems to me that whether you love, hate or are indifferent to spiders, killing remains the worst response, since a squished spider makes a mess and phobics then have to either stare indefinitely at the decomposing cadaver or become re-traumatised by tweezing bits of mangled spider leg off their slippers. I'm strongly against it and consequently I've never deliberately killed one. So here's the best, most humane and contact-free technique for evicting an arachnid from your home.

49

> 1. Place a glass over the spider (if the mere sight of the creature inside might make you hysterical, use a mug).
> 2. Take a piece of robust paper – thicker than a newspaper, which will crumple, but thinner than stiff card, which can disable the poor thing's legs, and slide it under the mouth of the upturned glass.
> 3. Carry the glass, now sealed with paper, to a window or front door. Place the whole thing in the open air, lift the glass and set the spider free.

How to repair wood scratches

Do not spray with furniture polish – it coats and smothers the wood and just makes it harder for any proper repairs to be done later. Instead, crack a walnut and gently rub the unshelled nut against the scratch, back and forth, to make it seem less obvious. If it's something really beloved, bite the bullet and seek the expertise of a restoration service or French polisher.

How to clean a lavatory

My friends tease me about it, but I have an almost maniacal hatred of toilet brushes. I loathe them, won't have them in the house and would never voluntarily touch any part of one in a hotel or holiday accommodation. There's something absolutely revolting about a brush used to clean poo that sits in a small puddle of stagnant water in the corner of your room, as though this is a sanitary and even remotely acceptable practice in modern life. I quite understand that people diligently dunk the bristles in bleach solution and so forth, but no one would keep out the same kitchen sponge for years on end, however often they cleaned it – and that only wipes food from your worktops. And so I apologise in advance if you'll countenance no other way of cleaning a lavatory, because I won't use one. Household members should clean up after themselves before leaving the bathroom in the first place. Woe betide anyone who decides it's mine or anyone else's job to make a much more effortful job of it later.

First, don household gloves. I have an allergy, so I always use the latex-free sensitive-skin Marigolds or similar. Lift the seat and squirt some bleach under the rim, allowing it to drizzle down to coat the entire bowl. Leave it for a bit while you clean the bath or stare at TikTok. Next, take a bathroom spray or hot soapy water and, using a washable microfibre cloth or kitchen paper, spray and wipe all around the outside of the loo (including the handle and the pedestal, which attracts lots of dust), then both sides of the toilet lid, then the top of the seat and its underside. Get around the back to clean around the hinges, where dust and grime can gather. Your bowl should now be clean – if it's not, you'll need to get your gloved hand below the waterline and scrub. Flush the toilet to be sure, and use the microfibre cloth or loo paper, and elbow grease, to shift anything that remains. Put the cloth in the wash. Finally, squirt a drop of bleach into your gloved palms and rub them together as you would hand soap on skin. Rinse under the tap, remove and stow away for next time.

While we're in this part of the house:

Buy a bathroom recycling bin

Most people in Britain recycle their kitchen waste, but less than half of us bother with the bathroom. Bathrooms contain heaps of disposable packaging, a great deal of it now recyclable. Get a small bin for shampoo and conditioner bottles, skincare packaging and loo-roll middles and build this into your recycling routine. Remember that pumps are practically never recyclable (on account of the coiled spring and tube being indivisible), so remove these before disposing of their bottles and screw into the new one if possible (Aveda and The Body Shop sell their bottles and pumps separately). The best facial cleansing is done with washable flannels anyway, but if you like cotton pads for eye makeup removal and the like, you can buy reusable ones very cheaply. Mine are from Superdrug and I just throw them in a laundry bag and machine wash (put them in the legs of tights if you don't have a bag). Switching to bar soap is a more sustainable way of washing hands (though aluminium cans and glass bottles of handwash are available, for variety) that is every bit as effective. There's also something very glamorous about bar soap, especially since it affords the opportunity to choose a beautiful tray for it. Mine's from Anthropologie and always elicits compliments from visitors.

Recycling symbols

Short-term household items will display a symbol signalling how best to dispose of them, but few people in Britain know what they mean. Taking a moment to acquaint yourself will save a mountain of household waste.

A looped, leafy plant

The item is compostable. Do not put it in the recycling, where it can't be processed and messes with the system. Deposit it in your compost bin with food waste.

A green square with a white semicircle with a love heart at its tip

This material is widely recycled by at least three-quarters of local authorities.

The same symbol in black

Less good. This material is recycled by 20–74 per cent of local authorities, so you'll need to check with yours.

Three green arrows in a triangle

Otherwise known as the Mobius Loop, this increasingly common symbol is letting you know that the item can be recycled. Remember that this doesn't necessarily mean it can be tossed into the recycling whole – different components and materials should be detached and separated before being sorted into the appropriate bin.

Circular arrows and the letters ALU

Aluminium – hooray! Widely and infinitely recyclable. Help your local authority by lumping your washed aluminium together – scrunch up your tinfoil (don't leave it in sheets), crush your cans and metal takeaway trays. Big old lumps are easier than scraps.

Number inside the green arrows

This number is telling you what percentage of the item's packaging material has previously been recycled. For example, a number 50 means that half of the materials have already been recycled.

Two interlocking green arrows – one dark, one light

This shows that the manufacturer makes a financial contribution towards recycling services. It does not necessarily mean the item itself is recyclable, so check the accompanying symbols.

A tree and the letters FSC

The material is made from wood sourced from responsibly managed forests, according to the independent guidelines set by the Forest Stewardship Council.

Black arrows forming a triangle

This plastic can theoretically be recycled. The number inside the triangle relates to a categorisation of this specific type of plastic material, and how easily and widely recyclable it is. Here's what each means:

1. Polyethylene terephthalate (known commonly as PET). Widely recycled by local authorities.
2. High-density polyethylene (HDPE). Widely recycled by local authorities.
3. Polyvinyl chloride (PVC, like the mini skirts and double glazing). Recyclable but not by all local authorities, so you'll need to look up Environmental Services to confirm.
4. Low-density polyethylene (LDPE). Recyclable, but not as commonly as the high-density kind, so check.
5. Polypropylene (PP). Used in things like airtight containers, mixing bowls, plastic measuring jugs and party cups. An absolute bugger to recycle. If you can, buy glass or paper instead or, if you must buy it, reuse it for as long as is practical.
6. Polystyrene or Styrofoam (PS). Another material that is very hard to recycle, so it's best to avoid it. As an alternative, use those starch packing peanuts that look like Quavers, which protect your parcels, then dissolve in the sink. This material is also used in disposable coffee cups, so carry a thermal mug; and in plastic party cutlery, so use your regular knives and forks, or buy bamboo.
7. 'Other'. A catch-all for myriad plastics that are a huge pain in the recycling plant's bum. Avoid them wherever possible.

When to save and when to splurge on household items

Spend

Mattress

You spend a third of your life lying in bed, so you'd be mad to voluntarily scrimp on your mattress. The good news is that brilliant 'expensive' mattresses are no longer anything like as dear as their equivalents of yore. Disruptor brands like Eve, Casper, Emma, Allswell and Simba (of which I own two, but I've come to believe they're all much of a muchness) make hybrid spring or memory foam mattresses that arrive conveniently in a box and gradually unfurl in a deeply satisfying manner, over a

'Your sofa is one of your home's vital organs and it needs to be right.'

twenty-four-hour period. They're wonderfully comfy and, unlike the memory foam of the past, not at all cloying and sweaty. I like a firm, traditional spring for my own bed, so mine came not in a box via courier, but carried up a staircase by two extremely grumpy men moaning about local traffic – but it was worth it. Whichever you go for, it's always worth pushing your budget. And buy a mattress cover – it makes the world of difference.

Bin bags

Cheap black refuse sacks – just don't do it. They are the ultimate false economy. Even double layered (and therefore double the price), they will stretch, split and leave bin juice all over your floor, making you furiously curse whoever it was that tried to save twelve pence on the roll.

Kitchen fitting

The most important money you will spend in your kitchen. A cheap kitchen fitted expertly will look way better than a luxury kitchen fitted badly. There are no exceptions. Good fitting is what makes a kitchen.

Pillows

I am now a middle-aged woman whose neck is banjaxed every few weeks. I cannot stress enough the importance of good pillows that hit the sweet spot between soft and firm, don't divot over time and support your head fully (not your shoulders – these should never be on the pillow). If you're vegan, this no longer means settling for an inferior pillow. There are now excellent feather mimics available for the same price as good-quality down. One cannot tell the difference. Wherever your preference on the soft–firm continuum, you will feel every extra penny spent.

Sofa

There is simply nothing less welcoming and more dispiriting than an uncomfortable couch. Your sofa is one of your home's vital organs and it needs to be right. The ideal sofa is squishy, nappable and roomy enough for cuddling the child, pet or adult of your choice, but also firm enough for seat cushions to retain their shape and for you to sit up with a laptop and work. Washable covers are a bonus.

You can scrimp on any decorative item as long as this is dead right.

Flooring

So you may not have a choice, of course. I had the floor I was given for many years and whether it was noisy laminate, splintery boards or carpet that was hard to keep clean, it was invariably the one part of the flat I disliked most. If you're in a position to choose or renovate, it's worth pouring money into flooring – both the materials and, even more importantly, fitting. This feature takes up more space than anything but the walls, and has the most transformative effect on a property.

Curtains

Properly measured and made curtains add something to a room that those which arrive in a packet rarely can. Mass-produced curtains often look thin, flimsy and generic, especially those with the shoelace-hole-style gaps at the top for a pole. High-quality curtains are always worth the money, and don't have to mean spending a fortune. Very posh curtain panels come up constantly on second-hand sites, and paying a seamstress to alter them can cost little more than a set from IKEA.

Taps

No one wants to change their taps every few years. Every ten is a reasonable expectation, and this costs money. Kitchen and bathroom taps are turned on many times a day. Bottom-of-the-range ones just will not go the distance. High-quality taps and fittings are also a clever way to make a cheap bathroom suite look luxurious.

Towels

When in M&S, John Lewis, IKEA or similar, it is always worth buying the heavier, fluffier, luxury towels over those on the value shelf. A few quid more will mean they stay flat instead of puckering at the ends, never become threadbare, stay soft and bouncy, and absorb moisture more satisfactorily.

Save

Paint

Anyone who's ever handed their decorators a load of overdraft-stretching Farrow & Ball will know that the professionals would rather work with something costing half the price from the builders' merchants. I have been there on more than one occasion. What pricey brands like Farrow & Ball, Little Greene, Fired Earth and Paint & Paper Library do absolutely beautifully, is colour. If your heart is set on a specific hue, buy a sample pot and take it to a trade shop to be mixed up in a cheaper formula.

Lighting

Houses are lit by lightbulbs and electricity, not by light fittings, and so exactly the same effect can be achieved on both high and low lighting budgets. High-street and out-of-town stores have terrific-looking lighting for less, as does eBay, which sells heaps of reconditioned and professionally rewired chandeliers and pendants (get an electrician to do it for you if not).

Picture frames

Silver photo frames are lovely heirlooms, but a monumental pain to keep shiny, especially when you've lots of them. Whether you favour a consistent aesthetic or an eclectic mismatch, high-street brands like H&M, Zara, M&S, Paperchase and Next do beautiful, stylish, low-maintenance frames that can be adapted cheaply with any redecoration.

Vases

Unless an expensive vase is some unique or distinctive *objet d'art*, then I simply cannot see the point in splashing out. A glass vessel is a glass vessel and eyes should be drawn to the flowers it hosts, not to the barely perceptible qualities of spendy glassware. Besides, as I know to my mercifully inconsiderable cost: vases smash.

57

Rugs

I feel slightly torn in saying this because expensive, handmade rugs are beautiful and really cheap, mass-produced rugs are often not, but there is a sweet spot where a rug is woven with some natural fibres, not printed on nylon, but is still affordable enough for children and animals to run carelessly across it without you suffering an aneurysm. I'm talking about Next, Made.com, John Lewis, Habitat, La Redoute and the like, as opposed to high-end design specialists charging thousands. All sell at prices just about low enough to give you some peace of mind, particularly in high-traffic areas such as the living room or a child's bedroom. I write as someone whose dream rug is over £3,000. Every time I daydream about owning it, I think of my dog emptying her bladder on its hand-tufted beauty and feel immediately better.

Toasters

The less your toaster looks like a vintage Winnebago, the more likely it is to live a long life of toasting bread properly. I have been through a handful of very pretty but very spendy toasters from KitchenAid, Sage and Porsche, returning one after the other, before concluding that none worked anything like as well as their distant predecessor by Russell Hobbs.

Cushions

The joy of cushions is that their covers can be swapped out quickly and economically, whenever you feel the itch to change up a room. To buy expensive cushions is to tie yourself to a scheme you may tire of. Spend money on the big stuff, then scatter cheap decorative items, like cushions, with abandon.

Kitchens

You absolutely can make an inexpensive kitchen look extremely high-end by adding good taps and worktops and getting the best fitter you can afford to install it all. The same applies to bathrooms. It's all about the accessories. Kitchen unit carcasses and bathroom furniture are much of a muchness.

Sheets

I know it's very much the done thing these days to quack on about thread count, but I am wholly unconvinced. At this stage, I'm fortunate enough to have slept in many a posh bed in multiple countries, and I can't really tell much difference between the sheets of the rich and famous and my own bargain bedding from Dusk. I no longer buy sheets from anywhere else. The most important thing is that your bedding is made from natural cotton or linen (anything manmade gets hot, sticky and cloying), fits your bed properly and is changed regularly.

How to build a fire in a fireplace

If I were in the wilderness without firelighters, I would probably freeze to death, but I've been building fires at home, in a fireplace, since I was about seven. Most children learned relatively young at that time, since coal fires were very much the norm in the South Wales valleys, and one watched one's parents or grandparents build the fire daily. There are doubtless more modern and eco-friendly ways to start a fire, but I only know my family's method, and it keeps you as warm as toast.

1. Get an old newspaper – broadsheet works best – and lay it open at the centre page, on the hearth (the flat bit at the front of the fireplace), between your knees and the grate (the metal cradle at the heart of it).
2. Take your fireplace shovel – or just use your firegloved hand – to rake through any old ashes from the hearth or grate. First be

absolutely positive that they are cool (embers can remain warm for well over twenty-four hours). If there are any intact embers, i.e. chunky grey and black bits as opposed to dust, set them aside for later. Don't worry if there aren't many – you'd usually struggle to fill a baked bean can, but they will prove extremely useful later on.

3. Sweep the small, greyish-white ash into the opened newspaper. We need it out of there. Pull up the two top sheets of paper around the ashes to form a Dick Whittington bundle, and discard. If you're not precious about your vacuum cleaner, you can skip this part by simply hoovering up the ashes, but be warned that there will be a good third-to-half of a carrier bag full.

4. From the remaining newspaper, tear each page off, one by one, crumpling it up and tying it into a knot, a bit like a pretzel, with the ends tucked into the knot to form a vague ball shape. Don't take too much care over this – it should take seconds. If you can't get the hang of it, just crumple each page to form a ball as you might before throwing something across the room to a wastepaper basket. Repeat this until you have a good ten or so newspaper balls.

5. Place the balls, clustered together, in the fire grate.

6. Place two firelighters (little white blocks of solid flammable material) on top of the newspaper balls. If you don't have firelighters, don't worry – skip this step.

7. On top of that, place your kindling firewood (about ten to twelve smallish sticks of pale wood), which must be bone dry, into a sort of criss-cross framework. The firelighters, if you're using them, sit in the heart of that frame.

8. Onto your nest of wood, place your reusable embers – those clumpy, solid chunks you found at the beginning. These get hotter faster than anything else and really help the fire to get going.

9. Pick out small chunks of coal (around the size of a new potato) and place them strategically into any gaps in your fire, yet not so much that you can't see through them. What you want is to loosely fill any gaps but not plug them, blocking the ventilation. Don't overload here – the flames must have space to come through.

10. Twist another sheet of newspaper to form a baton, light it with a match or lighter and use the flaming baton to ignite the firelighters.

11. As the paper burns, your fire will start to collapse and drop. Don't be disheartened. Just keep adding coal into the new holes, still giving it

room for air to rise through the fire, being careful never to smother it, to build the fire back up to its original height. Essentially you are now replacing the paper at the bottom with coal at the top.

12. Your wood should be burning well by now. It might take five to ten minutes before the coal and the ashes take over and sustain their own heat.

13. This part is optional, but with careful handling it works a treat. Place your poker vertically against the mouth of the fireplace, between grate and hood. Rest a broadsheet newspaper page against it to create a vacuum. This sucks in the air through the bottom of the grate and causes the wood to burn more ferociously. You should hear the wood crackling on the other side of the paper partition.

14. There should now be quite a blaze. Allow it to become well established before meddling too much. It needs to have been burning merrily for a good half-hour before you attempt to place a log on it, for example.

15. Place a fireguard across the fireplace. It's very important to own a fire extinguisher, whether or not – but especially if – you have an open fire in your home. Keep it within easy reach and ensure everyone in the house knows how to use it.

60

How to manage the crap drawer

The crap drawer. Don't pretend you don't know what I'm talking about. It's the drawer in your house – often in the kitchen, perhaps in the living room – that houses disparate items with no other friends and nowhere else to go. I have just sent my son to photograph ours and at the time of writing (and, realistically, for the foreseeable future), it contains:

- Three flower food sachets.
- Two small rolls of sticky tape.
- A cup-and-ball magic trick from a Christmas cracker.
- An old debit card that my husband uses for ID when collecting parcels for me at the sorting office.
- Cook's matches.
- A packet of Rizla papers, cleared up after a party and kept optimistically, if tragically.
- Two dice.
- Metal tape measure.
- Soft tailor's tape measure.

*'A crap drawer
is a domestic
inevitability. But
the virus must be
contained.'*

- Three hand sanitiser gels.
- Nine lip balms, assorted – five of them bound inexplicably together in a rubber band.
- Five black Biros.
- Mosquito bite clicker device.
- Packet of seeds, ancient and ungrowable.
- Small Maglite torch, battery missing.
- Large tube of Body Shop hand cream.
- Small tube of Aveda hand cream.
- A pair of cheap sunglasses, owner unknown.
- Tic Tac dispenser, almost empty, hated by everyone in the house.
- A home-burned compilation CD.
- Minion figure from the film *Despicable Me* (last watched by my children circa 2012).
- Single white shoelace, origin unknown.
- Personalised tin of Vaseline, unused.
- Plastic executive toy puzzle, unsolved, from Christmas cracker.
- Reel of cotton, beige.
- Reel of string.
- Expired offer code card for fresh flower delivery.

- Three coloured rollerballs.
- One pencil.
- One yellow felt-tip pen, barely working (the yellow is always barely working).
- One black fibre-tip pen used to mark out previous ear piercing, then handed to me to keep, for hygiene purposes.
- One green whiteboard marker (location of whiteboard unknown).
- One Brighton souvenir pen won on a pier stall and gifted by my then-young son, which writes horribly and leaves blobs of messy ink all over the paper, but can now never be thrown away.
- One Sharpie marker nearing death.
- Packet of 'Magic Snaps', a retro and slightly illegal-looking toy that (nominally) adults throw against the pavement to cause tiny, noisy explosions. How this came into my possession is unknown, but my son assures me he was in primary school at the time. He is now at college.

At this juncture, you may be thinking that with this volume of useless crap in my kitchen drawer, I'm the last person who should be giving advice on crap-drawer management, but here's the thing: resisting one crap drawer is futile. A crap drawer is a domestic inevitability. But the virus must be contained. Overcrowding one crap drawer and overspilling into another is the beginning of an outbreak that will result in a crap house.

So, every six months you need to skim off the fat of the crap drawer. Take out the bits that have a legitimate home elsewhere but have been swept lazily into purgatory. Remove the things you've identified as Not Strictly Crap whenever you've opened the drawer, and finally do something about them. You may have a purpose in mind for them, like a repair, relocation or redeployment. They cannot wait interminably for you to come good without ultimately overflowing. So seize the day and halve the crapload. What remains is undeniable crap-drawer crap, which can now live without overcrowding or the risk of boundary breaking.

Cooker hoods

Most cooker extractor hoods are rendered utterly useless because people don't change the filter inside from one year to the next. When they work, they are extremely effective at absorbing cooking smells and grease, and when they don't, they are a heavy hunk of pointlessly unattractive and expensive metal squatting in your kitchen. Unscrew and open yours: if you cook often and haven't cleaned it in over six months, I guarantee it will be disgusting and operating below par. This is why your cooking smells linger and taint your clothes. The optimal cleaning method can vary wildly from hood to hood, brand to brand. Most modern filters can be removed and thrown into the dishwasher on the hottest setting. Some need to be washed in a bowl or bucket with washing-up liquid or vinegar and bicarb. Others are disposable and simply replaced with new. The hidden nature of filters means that they are very often out of sight, out of mind, so set an alarm on your phone to remind you to do it regularly – every three months should do it.

63

How to clean stair carpets

Stair carpets get trodden on more than anywhere else in the house, and by the most people, meaning that fluff and hair get bedded firmly into the pile. Buy yourself a nit comb from the supermarket or (cheaper) a flea comb from a pet shop and use it to gently rake the carpet. This only works on non-loop-pile carpets. Alternatively, you can buy a lint remover tool (about a tenner from Amazon), which is even quicker. All will release a mound of fluff and hair without damaging the carpet – just be especially careful at the tread joins, so you don't pull the carpet away from its track.

Which pram you should buy

When pregnant for the first time, I know you will want the beautiful pram. I wanted the beautiful pram and so did my then-husband. We felt so proud of our bright-red, celebrity-endorsed, style-magazine-celebrated, hipster loft apartment on wheels that cost more than our annual gas bill. But seventeen years down the line, I can tell you for sure that very soon, you will no longer give a stuff about the pretty pram. You will resent how complicated it is to fold into a car boot. How hard it is to fit on a bus. You will hate how it knocks clothing off hangers on the one day you decide to shop for yourself. You will despise how much space it consumes in the hallway, how heavy it is to haul up the communal stairs. You will realise that you are not, after all, the kind of mother who needs a smoothie holder and yoga mat shelf. You're not, it will turn out, going to jog across multiple terrains, pushing a baby wearing matching lululemon spandex. You will realise you're a mother who needs something, just one sodding thing, to be easy in a life that is tiring. And you will buy an uncool, unpretty, undesirable Maclaren buggy for a hundred-odd quid. And as you collapse the thing one-handed in half a second, run with it dangling lightly from your pinky finger, unfussed baby under your arm, and onto a crowded train, before slinging the buggy carelessly in the luggage rack with no thought of any scratches or depreciation to its resale value, you will feel clever, rejoice, and mentally spend all your eBay cash from the Bugaboo.

A basic DIY kit for most jobs

Owning these items imparts an incomparable sense of gratification.

A small set of screwdrivers

Various sizes in both styles – flat and Philips. You can buy a set of complete screwdrivers, or one handle with multiple head attachments (either manual or electric). Either works, but an electric screwdriver is a great investment and has you covered for anything. Whichever you choose, what is essential is that you have multiple sizes for any job – never

'You will realise that you are not, after all, the kind of mother who needs a smoothie holder and yoga mat shelf.'

persevere with the wrong size of screwdriver, as it will keep slipping and very often mess up the slot in the screw head and ruin it.

Two pairs of pliers

It's amazing how often I need to reach for pliers. They are invaluable in most DIY jobs (pulling out pins, Rawlplugs, bending, twisting, wire cutting, gripping and removing pins, and so on), but also for all manner of unrelated jobs, such as opening hardened nail polish bottles, re-straightening earrings that have become bent, closing necklace links that have come open and more. I suggest buying long-nose pliers for most little jobs, but also some slip-joint pliers for bigger jobs (and jar opening). Remember with all pliers that the handles are as useful as the noses. Just turn your pliers around for a sturdy but softer grip on your item.

Stanley knife and cutting mat

Endlessly useful for cropping photos to size, craft projects, making photo mounts, opening boxes, slicing through plastic packaging ties, trimming wires, rubbers and plastics. Wrap dead blades in tape to prevent injuries to foxes, refuse collectors, etc. The cutting mat may seem excessive, but a smooth, flat surface with integrated measuring guides is worth the extra few points to protect your surfaces. That said, you still need . . .

Metal ruler

Don't bother with plastic. When you're cutting a straight line, it's too easy to cut into the plastic and acrylic versions and throw your line off kilter.

Claw hammer

Mine is 16oz and suits my frame and purposes. Useful for picture hanging and basically anything involving nails – one side bangs them in, the claw on the other removes them.

Fat, soft pencil

I loathe writing with pencil (it sets my teeth on edge) so I rarely have many to hand. Keeping one in a permanent kit means you'll always have one for marking out measurements and screw spots.

Chisel

For cutting, trimming, paring and scraping wood, and the one thing in my kit that I've never once needed, since I was atrocious at woodwork at school and would always now call on someone more competent. But I'm still glad I have it and it takes up little room.

Small hacksaw

For when materials are too thick or solid for scissors or a Stanley knife. I also have a small wood saw but never use it for the above reasons (my third-form wooden pelican ornament would explain this further, but I suspect a member of my family sensibly repurposed it as firewood).

Lump hammer

For achieving a dull, blunt thud of a bang. It's usually best to put something soft like a towel or firm like a chunk of spare wood between the hammer and its target, to stop anything becoming dented or otherwise marked.

Allen keys

If you would like to avoid opening your IKEA bed frame, having already returned the car you borrowed to drive to Croydon to get it, to discover the Allen keys are missing and all the shops are closed on a Sunday night, and consequently having to sleep on the floor, then have a full set up your sleeve at all times. I learnt the hard way.

Assorted screws, nails and Rawlplugs

You don't need heaps. Ask your hardware shop for a basic selection – staff are extremely helpful and expert, in my experience. Genuinely, there is no hardware-related question the men and women of Dockerills Brighton have failed to answer me.

Why you need a Swiss army knife

My mother, always a reliably excellent gift-giver, gave us all a Victorinox knife for one Christmas or another and I've only had to replace mine once for an identical model in thirty-five years. My preferred model is now called the Swiss Champ, a compact but weighty pocketknife with thirty-three different tools, from a magnifying glass to a bottle opener. I am devoted to it, keep it close to hand at home and always take it on work trips, both domestic and abroad (in my checked luggage when flying, of course). It means that you can always open a bottle of wine, however ill-equipped your surroundings. You always have a toothpick with which to extract stubborn lemon pith, a pin and tweezers for removing splinters (my favourite activity), screwdrivers and wire cutters for the emergency changing of plugs or fuses, and myriad other quotidian heroes. They make the most brilliant presents for men and women, and you can have the blade engraved or the outer shell personalised. Just don't buy women the models marketed at ladies, since they seem to have little beyond some nail scissors and one knife blade, which, ironically, is the least-used element of a Swiss army knife. I always opt for the chunkier models in classic maroon and every recipient has been wholly surprised but delighted. Lots of people prefer the pricier American-style Leatherman knives, but in my, admittedly limited, experience, these seem to be more work-oriented and useful for people who need to complete lots of handy jobs daily, as opposed to someone who needs tools to call on in any emergency – so whichever suits you.

Essential household maintenance items

I have a pathological fear of running out of essential household items. Here's what I always have in, without fail:

Superglue
You will always need superglue. There's nothing that mends broken items better and faster.

Lightbulbs
At least two of every type I use because it's easy to smash one while replacing.

Batteries
Plenty of AAs for remotes and AAAs for smaller gadgets, four each of the charger sizes and a couple of the more unusual sizes needed for specific items. I replaced most of these with rechargeable versions a couple of years ago, and despite the initially higher outlay, it is well worth doing – financially and ethically.

Lint roller
It's amazing how fast you can make things look better with a lint roller. A quick once-over of the sofa, armchairs and throws makes everything look much smarter and cleaner.

Torch
In case of power cuts, stopcock issues and rescuing items from behind unmovable furniture. Gets removed annually for Glastonbury. I use a Maglite, the US police officers' torches. They are quite literally brilliant and, I always imagine, a useful weapon of self-defence.

Why you must own WD-40

My stepfather and brothers, who were constantly working outside, repairing and rebuilding cars, drummed into me a deep reverence for WD-40, which my first husband also shared, so there's scarcely been a time in my life when I haven't owned a can of this almost magic water- and oil-displacing spray. You need some too, because, well, how long have you got? This is what WD-40 does:*

- Stops shoes, and most other things, from squeaking.
- Removes water marks from glass.
- Cleans white trainers (though I prefer a Magic Eraser sponge, available from hardware stores).
- De-ices cars.
- Removes cup stains from many woods.
- Loosens stiff-hinged metals, such as pliers, scissors and padlocks.
- Releases too-small rings from your fingers.
- Un-jams zips.
- Cleans away stickers and their annoying residue.
- Removes chewing gum and many stains, including lipstick and crayon.
- Shifts excess glue, even superglue.
- Shines silver.
- Adds slip to any items stuck together, such as Lego bricks, stacked beakers, pint glasses and so on.

*I apologise to any mechanics or DIY experts for the likely dozens more uses I've omitted.

Know your stopcock!

However little interest you have in household maintenance and however swift you are in 'getting a man in', I insist you know where to find your stopcock. I say this as someone who once stood alone in my son's newly renovated bedroom, hair and clothing soaked, holding huge laundry buckets filling rapidly with a deluge of water pouring through the ceiling and into the kitchen below me, while I waited both for an emergency plumber to arrive and for my husband and sons to, just this once, answer their sodding phones. I would have warded off some of the psychic scars had I known what I know now: that we have two stopcocks – one under a trap in the hallway and another outside in the street. Where's yours?

69

You might assume, as I did and as most people do, that it is under your kitchen sink. But you may very well be wrong, so do acquaint yourself now so that in future, you can put an almost immediate stop to leaks at the pull of a lever. It is too late when your house is flooding and you're all alone. I needed a whole new ceiling and major redecoration.

Books don't have to be for ever – please hear me out

At the risk of encouraging you to throw this book into the recycling: people need to become more ruthless about books, or at least, permit themselves to entertain the possibility that they may need to let some go. Let me be clear, I love books. I have countless novels and film books well over twenty-five years old, buy almost all non-fiction in print format, and own every edition of *Just Seventeen* from 1984 through 1989. I attach absurd sentimental value to objects and always have.

Books can be beautiful and frequently worth treasuring. But what separates them from much other great art is that they are interactive, living, usable texts, not static museum pieces too precious for everyday life. Some are bound to be keepers, their ideas so apposite, meaningful or influential that just knowing they are near is of comfort. Everyone has physical books that mean so much more than binding, spine and paper. But books don't need to matter forever to matter at all. They can serve their purpose – whether to entertain, thrill, offer practical guidance or insight – then be moved along to make way for new memories.

Having grown up in squalor with a father who never threw anything away – from clothes and books to newspapers and plastic bags – I do know that if you keep everything, you value nothing. Special items, like a trinket belonging to your grandmother, a book given to you by an important teacher or great love, an ancient mixtape made painstakingly by a school friend – none are honoured appropriately and deservingly, because they're jostling for your attention alongside a sand-filled bonkbuster and a lamp you'll never fix.

A few years ago, I almost convinced myself that, in throwing away a double CD of Morcheeba's *Big Calm*, I was discarding with it a late-1990s period of deep personal meaning – even though I no longer play CDs or smoke weed, have little desire to listen to folky trip-hop again, and have long since parted company with almost everyone who listened to it with me. They, like it, mattered at the time and, to an extent, always will, but that doesn't mean I should live with them. A fond memory of a book, song, record, painting, person or anything else should not automatically grant it permanent residency in your home unless you prize the past over the future.

Disguising everyday items

I have very consciously not told you what I personally loathe in interiors. I've done this partly because, well, who cares? Your taste is your own and whatever makes you happy is exactly how you should live. But also because I am instinctively resistant to rules and know many of you will be too. You are always the boss, so please, go forth and enjoy a single lily pushed into a tank vase of pebbles, an accent wall, a grey crushed-velvet ottoman bed, a mirror in the shape of a paned window in a rural church, or whatever else I'd never choose to live with myself (often for wholly irrational reasons). But for my own sanity, I must say this here, even if I am roundly ignored: please don't disguise everyday items as something somehow less shameful. Your telly doesn't need to be hidden away behind a reproduction Chippendale cabinet, as though you actually spend your leisure time reading poetry and drawing likenesses. Your washing-up liquid does not need to be poured into a hip ceramic handwash dispenser. Your real towels needn't be hidden away behind some posher display ones, so scarcely used that they leave fluffy filaments all over your guests' faces. Your loo paper is allowed to be stacked in rolls and be seen for what it is, because everyone who ever visits your loo is already more than acquainted with its purpose. Your marmalade is packaged well for its purpose and Marmite looks very lovely in its jolly, yellow-topped jar and both suffer from being decanted into an anonymous dish. Tunnock's Wafers are more thrilling freed from their stripy foil than they are picked up from a chintzy vintage china plate of anonymous chocolatey bricks. Milk jugs are nice; milk bottles are nicer. Mundane household items are universal and pleasing. I hate finding them hidden away on the apparent assumption that living ordinarily and keeping house is somehow unstylish, or, worse still, a bit below-stairs and common. I thought the age of storing VHS video tapes in leatherette cases got up to look like the works of Shakespeare was well over. But Instagram demonstrates that the sentiment lives on.

Food & Drink

'I want them to know the joy of expressing love for a friend or partner with a thoughtfully cooked plate of food.'

I'm sure I don't need to tell you that I'm not a chef, nor even an experienced food writer. My late mother once said about her talent as an artist, 'I am someone who knows how to draw rather than a person who does not. That doesn't make me anything close to an artist.' I know exactly what she meant. I know how to cook as opposed to not knowing how to cook, just as you may understand how to swim, or assemble flatpack furniture, while I resolutely do not. As a result, I'm a decent home cook, a just about passable baker and a good host.

My upbringing was somewhat chaotic. My mother (with whom we lived from when I was about seven, and who was a good and resourceful cook when the mood took her) frequently either forgot to go food shopping or had run out of money with which to do any. The unpredictable human traffic, unplanned events and work/sleep patterns of the very open family home meant that mealtimes were sketchy at best. We rarely sat down all together unless at Christmas, and if we did, it might be at 1 a.m., to eat a chilli my teenage brother had just cooked. Every family member sort of ran their own schedule and saw to their own needs, both complex and basic.

The unhappier side of this is that I felt frequently insecure, lonely, unsupported and unrooted. The positives are that I grew to be independent and self-sufficient, always pay my utility bills and haven't run out of toilet paper since 1992. I also know how to cook for myself and others a nice dinner, even if the cupboards are almost bare. It's a skill that has brought a great deal of happiness and satisfaction to my life, as well as having allowed me to survive during some tough times when resources were extremely limited.

I live an unrecognisably different life now (I'm a vegetarian, for a start, albeit a meat-cooking one), but the resourcefulness learned during my childhood at home in Wales and adolescence alone in London has stayed with me and will, I hope, be passed on to my (carnivorous) teenage sons. I want them to know the joy of bringing home carefully chosen and budgeted supplies, of making themselves something lovely to eat, of feeling the warmth in expressing love for a friend or partner with a thoughtfully cooked plate of food. My eldest son is already older than I was when I left home and has none of the worries I did. But I still want him to know how to stock a freezer, roast a delicious chicken for his housemates, mix a killer Martini for a date and waste nothing valuable on the dustbin, not least because not being able to cook is quite embarrassing and not really justifiable in someone physically and mentally capable. No one needs to be an expert, thank goodness. But everyone does need a few tricks, tips and good dinners up their sleeve.

'Not being able to cook
is quite embarrassing
and not really justifiable
in someone physically
and mentally capable.'

How to perfectly scramble/poach/fry/boil eggs

Scrambled eggs

If you're having toast, plunge it now. Crack the eggs into a cold pan. For every three whole eggs, add one extra yolk and put the white into the freezer for another day. Add a tablespoon of cold water and beat everything together with a fork or a small whisk. Throw in a knob of butter, and add a little grated cheese or cayenne pepper if you like (I like). Put the cold pan of eggs on a medium–low heat and leave for a few moments. As soon as the eggs show the slightest signs of scrambling, grind in salt and pepper, stir with a wooden spoon and turn off the heat. If they're done, serve. If they need a little longer, turn off the heat – the residual warmth of the hob will see them over the line. No milk. Never milk.

Poached eggs

There are two methods, and which you use depends entirely on how fresh your eggs are. Neither involves an egg poacher, since these essentially dry-fry an egg until it's spherical and rubbery. Fine if people like the result, but they've really no business calling them poached eggs.

How to determine how fresh your eggs are

Fill a jug or bowl with cold water and lower an egg into it. Very fresh eggs will immediately sink to the bottom and lie horizontally on their sides. Eggs that are around a week old will do the same, but their fat ends will lift slightly. Old eggs will have their bums pointing upward, so they're almost vertical in the water. I wouldn't poach these, personally – it's asking for trouble. Fry or scramble them, or use in a recipe. Rotten eggs will float to the top, as oxygen has built up inside. Throw those away.

For very fresh eggs

Half-fill a saucepan with boiling water from the kettle and keep on a low heat – the water should be relatively still, not at a rolling boil. Crack your egg into a mug with a handle and with the china dipping into the simmering water, tip in your egg. Don't panic. Let the white start to chase itself. Cook on this low heat for 3 minutes (if you love soft yolks but hate snotty whites, as I do, you can do a minute shorter or longer, according to preference). Remove the egg with a slotted spoon and prod gently to see if the white is firm but the yolk soft – the joy of poached eggs versus boiled is that you can easily pop them back in if you've underdone them. When satisfied, place on some kitchen paper to absorb excess water, then serve.

For less fresh eggs

Half-fill the saucepan with boiling water and keep on a low heat. Crack your egg onto a small plate. There will be a bulky mass in the middle and some wateriness around the outside. Use kitchen paper to mop up the watery white – you can't poach it, as it will just make a mess. Use a spoon or chopstick to briskly stir the water into a whirlpool and while it's still whirling, dip the plate into the water and ease in the egg. The current should wrap any stray white around the egg. Cook as described opposite.

Perfect fried eggs

When everything else in your breakfast is ready and your toast is toasting, heat some groundnut oil in a non-stick frying pan. If you've a nut allergy, use vegetable or corn oil. Heat to a medium–high temperature and crack in your egg. Allow a golden frill to develop around the outside, then reduce the heat and leave for a couple of minutes until mostly set. Finish cooking the white by spooning some of the hot oil over the top, until the white turns translucent. Remove with a slotted spatula or a fish slice and drain on kitchen paper.

Boiled eggs

Start with room-temperature eggs – cold eggs crack and leak in boiling water and are impossible to time perfectly. Pour boiling water into a pan and place on a medium heat to simmer gently. Place an egg on a slotted spoon and lower carefully into the water. When it returns to the boil, turn down to a low heat and boil for:

4.5 minutes

Firm white, runny yolk – perfect for dipping.

6 minutes

Firm white, soft, but not runny, yolk – perfect for topping a ramen or chopping for kedgeree.

8.5 minutes

Hardish boiled but not chalky and grey, ideal for making egg mayonnaise sandwiches (for which you'll need one extra yolk for every three whole eggs, so discard the fourth white).

Extra-large eggs will take a little longer. As soon as your preferred time is up, remove with the slotted spoon and run the egg briefly under the cold tap. Crack and eat immediately.

How to make the perfect baked potato

A properly baked potato is possibly my favourite meal of all time. There's not much that beats a huge crispy shell of skin filled with light, fluffy mash drinking up wodges of cold butter and salt. (I once cut short a telephone interview with a supermodel in New York because the huge potato I'd been baking for two hours had reached its peak condition and I could wait no longer to tuck in.)

Doing a potato justice is the ultimate exercise in patience – rush and you'll ruin it. And that includes any intervention whatsoever from a bloody microwave. I'm all for convenience and time-saving in practically every other area of life, but I will not entertain any form of 'hack' (that's tip to anyone over thirty-five) involving a baked potato. The entire point is that it takes ages. It demands nothing of you but time, so don't try to cut it short – just have something different for supper.

Method:
1 Preheat the oven to 220°C/430°F.
2 Rub the largest floury potato you can find with water or oil (I favour water, as it gives a flakier skin texture. My husband favours oil, which is crunchier, so your call).
3. Pat the moistened skin with sea salt crystals and skewer the potato lengthways with a metal barbecue skewer (sold in any supermarket or hardware shop).
4. Place on the middle oven shelf, close the door and immediately reduce the temperature to 200°C/400°F.
5. Leave for a minimum of 90 minutes, maybe even 2 hours for a whopper.
6. Remove from the oven, extract the skewer (protect your hands), then quickly place the potato on a chopping board. Cut a cross shape into the top and, with a tea towel to protect your fingers, use both hands to pinch the potato upwards, releasing all the steam. This makes the potato extra fluffy (never leave baked potatoes uncut – the steam will reabsorb and they go damp, soft and somehow gritty-tasting).
7. Place cubes of cold butter in the cavity (I don't hold with room-temperature butter on a potato), with salt and pepper. At this point, I can't help but suggest stirring in a teaspoon of Marmite and topping with a large heap of grated Cheddar. But that's just me.

'I once cut short a telephone interview with a supermodel in New York because the huge potato I'd been baking for two hours had reached its peak condition.'

'There are three ways to bring things back from the brink: add water, acid or bulk.'

How to chop an onion

When I need stacks of super-fine onions, I'll generally process them to save time (or use pre-chopped frozen), but to finely dice an onion or two, I use this method:

1. Chop the ends from the onion and peel.
2. Wet your knife under the tap. This will help stop crying (Mrs Davies, my secondary school cookery teacher, was absolutely right).
3. Slice the onion horizontally into two halves and place each half flat on the chopping board.
4. Using your cook's knife, slice horizontal slits into the onion, stopping a few millimetres from the root end, so it stays intact.
5. Make perpendicular slits downwards, in vertical lines.
6. Chop at the ends as though you are slicing the onion for rings. Fine, even dice should now fall away instead of slices.

What do I do if my food tastes bland?

It sounds so obvious, but the answer is almost certainly to season it better. Simple seasoning makes food taste not of salt and pepper, but of itself. There's no use grinding pepper and sprinkling salt onto a finished dish – you need to season your cooking throughout, almost in layers. That means a little salt and pepper as you fry your meat, a little more when you add wet ingredients, a little more when everything is simmering away happily. In fact, you are least likely to need seasoning at the end, upon serving. The work is already done. Seasoning properly really is the most important thing you will do.

What if my food is too salty?

Okay, so over-seasoning is, of course, a thing, which is why it's safer and better to layer it gradually, tasting along the way. But if you've overdone it, there are three ways to bring things back from the brink: add water, acid or bulk. Rinse off over-seasoned meat, then return to the cooker, or add water to an over-salted pot of food and simmer gently. Acid, in the form of lemon juice or a dash of vinegar, is also good for cutting through a pot of salty curry or soup. If either fails, bulk up the recipe with more ingredients: potatoes, vegetables, meat or pulses, as appropriate.

Why does my stew taste like boiled shoes?

My friend Jenny asked me exactly this when she heard I was writing this book, so I felt I should answer it. Beef stew is the most delicious dinner only when the following elements are in place:

1. Appropriate stewing or braising steak is used. That means good fat content that becomes soft and extremely flavoursome when cooked over many hours. The lean stuff (usually more expensive) becomes tough and doesn't have a great deal of flavour.
2. The beef is sealed before adding to the stew. Throwing raw meat into a stew will just boil it sadly and colourlessly, and you'll miss out on all the flavour. I toss my beef cubes in a little flour seasoned with salt and pepper. I then fry it in fat, in a very hot frying pan, in small batches of between 10 and 14 well-spaced pieces at a time. When each batch is brown, I transfer it to the main stewpot, and start on the next batch in the frying pan. When all the beef has been browned and transferred, I deglaze what is now a very mucky frying pan with a glug of wine, to catch all the delicious burnt bits, then pour that into the stew, too.
3. The stew must cook for ages. That's the whole point of it. If you don't have at least 4 hours (preferably 6) for the stew to slowly glug and gurgle away on its own, make something else for dinner and save stew for when you're freer.

Intermittent fasting

You will have heard lots about intermittent fasting (IF) in recent years. There are piles of books by doctors and dieticians, as well as by those, like me, who are infinitely less qualified to offer significant nutritional advice. I have no opinion on how much anyone weighs and I have neither the expertise nor the interest to form one that's worth listening to. All I can say, as a non-qualified person who loves food, eats large portions, loves the clothes she already owns, and has never maintained a diet for more than a few days without becoming sad, hopeless and quite angry, is that intermittent fasting is how I very happily eat, almost all of the time. And – give or take the standard half-stone swing in either direction – I have remained the same dress size for my entire adult life. I obviously expect that to change at some point, but more importantly than anything weight-related, IF makes me

'Diets make
me cross and
miserable.
Intermittent
fasting makes me
relaxed and well.
I expect to do it
for life.'

feel so, so much better. I don't bloat uncomfortably like I used to, and I've nothing like the digestive problems I'd always assumed in my twenties were permanent. I don't wake up starving and I don't constantly crave all the sugar that made me sleepy within minutes. I'm able to feel satisfied at the end of a meal. IF living may not ultimately be for you – just as calorie counting, low-carbing, slimming clubs, 5:2, paleo and reconstituted protein shakes costing more than a decent bottle of wine will never be for me. It is certainly not appropriate for anyone who has ever suffered from disordered eating or other mental health issues relating to body image and weight. But if you're curious, and are in suitably good health, this is all I do: I eat for only eight hours a day. Then for sixteen hours, I fast. During my 'eating window', I deny myself nothing. I have no forbidden foods. Nothing is 'good', 'bad' or 'a treat'. Then, during my 'fasting window', I drink only water, tea or coffee (lots of fasting gurus forbid this. I'm afraid tea is a non-negotiable for me and I reject their rules with no ill effect, possibly because I take such minuscule amounts of milk). I probably consume fewer calories automatically, but I pay no attention to counting or even thinking about them. I track my timings in a free app, which I hesitate to recommend because a small child could have developed it (there are heaps of them in the App Store). That's it. It feels very logical to me that working up an appetite is better, and more natural, than it was to never allow myself to get hungry. But the biggest joy of IF, for me, is that every cycle is just a day. If you have a sociable Saturday, you can just rejig Sunday. If you're on day twenty-six of your cycle and all you want is a drip feed of ice cream and sixteen episodes of *Say Yes to the Dress*, so what? There'll be no self-destructive wailing that you've 'messed up' some arbitrary weight-loss plan and failed 'yet again' – you'll just get back on the clock when you're feeling better. Diets make me cross and miserable. Intermittent fasting makes me relaxed and well. I expect to do it for life.

Essential equipment for all kitchens

Palette knife

Not really a knife, more a thin, blunt spatula for smearing, spreading, unsticking, lifting and flipping small or delicate foodstuffs. You don't need it all that often, but when you need one, you really need one. The (often more expensive) silicone and plastic ones are not fit for purpose – get one with a metal blade.

Balloon whisk

Essential for sauces. I use a Good Grips (silicone handle, steel whisk) and it's the best I've owned.

Silicone spatula

For scraping every last scrap from your mixing bowl or saucepan, without making a racket or damaging either.

Wooden spoon

For crushing garlic (place clove on chopping board, sprinkle with sea salt, cover with wooden spoon and slam down your fist), and for stirring everything from cake batter to beef stew.

Measuring spoons

Spoons in cutlery sets are not the same thing, since 'spoons' are, in fact, exact measurements. Teaspoon = 5ml, Dessert spoon = 10ml, Tablespoon = 15ml. If you really can't accommodate a set, then use a Calpol spoon (5ml) and multiply accordingly.

Measuring jug

For stock, milk, liquids for baking and so on. I favour a glass Pyrex with measurements printed on the outside.

Spatula

For frying eggs, flipping burgers and tossing pancakes without tears. Buy a silicone one to protect your non-stick pans from scratching.

Two chopping boards

If you can keep a dishwasher-safe plastic board for meat and fish, and a wooden board for everything else, that's ideal.

Knives

I feel very strongly about knives. You can amass as many as you like and if they're great quality and kept razor sharp, you'll always love them. But I guarantee there will be three you reach for most often. If pushed for space or money, I would direct my available resources towards a cook's or chef's knife, a paring knife and a serrated knife. A boning knife is all well and good, but for better or worse, most fish is bought filleted.

These are the three knives that I can't do without in my kitchen:

Cook's knife

The most important knife in the kitchen, this can be used to cut, chop, dice, slice or mince practically everything but bread. They are usually about 15–30cm long (mine's 15cm because I'm small – just choose one that feels comfortable in your hand) with a smooth blade that tapers upward at the tip to allow for a rocking action when slicing and chopping. The blade on a good-quality cook's knife will go all the way back, filling the handle, rather than stop where the handle starts. This even weight gives a much better chopping action and means the blade won't fall out as the knife ages (anyone who also had to furnish their first place on pennies will know what this looks like.

Paring knife

Smooth, wee, a bit like a mini version of the cook's knife, for smaller foods. A more petite knife can be used more safely for jobs like peeling apples, coring fruit and vegetables or slicing garlic. Can work in place of a cheese knife, or even utility, fillet and boning knives.

Serrated knife

An essential for slicing bread and chopping softer foods or those whose chemical makeup damages or blunts smooth blades quickly, for example tomatoes and lemons (truly, these are knife kryptonite).

Knife sharpener

There's no point buying quality knives if you don't sharpen them regularly. I've never got the hang of a traditional whetstone, and I'm too cowardly for the long tubular sharpening steels such as my grandfather used, impressive as they look. Instead, I use a MinoSharp type – a small plastic-encased sharpener you fill with water, then draw the knife back and forth through the slit. They're safe, fast and fit in a kitchen drawer.

Colander

For draining pasta, washing fruit and vegetables, shaking lettuce and a million other uses. I use a Joseph Joseph plastic one with a handle, since the traditional two-handled metal versions, though prettier, only work if your sink is empty enough to sit them safely down, which mine rarely is.

Hand/immersion blender

I adore my full-sized Magimix processor and wouldn't be without it, but it's expensive, a pain to wash, and so hefty that many people wouldn't be able to accommodate it in their kitchen. For convenience and out of sheer laziness, I now find myself reaching more often for my hand blender – and that impulse is entirely down to buying a Bamix a few years back, because it is so infinitely better than any other I've ever owned. I chop onions, garlic and chilli in the little chopper attachment, froth milk, whip cream and stiffen egg whites with the beater attachment, and blend soups in seconds with the main blade. It washes up almost instantly by being switched on with its head submerged in hot soapy water. It is utterly brilliant and worth every penny of the higher price point. I am unendingly grateful to whoever it was on Twitter that first encouraged me down to Lakeland to buy it.

Sieve

For refining, smoothing, airing or draining everything that's too fine for the colander – flour and rice, for example.

Grater

I love the Microplane-type graters in different sizes, for everything from coarse-grated Cheddar to a fine dusting of nutmeg. But if budget or space are an issue, get a box grater with multiple surfaces. Those rotating graters with a handle seem brilliant, but I've never found one that does the job as fast as the traditional model.

Scissors / kitchen shears

For opening parcels, trimming fat and gristle, chopping herbs quickly and spring onions lazily, snipping leftovers for the dog's or cat's bowl, breaking into maddening food packaging like that of bacon, and even slicing pizza.

Peeler

The Y-shaped peelers (I use Good Grips) are much quicker and less achy on the wrist than the traditional straight ones.

Non-stick frying pan

If you can accommodate several, great. If not, you need at least one for omelettes, fried eggs, bacon and whatever else. If it's big enough to accommodate a slice of bread, you can also make toasted sandwiches without having to store a toastie machine. I have both cheap pans and very expensive ones and not one of them gets used as often as my Earthpan – eco-responsible (it's recycled and recyclable), never sticky and, while not at all cheap at £40-odd, much less expensive than the posh pans recommended by chefs (I also throw mine in the dishwasher with no ill effects, though Earthpan don't recommend this themselves).

Three lidded saucepans

A large pan for pasta and potatoes, a medium pan for vegetables, a small pan for reheating a sauce and scrambling, boiling or poaching eggs. I've bought extremely expensive, well-reviewed, heavy German pans in the past and ended up resenting them bitterly for needing a hand wash. Now I use them only for cooking things that can be cleaned away waterlessly with the wipe of some kitchen paper (vegetables, omelettes and the like). For everything else, I use Tefal and Salter, because I own a dishwasher and life is finite. Congratulations to anyone who can cope with those chef-approved and apparently superior stainless-steel pans – I find they stick, both on the hob and in the dishwasher.

Steamer

If you can find a large pan (as above) with a matching steamer layer, then marvellous. If you can't, or if space is tight, get a collapsible metal steaming nest from any kitchenware shop or site.

Tin opener

Much as I could probably fight my way into a Heinz tin if craving beans on toast badly enough (frequently), you'll need this for tinned tomatoes – the cornerstone of many great dishes – and sweetcorn, lentils and anything else without a ring pull. I use Good Grips, as it keeps knuckles well away from the action.

Heavy-bottomed stew/casserole pan

This is a big pan whose lid and handle can cope with being transferred from the hob to the oven, and staying there for some time. Can be used for stews, chillies, soups, curries – anything in which many ingredients are thrown into one slow-cooked dish. I use a Le Creuset, but anything oven-safe with a heavy bottom works.

Cast-iron pan (skillet)

If you're a vegetarian, you can probably live without a skillet (though they are the best for frying mushrooms), but for when you need to sear steak or chicken, and really conduct the heat, this is a must. This is also the best pan for frying sausages. Only ever handwash it (and I'd only bother washing it at all if I'd been cooking meat or fish), and rub in a little oil with kitchen paper after cleaning to stop any rust or sticking.

Wok

Ideal for very fast meals cooked briskly on a very high temperature. Storage of a full-sized wok is a pain, but you can buy half-sized woks easily enough, and they're sufficient to feed two people with a large stir-fry.

Baking tray

For baking, catching drips from above, crisping bottoms and heating frozen foods.

Roasting tin

For roasting vegetables, potatoes and meat.

Electric kettle

This may sound obvious, but I'm staggered by how many people attempt to boil water in a pan, on the hob, with no lid, for cooking purposes. You'd be quicker waiting for a cat to fetch a stick. Unless you're in a power cut, always heat pasta, rice, egg and stock water in the kettle, then transfer to a pot and bring back up to the boil.

91

Can I use something after its best-before date?

Yes. Think of 'best before' as some friendly advice given to maximise your enjoyment of food, not a warning to prevent you from dying. Anything past that date probably won't taste as good as it once did. It may not work in the way you'd expect (old bread flour doesn't rise properly, for example). But it will not make you ill or pose a risk to your health. 'Use by', on the other hand, acts as more of a warning, but is also there to cover the backs of food retailers, who don't particularly want a lawsuit should their eggs cause you to be sick throughout your driving test or wedding day. So I take it seriously, but not neurotically, and would generally allow most foods an extra few days' grace, understanding, of course, that on my head be it. I judge fruit and vegetables by sight, regardless of the date.

Five ways to feed several hungry children very fast

Pretend macaroni and cheese (12 minutes)

Boil macaroni in water. While it cooks, warm double cream in a saucepan, season, and melt in a fistful of grated cheese. Fold in the cooked and drained macaroni, transfer to an oven dish, and grill under a high heat for a couple of minutes.

Egg-fried rice and greens (5 minutes)

Crack an egg into a bowl and beat it with a fork. Dash in about a teaspoon of soy sauce, then empty a pouch of microwavable rice into the oil and egg mix. Stir. Heat a wok or frying pan to a high heat, then add a little sesame or groundnut oil and swirl it around the base. Throw in any one or more available vegetables – broccoli, spring onions, green beans, peppers, carrots, anything – and fry briskly. If they need more softening, dash in some water and cover with a lid for a minute. Empty the eggy rice into the wok, turn off the heat and stir the whole mixture with a fork to cook it. Season.

Almost-instant fish pie (8 minutes)

Cook a whole packet of frozen mash cubes (cheap and available in any supermarket) in the microwave. Turn on the grill. When the mash is ready (in around 3 minutes), transfer to an ovenproof dish, throw in a tin of tuna, another of sweetcorn, two handfuls of microwaved frozen peas and a large fistful of grated cheese. Combine everything with a fork and top with more cheese and a drizzle of oil. Place under the grill for a couple of minutes to brown. Serve with baked beans.

Garlic spaghetti (11 minutes)

Place the spaghetti in a saucepan of water and cook according to the packet instructions. Heat a tablespoon of garlic-infused olive oil (available quite cheaply everywhere) and snip in a few rashers of bacon to fry. When the spaghetti is cooked, either throw the garlicky bacon dressing over the pasta and coat, or – if your children need pasta to be red – add a carton of passata to the frying pan, heat through, then toss in the spaghetti to dress. Serve with grated cheese.

Noodle soup in a cup (5 minutes)

Pour boiling water into a jug to make 2 litres of vegetable stock (Marigold powder is my favourite and comes in a reduced-salt version suitable for little children). Pour into a saucepan and simmer on a medium heat.

Throw in any vegetable to hand (frozen peas work perfectly fine, as does tinned sweetcorn – just add them nearer the end). Smash a large handful or two of noodles in their bag with a rolling pin to make them smaller (and quicker to cook). Add to the stock and cook for around 2 minutes – taste one to test if cooked. Pour soup into mugs and serve with a teaspoon – children seem to find this fun. I can only assume it's the same thing that makes sleeping in a tent in the garden fun when they've perfectly comfortable beds inside.

How to make a no-lumps white sauce

I learned how to make a white roux in a home economics lesson when I was eleven, and I'm pleased to have done so. I made it for years whenever I needed a sauce, feeling very clever and thinking that's just how it was done. But then I learned this infinitely simpler all-in-one method in my twenties and I'm pretty sure I haven't gone near a roux since. For most home cooks, this will be everything you'll need in a white sauce without a single lump or moment's frustration, and it will serve you very well throughout your cooking life. I use it for macaroni cheese (the proper kind, not the super-fast emergency kind opposite), lasagne, fish pie, moussaka – anything that requires a white sauce – and I can promise you that it never, ever goes wrong, provided you follow the rules and use everything but the flour cold from the fridge. The recipe is, however, a true chef's nightmare, since it mixes imperial and metric measurements, but what can I say, other than that the '4040 pint' is easy to remember and the quantities work just perfectly?

93

Ingredients:
40g cold unsalted butter
40g plain flour
1 pint of cold milk (full-fat, ideally. Semi-skimmed is fine. Definitely
   not skimmed)
Salt and pepper

Method:
Put everything into a cold pan at the same time, and place on a low-medium heat. Using a balloon whisk, stir the ingredients continuously, ensuring that the whisk is touching the bottom of the pan at all times. Do not stop whisking as all the butter melts, the sauce gradually thickens

and approaches the boil. Season with salt and pepper (doing this too early makes the sauce a bit grey). Turn the heat right down to stop it bubbling over, until you're ready to use it.

For cheese sauce, follow everything above, adding a pinch of either cayenne pepper or mustard powder with the rest of the ingredients at the beginning. When the sauce is finished, remove from the heat, grate in a little nutmeg, and add fistfuls of coarsely grated cheese (whatever mixed offcuts are looking a bit sad and dry in the fridge drawer). Stir until melted.

I almost always make double quantities – 80g × 80g × 2 pints – and freeze half for my kids to make themselves macaroni at a later date. It freezes beautifully for a good couple of months.

How to keep Champagne, Crémant, Prosecco or similar fizzy

There are a hundred different gadgets for this purpose and I've bought a couple of them myself, but they're ugly (usually got up to look a bit like an executive toy for men – all matte-black plastic and ugly faux Perspex), invariably fail to wow, then get a bit sticky and lost in the back of the drawer. Instead, I now save my money and defer to the maître d' in a very grand Parisian hotel I was lucky enough to visit several years ago. He always popped an upturned teaspoon into the open bottle, its handle dangling inside, its round resting on the bottle neck – the metal of which deterred any gas leakage from the interior, he assured me. I can't tell you if the science stacks up, but I can say that the method really does, and so in the rare event of unfinished bubbles, this is precisely what I always do.

How to make risotto

People are terrified of making risotto in the same way they are scared of soufflé, yet in fact it's very easy but just needs your patience, focus and attention. This is not a dinner you can leave to look after itself. You must stay with it throughout in order for it to work. But honestly, on the right evening, this is a pleasure. I find the repetitive but untaxing pattern of hydration-stir-hydration-stir quite calming. I feel in control and free to think about other things, while being unable to leave the risotto and actually assist anyone with anything. Eating risotto is similarly unchallenging. One piece of cutlery, one creamy mass, a delicious vehicle for leftover meat, vegetables or wine. Give risotto half an hour of your

'Give risotto
half an hour of
your time and
it is effortless
thereafter.'

time and it is effortless thereafter. This recipe is for mushroom risotto, as it's the most commonly asked about (and my most frequently made), but when you understand the basic cooking method, you can adapt it to any risotto – some ideas below.

Ingredients *(serves 2 greedy people):*
½ pack (about 15g) of dried porcini mushrooms
2 celery sticks
1 fat garlic clove
Olive oil, for frying
25g unsalted butter (vegans can just leave this out)
A sprig of thyme
1 litre vegetable stock (I use either Marigold powder or Knorr Concentrated Liquid Stock; non-vegetarians may prefer to use chicken stock, which works well)
½ 500g box of risotto rice (Carnaroli, Vialone Nano, Arborio or similar – risotto will not work with regular rice)
1 glass of any dry white wine
Salt and freshly ground black pepper
250g mushrooms of your choice – portobello, chestnut, button – anything, or a mix of 2 or more
A large handful of fresh flat-leaf parsley or fresh basil
A large handful of Parmesan or pecorino cheese (vegetarian versions are available)
1 tablespoon cream or crème fraîche (vegans can skip or use soya cream)

Method:

An hour or two before you start, drop the dried porcini mushrooms (if you can't get these, use dried wild mushrooms) into a 1 litre measuring jug and add boiling water to the top. Leave until you're ready to cook.

When ready to cook, return to the jug. The porcini will have plumped up and the water will be brown. Scoop the porcini out of the mushroom stock and set down on a chopping board, keeping the stock in the jug. Chop the porcini coarsely.

Blitz together in a processor the celery sticks and garlic.

Take a heavy-bottomed pan and add a dash of olive oil and a knob of butter, if using. Throw in the celery and garlic and fry together on a medium–low heat for 3–4 minutes. They must not brown, so keep an eye on your heat. If they start to brown, throw in a tiny bit of tap water.

Toss in your chopped porcini and thyme and fry for another minute.

Get a large, empty saucepan. Back in your jug, you'll be left with porcini stock that is a little gritty, so pour it through a sieve and into the empty pan. Rinse out the jug and make up a litre of vegetable stock. Add that to the pan of porcini stock. Pop this large volume of liquid on a low heat and keep simmering. This is what you'll be using to cook your risotto.

Return to the heavy pan containing the mushrooms and the celery mush. Add the uncooked risotto rice. Stir well so the rice gets nicely coated in oil and flavour. Do this for a minute or so.

It's worth turning up the temperature a bit at this point. Still stirring the rice, pour in a generous glug of white wine to deglaze the pan. It will sizzle and the rice should absorb it quickly, but stir until all the liquid has gone and the alcohol has been cooked off. Grind in some black pepper and a little salt, but don't go mad on the latter as the stock will be salty.

Now to make your risotto. Have your pans – the rice and the stock – side by side at the cooker, both on the heat. Take a ladleful of stock and tip it into the rice mix, stirring the rice with a wooden spatula or spoon until all the stock has been absorbed. Only then can you return to your stock for another ladleful. It is absolutely essential that you do this ladle by ladle, adding more only when the last ladleful has been absorbed by the rice. The continuous stirring is also essential – you don't ever want a reservoir of stock in one part of the pan. The stirring ensures that all the grains of rice are cooked evenly – no hard bits in mush.

Repeat over and over: ladle of stock – stir until gone – ladle of stock – stir until gone. Do this back and forth until the rice is cooked, but with a little bite (generally around 25 minutes, but frequently more or less, depending on the rice).

While this is happening, heat a frying pan and fry your heap of fresh mushrooms in a little olive oil. There is nothing at all fancy about this – just fry them quickly until their water content has evaporated and they've browned a bit. I only do this separately because throwing them into the risotto raw means they steal all the rice's cooking stock and the whole thing takes much longer. Set the cooked mushrooms aside for later.

At this point, the risotto is probably nearly ready. You've probably run out of stock. If this is the case but the rice still needs a few more minutes, just add some boiling water from the kettle to see it over the line.

Throw in your cooked mushrooms. Add some sort of soft herb – flat-leaf parsley works very well; basil is also great in risotto. Stir.

The risotto should now be quite creamy and sloppy because of the starch, but if you like it even more babyfood-like (I do), grate in a handful of Parmesan or pecorino and stir in either a knob of unsalted butter and/or a spoonful of cream/crème fraîche. Check the seasoning and add more salt and pepper if necessary.

Serve with more Parmesan.

Other risottos – the one ladle of stock at a time method remains exactly the same for all:

Classic: Use a small, very finely chopped onion as your savoury base, instead of celery and garlic. At the white wine stage, add a pinch of saffron threads. Finish with butter and Parmesan, as before, but don't add parsley and cream.

Lemon: Use the same savoury base and vegetable (or chicken) stock, but omit all the mushroom ingredients. When the rice is almost cooked, add the juice and grated zest of a lemon, and some frozen peas if desired. Finish with parsley and Parmesan, as above.

Chicken: Use the same savoury base as for the mushroom risotto, and use chicken stock. Omit all the mushroom ingredients. When the risotto is ready, throw in every shred of roast chicken you can tear from the leftover carcass of a Sunday lunch. Works nicely with some cooked frozen peas stirred in, too (just zap them for a couple of minutes in the microwave and throw them in just before serving).

No risotto freezes well. However, it reheats fine from the fridge in the microwave. It'll be a little claggier, less creamy, but still delicious. If too stiff, loosen with a little vegetable stock and stir before heating.

Kitchen gadgets that no one needs but that I love all the same

Bread maker

Sales of these have soared since the Covid-19 pandemic and they were out of stock everywhere for months. I'd never been more pleased to have my trusty Panasonic, still going strong after fifteen years of continual use. Bread makers are bulky, not very attractive and have the air of something that will be used for a month, then abandoned to gather dust. But truly, mine has been among the most useful bits of kit in my kitchen. They are the easiest things in the world. My husband can make a loaf while he's waiting for our bed tea to brew – one just throws in yeast, flour, butter, salt, sugar and water and sets the timer. When we wake the following morning, the house is filled with the aroma of warm, freshly baked bread. It also makes terrific pizza dough and cake. My old, middle-of-the-range machine cost about £120 when it was given to me for Christmas, and has saved me fortunes over the fifteen years since. If you can accommodate one in your kitchen, you won't regret buying.

Boiling-water tap

A huge extravagance and one I couldn't justify for years, until our sixth expensive kettle in eighteen months conked out and my fury caused me to finally pull the trigger (we drink a lot of tea, but still). After shopping around, I went for a Quooker (less money than the nearest competitor) and now I think I'd rather sell off my jewellery than be without it. It's brilliant for tea, of course, but also saves so much time in cooking. I have instant pasta water, stock on tap for soups and risotto, and can boil up a pot of mash in no time. My model of Quooker also dispenses filtered water and includes a removable hose for filling vases and buckets without having to wedge them into the sink. I love it.

99

Breville sandwich maker

A bulky gadget that performs only one function is unlikely to take priority in a small kitchen but oh, the peerless joy of biting through the chewy, triangulated seams of a Breville toastie, molten cheese immediately dripping down one's chin, feeling too impatient to wait for tomatoes to sufficiently cool to leave the roof of one's mouth intact. There's nothing more delicious. Whatever my circumstances and wherever I've lived, I've always found space for a Breville (the same £15 model I bought from Argos twenty years ago, in fact). Don't be tempted by posher sandwich toasters. They are perfectly fine in their own right, but absolutely cannot replicate the very specific ecstasy of a Breville.

How to host a dinner party

I love cooking, hosting and socialising, but never at another's expense. There's nothing more awkward and boring for guests than sitting behind a closed kitchen door as you stress over a labour-intensive meal that not one of you would cook under any normal circumstances. It's completely

'If people come round, they're coming to have fun with you, not to judge MasterChef.'

mad. Let a proper chef do it when you go out, while you sit calmly and unsweatily, pausing the conversation only when a nice server tops up your wine glass. If people come round, they're coming to have fun with you, not to judge *MasterChef*. What Covid surely taught us, once and for all, is that being with people we love is what makes us happy, so make the most of your guests, lose the starter and just open a bottle instead. Make one slow-cooked course during the day, ideally in one large pot – a delicious stew, Indian or Thai curry, a rich, flavoursome chilli or lasagne – and just whip up an easy accompaniment: rice, mash or pasta. Or roast a big chicken and serve it with a salad and crusty bread. By all means, serve a second course, but make it something that takes moments to free from its packet – ice cream, a couple of good cheeses and crackers, a bakery tart that needs three minutes in the oven to warm through, dolloped with cold crème fraîche. You can still make the whole thing lovely by dimming lights, burning candles, preparing a great playlist in advance and whacking on a red lip.

How to make hollandaise

If you have eggs to poach and muffins or nice bread to toast, you might as well whip up a hollandaise for eggs Benedict (with ham) or Florentine (with spinach). I say whip up because, contrary to widespread opinion, homemade hollandaise sauce is extremely quick, easy and very delicious. I feel that perhaps boutique hotels and gastropubs have convinced people that something very simple is way beyond a civilian's capabilities. The key to a silky, ungreasy hollandaise is never overheating, adding fat very slowly and maintaining a continuous whisk. Takes five minutes.

Ingredients *(to serve 4 greedy people)*:
2 eggs
1 tablespoon white wine vinegar
225g packet of butter
Sea salt and freshly ground black pepper
½ lemon
A handful of chopped fresh tarragon (optional)

1. Take a smallish saucepan and pour in enough boiling water to reach about 3cm above the bottom. Put it on a medium–low heat so it's simmering steadily, never bubbling over.
2. Crack 2 eggs, separate them by passing the yolk into the shell halves, and throw the whites into the freezer for another day. Place the egg yolks in a glass Pyrex dish, whisk well, then add the tablespoon of vinegar.
3. Open the packet of butter and place the whole lot in a jug. Microwave on a low temperature until melted. Set aside.
4. Place the Pyrex dish containing the egg yolks and vinegar over the pan of simmering water. It's important to use glass so you can see the water beneath and ensure that it absolutely never touches the bottom of the bowl – there must be a gap to avoid overheating.
5. Immediately start whisking the yolks and vinegar with a balloon whisk. After a minute, the mixture will almost double in volume and become a paler lemon colour. Get your melted butter jug.
6. Still whisking, very slowly drizzle the melted butter into the yolk mix – think of a stream about as thick as a phone charging cable. As you pour slowly with one hand, whisk the contents of the glass bowl continuously with the other. The sauce will soon thicken.
7. Grind in some black pepper and sea salt, and squeeze the juice of the half-lemon into the sauce. Taste a little and add more if it needs sharpening.
8. If you like the aniseedy taste of tarragon (I love it, many hate it) and you have some, throw in a few finely chopped leaves.
9. Pour the sauce over your eggs and muffins. To keep it warm for second helpings, replace the bowl on the saucepan, but turn off the heat while you eat.

How to roast a chicken

Disclaimer: All ovens are different. The way I roast chicken in my Brighton home is not how I roasted it in my old London flat, or how I learned to roast it in my grandmother's kitchen in the South Wales valleys. Birds vary, too – I find supermarket chicken a bit more watery than those from my local butcher and, as a result, the latter takes less time to cook and crisp up. You can only really tell categorically whether a chicken is roasted if you poke its thigh with the tip of a sharp knife and the juices

'I feel that perhaps boutique hotels and gastropubs have convinced people that something very simple is way beyond a civilian's capabilities.'

run readily, hot and clear, with no pink. That will happen sooner with some chicken/oven combinations than with others, so keep a keen eye and nose on proceedings.

1. An hour before cooking, remove the chicken from the fridge and its packaging and place it in a baking tray that fits it well – not tight, but not with acres of space to spare either (too much space causes smoking and burning). Dry the skin with kitchen paper.

2. Preheat the oven to 210°C/410°F (this is utterly essential – so many cooking disasters lead back to cold ovens and pans).

3. Chop a lemon and an onion in half. Pop half of each in the chicken's cavity (practically no shop-bought chickens come with giblets these days, but if yours does, you need to remove them first). You can put some herbs inside, too (you get all the flavour this way, but none of the burn). Rosemary or tarragon with a sprig of thyme and a bay leaf works well, but if you're not keen, just skip it.

4. Mix around 2 tablespoons of room-temperature butter and a glug of olive oil together in a bowl. Take a handful and massage it into the bird's skin. Remember not to ignore the legs and wings – get everything greased up.

5. Grind on some black pepper and crush some salt flakes over the skin.

6. Place the tray in the upper-centre part of the preheated oven.

7. Roast for 15 minutes per pound of chicken, plus 20 minutes for luck.

8. Half an hour into cooking, open the oven door briefly to spoon the hot fat collected in the bottom of the roasting pan back onto the skin of the bird. This usually only needs doing once. If this process causes the temperature to drop, don't worry and turn the dial to 200°C/400°F.

9. When the chicken's skin is golden and crispy, and a skewer inserted into the crease between thigh and torso produces hot, clear juice, it's ready.

10. Cover the cooked bird loosely with tin foil, taking care not to touch the skin, and wrap a warm tea towel around the outside. It's at this point that I normally sit it in the utility room on top of the tumble dryer, but anywhere warm with no draught is ideal. It will stay warm for ages – probably over an hour. Now you can get on with preparing whatever you're having with it: mash, roast potatoes, salad, chips, ratatouille, crusty bread, greens or whatever else you like.

How to get kids to eat vegetables

I'd love to give you an answer that didn't involve fraud and deception, since we all know that the rather condescending advice given by people who have clearly never had an inherently picky child is to keep putting delicious vegetables on a child's plate indefinitely, before clearing the table and, yet again, serving them to the dog. I have one child (now very nearly a man) who ate about four things for years, despite cajoling, standing firm, bribing with stickers, visiting specialists and every other doctor, and attempting academic-prescribed treatments. He still doesn't really do vegetables, and this is a man from a family of voracious and unfussy eaters, to whom at one stage we would have handed the contents of our pockets for eating a floret of broccoli. Why did I cave and resort to trickery? Because I felt sure he would faint from scurvy if the situation was allowed to continue.

Take a vegetable with a relatively bland flavour when unseasoned – butternut squash, cauliflower, courgette, spinach, sweet potato, pumpkin and so on – and steam until soft. Process with a hand blender to a smooth paste. Fill small freezer bags or pots with the paste and deep freeze. Do this with as many vegetables as you can, so you have a rainbow of colours to choose from. Get to a point where every time you cook anything saucy, you can throw in one of the purées in an undetectable colour. Cauliflower works a treat in macaroni cheese and fish pie, beetroot and pumpkin can be well concealed in Bolognese or shepherd's pie. I can hide a full five-a-day quota in a simple-seeming tomato pasta sauce. You can still serve with something on the side perceived by the child to be more benign, like frozen peas or carrots, so they don't forget what the real thing looks like. And buy plenty of multivitamin tablets.

What do I need to keep in the freezer?

I have a family of four, including two teenage boys and two greedy adults, and have a total inability to cook appropriately small portions (I'm one of five siblings). So for me, the freezer is vital. Though its contents have changed since my children were little (the fish fingers, potato waffles and Arctic Roll have mostly gone – though mmmm, Arctic Roll), most of the same time-saving staples remain, and I still pride myself on always being able to feed everyone from the freezer if we're all out of fresh food.

'To be never
more than three
minutes from
mash is surely a
state of grace.'

This is what helps:

Nuts

I love adding nuts to porridge, muesli, ice cream, stir-fries and curries, but their oil content means they go off very quickly and taste foul. Now I throw handfuls into a freezer bag as soon as I get them home, so I always have some to hand. They defrost in practically no time.

Chopped onions

Trust me. These are life-changing in that they are very often the difference between me thinking I can't be bothered to cook and actually making something delicious. Just pour them into a hot pan to get rid of any excess moisture, then turn down the heat and treat as you would fresh onions.

Soffrito mix

Same deal as the onions, but with the addition of chopped celery and carrots for a full savoury base. Add a bay leaf and some thyme, and you have a soup when you've very little else in (just add stock, spices and lentils), or whip up a cottage pie in no time, especially if you have . . .

Mash

Not as good as the real thing, but to be never more than three minutes from mash is surely a state of grace. Always buy one that contains only potatoes, butter, salt, pepper and maybe milk – no weird non-foods.

A supper

I always try to have at least one thing in the freezer that needs minimal intervention to become a proper family dinner – Bolognese, chilli, cheese sauce for macaroni, stew – anything you can either defrost in the microwave or throw solid into a pot and leave on a low heat.

Spinach

I love fresh spinach, but it feels as though it barely lasts enough time for me to put away the shopping. I now only buy it for salads, and keep frozen spinach permanently on hand for soups, curry and dhal. It comes in helpfully portioned cubes and defrosts fast when submerged in a sauce.

Bananas

There is always a banana or two on the turn and headed for the bin. Instead, peel them, throw in a freezer bag and keep topping up, for an instant source of smoothie, or for baking banana cake when more in the mood.

Broccoli

See spinach. For soups and the like, it's more than fine.

Pastry

I've just realised that I haven't made fresh pastry since Christmas Day 2018. It was delicious, but no more delicious than an equivalent pie made from Jus-Rol shortcrust. Certainly, I've never made a puff pastry that was a patch on frozen, and I've never attempted to make filo at all. Just buy all-butter varieties (swerve the margarine stuff) and run a bath instead.

Egg whites

I tend to use extra yolks in most egg dishes, so I always throw the whites into freezer bags in pairs, then make a huge Christmas or Easter pavlova.

Wine

My husband drinks white, I drink red, so there are frequently half-filled bottles of wine sitting on the worktop. I hate waste, so if I'm not going to drink it, I pour it into freezer bags to avoid opening a bottle specially for a recipe that needs a glass or glug to deglaze the pan. Defrosts in about 20 minutes.

108

Peas

No home should be without them. Endlessly useful for risotto, pasta, kids' suppers, dhal and soup. I mostly microwave them from frozen first, as they bring the temperature right down in whatever you're cooking (though this can have its uses). Also essential to take down swelling following a domestic fall or burn – just hold the full bag to the affected area.

Berries

I find berries peak for about a day before becoming rotten and in Britain, at least, they're so expensive that throwing them away feels almost criminal. Now I immediately decant half into a freezer bag to use for porridge, smoothies, granola and ice cream.

Vegetable offcuts

I know it sounds gross, but bear with me. Every time you chop the end off an onion, parsnip or carrot, or trim the leaves from a cabbage or leek, throw the offcuts into a large freezer bag. Top up the bag until full, then add herbs, a bay leaf and add to a pan with water to make vegetable stock. It's delicious with noodles, in gravy or soup. You could skip the freezing and just compost, of course, but not all councils (including mine) offer this service.

Herbs

My greatest cooking extravagance is herbs, because when I have parsley, basil, rosemary, mint and coriander, I can make something ordinary taste more interesting and special. I'm happy to use dried oregano, thyme, bay leaves and most spices, but for soft green herbs, ginger and lemongrass, a store of frozen fresh is much better. I also keep a store of frozen chopped chillies because it's easier to do a job lot in the processor once in a while than it is to go through the faff of protecting your skin and eyes each time you'd like some heat.

Lemon wedges

Cut lemons into wedges and freeze, so you always have fresh lemon where a recipe requires it, and instant access to a cold gin (or vodka) and tonic when you feel like one.

Ice

Amazingly, this is the one thing I have to consciously remind myself to keep in stock. When a girl needs a Martini . . .

How to make a perfect Martini

I loathe gin, which puts me out of step with pervading drinking culture, so I make this with vodka, but the recipe works either way. It's my friend Julia Raeside's recipe, but I think she originally stole it from Roger Moore and adapted it:

1. Tip a shot of dry vermouth into a Martini glass, swirl it around, tip into a second glass if making two, and repeat. Then pour into a cocktail shaker and swirl that around too. Place your glass(es) in the freezer.
2. Place a couple of ice cubes in the cocktail shaker, add one measure of gin or vodka per Martini, and shake a bit – no need for a workout – then place the shaker in the freezer. Leave for 15 minutes.
3. Retrieve the glasses, wipe around the rim of each with a lemon wedge, and pour the Martini through the ice strainer of the shaker.
4. Serve with a couple of olives on a cocktail stick, or a twist of lemon peel.

How to treat a hangover

There are five pillars of hangover management – water, salts, carbs, protein, sugar. If any one is missing, the entire day collapses into a pit of despair. When you've had enough sleep and have stopped being sick (where applicable), take a shower, then prepare the following:

1. A pint of water, sipped as it is, then refilled with a solution of either Dioralyte powder or an Alka-Seltzer tablet (the former marginally less revolting than the latter, but whatever you have).
2. A fried egg sandwich on any bread.
3. A can of Coca-Cola or Pepsi (never Diet Coke, Pepsi Max or anything else with sweeteners instead of sugar). Full-calorie Lilt also works well if you don't like cola.

Drink your water, make your sandwich. Sit down very quietly on the sofa. Eat your egg, drink your fat Coke and watch something banal and unchallenging on TV, like reruns of *Four in a Bed*. You'll be pondering the evening's takeaway in no time.

110

Why become a vegetarian?

It was a slow-burning decision. An accident, then a choice that made an almost negligible practical impact on my life. I'd always thought vegetarianism had to be driven by anger, righteousness, trauma, a pivotal moment where I witnessed some horrific cruelty that drove me to make a huge sacrifice for the sake of my principles, forgoing my beloved T-bone for the greater good.

But in the end, I realised this perception of heroism was stopping me making a terribly straightforward decision. It wasn't Simon Amstell's *Carnage*, a feature-length mockumentary none of my friends could persuade me to watch. It wasn't even the field of pigs I watched on a Suffolk holiday, each of them with sentient expressions I recognised as almost human, or the revelation that they were the lucky ones, that many meat pigs are kept underground, never seeing daylight, forced to give birth in cages that prevent them turning to see their new piglets before they're taken away. It wasn't the news that there is not enough land on Earth to farm all meat humanely. It wasn't the uncomfortable realisation that I adored my dog out of all proportion but gave no thought to the lambs and cows I ate with gravy, and it certainly wasn't the horrific scenes

'There are five pillars of hangover management – water, salts, carbs, protein, sugar. If any one is missing, the entire day collapses into a pit of despair.'

'What I never in a million years expected was what proved to be true: giving up meat is easy.'

of torture people felt the need to post between LOLcats and baby snaps on social media. For decades, I waited for a lightning bolt when in reality it was a light, constant drizzle that ultimately wore me down.

First, I did what people lucky enough to be comfortably off do to make themselves feel better: buy only organic and sustainable meat, and eat it rarely, like a posh bar of chocolate or ten-quid wine. Never mind that I was turning a blind eye in restaurants, or when I took my family for a Sunday roast, or when I was hungover and fancied a Pret bacon baguette. Never mind that I picked up a raw chicken as though handling plutonium, that the sight of offal made me gag, or that my posh meat made an enormous carbon footprint, guzzling water, grain and land. I didn't eat enough to make any difference, and besides, abstinence and deprivation weren't my style. I was a keen cook, libertarian and foodie! I had no desire to join a gang that would have the wellness Insta-charlatans and Morrissey for members. I could have it all ways – the occasional juicy steak or hearty pie – and still feel moral, moderate and zestful.

And so it happened while I wasn't looking. Not so much a moment of clarity as a gradual falling away of scales. There simply came a point when there were so many conditions and disclaimers attached to my diet – no pork, no veal, not intensively farmed, only organic, sustainable and insanely expensive – that it just seemed easier and more honest to step up and stop altogether. I had a hundred environmental and human reasons to quit, but only one to keep doing what I was doing: taste. It seemed petty and embarrassingly pathetic of me, when there were so many delicious alternatives, to allow something so small and self-serving to be a deal breaker. Things were born, caged, frightened, then killed, just for me. It seemed a wholly wasteful, needlessly extravagant and frankly impractical way to deliver protein to my diet.

As undramatic as the decision was, I was unprepared for how inconsequential the change would be. What I never in a million years expected was what proved to be true: giving up meat is easy. It's astonishing how quickly chicken, beef, lamb and pork (yes, even bacon) just become non-foods. I don't crave them in the way I once expected – I simply skim past them on the menu, as though they're written for someone else. My friends either didn't care or were intrigued, only a step or two behind me on the path to vegetarianism. My husband grilled bacon on the very first weekend and my Bisto Kid instinct to follow the smoky fumes and alluring sizzle had simply vanished overnight. The chicken curry on the table next to me held no appeal. Sausages didn't become some irresistible forbidden fruit I suddenly needed as though my very life depended on it. I felt no more hungry, restricted or less satisfied. I continued to eat greedily and giddily, looking forward to every meal in the way I always had. Perhaps even more so, since it is no longer a case of landing on mushroom risotto or goat's cheese tart and liking or lumping it. Every high street has multiple vegetarian options, many of them far more exciting, interesting and delicious than yet another burger or chicken breast. My culinary repertoire somehow expanded and meat suddenly, unexpectedly, seemed boring, unimaginative, queasy-making.

I said I would never become a vegetarian and I meant it. And maybe you feel the same. You may well be right, and I don't judge you at all. After forty-three years of enthusiastic meat eating, I hardly could. My sons eat meat and I cook it for them happily; my husband – meat-free in the week – always orders it on Deliveroo Fridays. I'm not about to become vegan because I'm far from perfect and it's hard. Maybe you've found the right balance for you – whether making an ethical gesture for the environment by engaging in meat-free Mondays, or being careful about the quality of the meat you eat, the farming you support. Maybe you live happily on KFC and never give the meat-free alternative a single thought. But there's also a strong chance that, like me, your friends are starting to jump ship, and you're tempted but pre-emptively defeated by the insurmountable challenge you believe lies ahead. And so I want to tell you, you can quit in a moment, and never look back, just as I did. I want to tell you that it's really not hard. I feel happy, in control, healthier and richer following my decision. There was no fire in my belly, no placard-waving in my head, no strong opinion on the diets of others, no belief that I had to be perfect to make a positive change. Just a realisation that my excuse was no longer good enough. I love animals, I love the planet and my fondness for mince should not be their problem. Vegetarianism is not a sacrifice, it's a simple, logical act, much like recycling bottles or rescuing a dog, and it matters. Why deprive yourself of the opportunity for the sake of a bucket of wings?

How to avoid fake meat

Here's the rub. I have a deep hatred of fake meat and unluckily happened to become a vegetarian at the same time all those hipster vegan burgers became standard in quality fast-food outlets (I long for the return of the traditional veggie burger, made of pulses or vegetables, with no creepy fake blood made from beetroot – only the Honest Burger and Smashburger chains continue to offer them). For cooking, this initially posed a problem. I refuse to make multiple meals nightly for different family members, but also am not keen on soya mince. Having tried every imaginable recipe and formula, I finally found the perfect solution: 500g of brown mushrooms, pulsed in the processor, plus two tins of green lentils, makes the perfect amount of vegetarian 'mince' for a huge family-sized vat of Bolognese, chilli or a large cottage pie. Add a teaspoon of Marmite to the pot for even greater depth and an extra hit of umami (I add it to vegetarian gravy, too – it's perfect). Before you say 'but I hate mushrooms', as so many unfathomably do, let me reassure you that you won't know. In fact, I type hoping my mushroom-loathing children never read this book and discover that they've been greedily gulping down my vegetarian mince for four years and counting.

How to make gravy

I will cut corners and save time with all manner of convenience foods, but I will not undo all the time and love I've given a Sunday lunch by drenching it in instant granule gravy, any more than I'd smother any other supper in ketchup. I don't understand why anyone would work so hard to make something lovely, then retire at the last, relatively effortless hurdle. Making gravy is easy and satisfying, especially if you make twice as much as you need and freeze half for a lazier day.

Ingredients:
1 tablespoon meat juices per person
1 tablespoon plain flour per person
A glug of white wine (for chicken or roast pork gravy) or red (for beef or lamb) if there happens to be some open (don't uncork specially)
1–2 litres stock (a litre is about right for up to 3 people)
Salt and freshly ground black pepper
Marmite, if you have some

Method:
When you've finished roasting your meat, lift it from the baking tray and place it on a chopping board or rack. Cover loosely with foil and wrap in a tea towel to keep warm while it rests.

If you're making a small quantity of gravy, remove any juices you don't need and set aside (I rarely do this – I'd rather use it all and make too much gravy so I can freeze what we don't eat). Place your roasting tin on the hob and turn the flame beneath it to medium.

When your juices and burnt bits of meat are sizzling in the roasting tin, add the flour and immediately start to combine the juices and flour with a balloon whisk. They should form a paste. Cook for a couple of minutes, stirring all the time with the whisk. If bits start to catch and brown, don't worry – this just intensifies the taste.

If there's wine on the go, pour in a splash to shift any remaining bits of roasting flavours stuck to the tin – if not, just use stock. Whisk the whole thing so everything is combined and becomes more fluid.

Now start adding your stock, bit by bit, ensuring all the while that your whisk is scraping the floor of the tin. Keep adding the stock and whisking, adding more and whisking, until it looks like gravy. If it's too thick, just add more stock or boiling water from the kettle.

Taste, then season with salt and pepper accordingly (remember your stock will be salty). Stir in a teaspoon of Marmite (even if you hate it on toast) to darken and enrich the gravy. Serve.

Freezes brilliantly, provided your meat didn't come from the freezer in the first place.

Thirty-seven things to have in your kitchen cupboard

Chilli flakes

I'm heat-addicted, so I put these in everything from soup to scrambled eggs, but even if you're spice-averse, chilli flakes are useful for when a dinner guest would like to turn up the heat without spoiling a whole batch for you.

Salt

Have the cheaper table salt on hand for pasta, rice or potato water, and pricier Maldon salt flakes for crisping potatoes, seasoning salad dressings, sprinkling on finished dishes and the like. There's no point boiling your cash in water that will be poured down the plughole in ten minutes. As for Himalayan pink salt, buy whatever makes you happy, but do know that in terms of health, salt is salt, is salt – however pretty it looks.

Black peppercorns

There is literally no point in the pre-ground stuff. Peppercorns are cheap and you can even buy them in a grinding bottle if you don't have a grinder in the kitchen.

Stock

My default stock comes from a bottle or tub. For meat stock, I use Knorr concentrated liquid, available in any decent supermarket. For vegetable stock, I more often use Marigold powder, which, incidentally, is genuinely delicious drunk from a mug when I'm full of a cold and self-soothing (cook some noodles in it if you need some bulk). If you're a vegetarian with the space and the budget, keep some dried porcini, too. They make delicious, rich, savoury stock, similar-ish to beef in flavour.

Olive oil

The world is now mad for extra virgin olive oil, but unless you're using it to drizzle, dress or finish a dish, that not-insubstantial cash is going up in smoke. I always have cheap olive oil for cooking, extra virgin for when it counts.

General cooking oil

I use groundnut oil for most other cooking, since it can get extremely hot without smoking. If you have a nut allergy, use vegetable or corn oil. I like the now extremely fashionable coconut oil for some things, but it doesn't have the lightness of groundnut and, to me, leaves a not always desired oiliness on the tongue.

Porridge oats

Obviously delicious for breakfast, but great for making crumble, flapjacks, biscuits and various easy baking projects for children, too. Also wonderful as a skin soother for eczema sufferers – scoop oats into a muslin cloth, gather and tie around the taps before running a bath.

Tinned chopped tomatoes

Much better than fresh tomatoes for anything red and saucy. Essential for any ragù and many a curry or soup. If you buy the finely chopped, slightly pulpy type, it will save you time. Incidentally, I rarely bother with tomato purée as it tastes slightly to me of blood – good tomatoes and proper seasoning are generally enough.

117

Passata

Essentially, these are liquidised tomatoes. Wonderful for soups, pizza toppings and for acting as an instant pasta sauce for a fractious child. Once opened, store in the fridge and use within a few days.

Plain flour

When storage is tight, just buy plain flour. You can always convert it to self-raising when needed (add 2 teaspoons of baking powder per 150g). I use plain flour constantly for pancakes, gravy, sauces, Yorkshires and stews. Invest in an airtight plastic container for storing it – flour weevils always make it through paper packets: harmless but deeply off-putting.

Curry powder

You can make your own, combining ground cumin, coriander, turmeric, chilli powder, ginger and pepper in a large jar, or you can buy excellent pre-blended curry powder in an Asian supermarket.

Oregano

One of the few green herbs I prefer when dried. Ideal for anything Mediterranean, like pasta sauces, risotto, moussaka and so on. Also works well in chilli con carne.

Thyme

Ideal for most slow-cooking recipes. Earthy and aromatic. Add early doors.

Cumin

Earthy and aromatic. I use it in Indian and Mexican food especially.

Coriander

Soft green herbs don't like being cooked for ages, so I tend to use dried coriander early on in recipes, then for a zingier and more reviving taste, add chopped fresh coriander leaves at the end. Important in Mexican and Thai food, in particular.

Chinese five-spice

Pre-blended spices that work in any Chinese dish and in many marinades and meat-rubs. Adds instant flavour to stir-fries, which can otherwise taste bland. Is best friends with soy sauce.

Marmite

The best thing for browning gravy and adding a deep savouriness to slow-cooked dishes. If you really can't stand to have it in the house, buy Geo

Watkins mushroom ketchup (which looks nothing at all like ketchup, more like black tea, and lives next to Worcestershire sauce in the spice aisle of a decent supermarket). Both are vegan.

Vinegar

You need some form of vinegar for making salad dressings and hollandaise, and for doing justice to chips (though I have a soft spot for the cheap and nasty non-brewed condiment for that specific purpose). White wine vinegar is a good all-rounder.

Soy sauce

Essential in all East Asian cooking and great for adding an instant savouriness, both as ingredient and table condiment.

Ketchup

Not a huge fan of it myself, but no home should be without Britain's favourite condiment.

Mustard

I like English mustard with Sunday lunch, most cheeses and in sauces, Dijon in salad dressings and wholegrain in mash, but it's a matter of personal taste and I could certainly live with only Colman's if I had to.

Tinned chickpeas

A day-saver when one must manifest a filling meal from practically nothing. With chickpeas, one can make delicious and cheap curry, wraps, salad, burgers, 'meatballs' and soups.

Tinned green lentils

Pre-cooked green lentils perform an identical function to chickpeas. Utterly indispensable for vegetarians, lentils are also great for bulking out meaty sauces, stews and pies.

Baking powder

For converting plain flour to self-raising, and for adding airiness to American pancakes and Yorkshire puds.

Sugar

Essential for making bread and practically any pudding. Even if you don't bake, good manners dictate that you should be able to make any visitor or tradesperson a cup of tea to their liking.

119

Pasta

At least two bags – a shape (like penne or fusilli) and a noodle (like spaghetti or linguine). I am never, ever without pasta. There have been a couple of periods in my life when I've been able to afford to eat little more than pasta and cheese, or potatoes and butter, for many weeks at a time, and my love for both has never waned. A bag of pasta means there is always something comforting to eat. Don't bother with the fresh stuff in the supermarket. It's watery, eggy, claggy and overpriced. Unless Nonna made it with her own bare hands this morning, dried pasta is usually better.

Rice

See pasta. Another cheap, essential carb with endless possibilities.

Noodles

Another carby godsend. Fast, simple and perfect for stir-fries, noodle soup (just throw into some stock with vegetables when poorly) and spicy Korean-style ramen. Particularly delicious with eggs.

Dried dhal lentils

An essential convenience food when you don't eat meat. I make a huge vat of dhal once a month, then feast on it for days. Delicious with fried eggs for breakfast, as a soup with flatbread for lunch, with rice for supper. I won't offer a prescriptive recipe, because the point for me is that dhal is an infinitely versatile, very forgiving vessel for whatever I have in the kitchen. My method (taught to me by my friend Daxita Vaghela, but adapted organically and sloppily over time) basically involves boiling up a large pan of pre-rinsed lentils and cooking with one whole chilli pepper, scored down the middle with a knife, in salted water until soft. While that happens, heat some oil in a heavy frying pan until smoking and cook mustard and cumin seeds until they pop. Add a couple of sliced onions and any other Indian spices you fancy (ginger, coriander, turmeric and the like), and cook until soft, golden and fragrant. Throw in any suitable leftovers like spinach, mushrooms, tomatoes – whatever's going, and cook for a few minutes. Blitz the lentils in their cooking water with a hand blender (I do chilli and all, but remove it if you don't like heat) until they're the texture you want. Add the juice of half a lemon – it helps with bloating. Some like soupy dhal, others like it thick – you can always add stock to thin it out. Then tip all that tasty oniony stuff from the frying pan into the blitzed lentils, and stir. Serve with fresh coriander leaves if you like (I love).

'Unless Nonna made it with her own bare hands this morning, dried pasta is usually better.'

Coconut milk

Handy for making many curries and soups, for flavouring rice, adding to smoothies and more.

Red kidney beans

These are handy in all sorts of recipes, but I mainly keep them on hand so I can whip up a quick minestrone when I need to clear out some ageing vegetables in a hurry.

Pesto

The king of convenience foods. Choose one that contains olive oil rather than sunflower or vegetable, if you can afford it.

Baked beans

When I want beans on toast, simply nothing else will do. I personally favour Heinz, but I know there's strong support among foodies for Crosse & Blackwell. Behind whichever label your heart lies, baked beans on toast surely represents the best deliciousness to effortlessness ratio in cooking, and is filling, nutritious and healthy.

Peanut butter

Delicious on toast, of course – especially with sliced banana on granary – but also extremely useful for Southeast Asian cooking, such as satay dishes and curry.

Tinned tuna

I can't bear it myself, but I'd still never be without it. Tuna offers dozens of possibilities, from pasta bakes and jacket spuds to sandwich fillings and quick, cheap tomatoey curries.

Chilli sauce

I love extra-hot sriracha, but any chilli sauce will do. For times when you need to turn up the heat in an instant.

Teabags

To calm anxieties, fuel conversation, ameliorate suffering and cushion any blow. Rich, malty builder's tea is what fuels my family, but whatever floats your particular clipper. Keep in plentiful supply – I'd sooner run low on oxygen.

Opening a bottle of Champagne

This makes people nervous and I understand why. No one wants to take someone's eye out or, worse still, waste the Champagne on the kitchen floor. The secret is always to twist, not push the cork from the bottle neck. Put your hand over the top of it and unscrew as you would a jam jar lid. If you're still nervous, place a tea towel loosely between the cork and your hand as you work.

How to chill wine in a hurry

Again, I defer to the experts. A waiter at Claridge's hotel in London assured me many years ago that by far the fastest way to chill wine is not to put it into the freezer, but to pop the unopened bottle into a bucket or washing-up bowl and fill with iced cold water. If you have one of those ice packs in the freezer, chuck that in too. Place the whole thing outside in the garden on cold days, if you have one. Should be drinkable in twenty to thirty minutes.

How to cook rice

Rice has a PR problem. It's an easy thing to cook that people think is much harder. For perfectly cooked, classic, white long-grain rice there are only really four things you need to remember: rinse, double, cover, leave. It doesn't make for a satisfying acronym, sadly, but it's worth committing to memory.

1. Put your uncooked rice (about 80g per person) into a measuring jug and notice where it hits along the measurement line.
2. Place your rice in a sieve and rinse in cold running water to get rid of the excess starch.
3. Take the empty measuring jug and pour in boiling water to exactly twice where the rice previously hit – for example, if your rice reached the 100ml mark on the jug, now fill to the 200ml mark.
4. Tip the rice and the water into a lidded saucepan and add some salt.
5. Bring back to the boil and stir once to separate the rice.
6. Cover with the lid, turn the heat down to low, and leave covered and undisturbed until cooked (see the packet, but around 10 minutes).
7. Taste some rice on a fork. If it really needs another minute, put the lid back on and leave.
8. Fluff up with a fork and serve. There should be no residual water, but if there is, drain it in a sieve.

How to stop avocados and guacamole turning brown

Prepare when you're almost ready to eat. Add a generous squeeze of lime juice (lemon also works, but the flavour doesn't go quite as well) and return the removed stone to the bowl, nesting in the middle of the avocado.

How to make inedibly hard avocados, peaches, nectarines or pears ripen more quickly

Place them in a bag with a sacrificial banana. They'll ripen overnight.

How to stop grapes rotting prematurely

Always remove the grapes you're about to eat by snipping their branch off the bunch with scissors. Pulling the grapes individually from the bunch, leaving their stalks on the vine, will send the remaining grapes rotten.

How to stop mushrooms becoming slimy

Mushrooms wrapped in plastic become slimy and fishy smelling quite quickly. Avoid this by removing them from the (utterly needless) plastic packaging as soon as you unpack the shopping. Decant the mushrooms into a paper bag and either refrigerate or store in a cool cupboard.

Perfect Yorkshire puddings

This recipe comes from my ex (a Yorkshireman). While I always cooked Sunday and Christmas lunch, he usually made the Yorkshires. Because, yes, they do go with all roast dinners – to eat them only with beef seems wilfully penitent. You may want to mess about with the recipe, drop the mustard (though it does give a nice colour), increase the seasoning and so on. What cannot be altered is the very high heat and a fat that can withstand it, i.e. definitely not butter or olive oil, which will burn.

Ingredients:
Groundnut oil (or beef dripping if you eat meat)
140g plain white flour
A pinch of English mustard powder
4 large, fresh eggs, beaten with a fork
200ml full-fat milk
Salt and freshly ground black pepper

Method:

1. Preheat the oven to 230°C/450°F.
2. Pour a little oil into each cavity of a large 4-hole pudding tray, or a small 12-hole muffin-style tray, and swirl around to cover the bottom. Place the oily tray in the top of the preheated oven and get on with your batter.
3. Put your flour and mustard powder into a mixing bowl and tip in the beaten eggs. Stir with a balloon whisk or use a hand blender to fully combine them.
4. While still whisking or blending, drizzle in your milk slowly until the batter is loose and lump-free. Grind in some salt and black pepper.
5. Put on an oven glove and open the oven. Your oil should be smoking. If it isn't, close the door and give it another minute. When smoking hot, remove carefully and place on the cooker.
6. Pour your batter equally between the holes. It should bubble and sizzle against the fatty metal sides. Place carefully back in the oven on the top shelf.
7. DO NOT OPEN the oven for the next 20 minutes at least. Look through the glass to see if your puds are puffy, high and golden, giving them a few more minutes if needed. Get everything else on your plate. Serve from oven to plate and eat on the spot.

These freeze beautifully, but wait until they're cool and never defrost them in the microwave (they'll go hard).

How to measure pasta

I wish I had an answer that didn't betray my gluttony, but I unfailingly make way too much and eat it all. For shapes, fill your bowl with dry pasta before tipping into the boiling water. This gives you the right amount for a full bowl plus some return-to-the-pan grazing of leftovers (mmmm, cold pasta). For macaroni cheese, fill the oven dish three-quarters of the way with dry pasta to measure. For spaghetti, I cook half a regular packet (not the extra-long or the family-sized short) for two greedy people.

How to stop pasta sticking

When pasta sticks to the pot it is usually because the pot is overcrowded, or the water was too cold. A large, roomy saucepan and a proper rolling boil of salty water is essential before you empty in the dried pasta. Then get it back up to the boil as fast as you can before reducing to an enthusiastic simmer. If you're cooking spaghetti or linguine, twist the bunch of pasta as you throw it into the pan to separate the strands as they fall, or snap the whole bunch in half (Italians, look away now). Do NOT pour olive oil into the cooking water. This stops sauces coating the drained pasta properly and I'm convinced it slows cooking time.

Water – a cure-all

I may be useless at drinking enough, but I rely heavily on water in cooking. It's such an underrated kitchen ally. A dash of water makes omelettes and scrambled eggs fluffy and light, makes dough or pastry more manageable, revives stale bread rolls while imparting a delicious chewy crust (just wet your hands, stroke all over the roll and throw into the oven for 5 minutes), thins out a soup or sauce, and stops onions, garlic or celery burning when cooking on a high heat. Even as a by-product, it's endlessly useful – the water in the bottom of the vegetable steamer makes the best gravy, and a cup of starchy, salty water scooped from the pasta pan does a peerless job of emulsifying the accompanying sauce and melding everything together beautifully. It's amazingly often the best thing for the job and it's practically free, so use it.

How to make almost any soup

In a world of useless, space-eating, dust-gathering gadgets, electric soup makers are those I understand the least. I can think of no need to employ specialist machinery to make what is embarrassingly easy and fast to make in a pan. And for so little skill and effort, the rewards are huge. When you know how, you can make a vast quantity of healthy, wholesome soup for very little money. Most soup stays edible for three to four days in the fridge, freezes beautifully and defrosts fast. It's a batch-cooker's dream.

Base ingredients for a large, family-sized vat of smooth soup:

Stick of celery, chopped
Large onion or 3–5 shallots, chopped
3–4 carrots, diced
Bay leaf or thyme sprig
Chilli and garlic
Knob of butter
A little olive oil
2 litres stock

Main ingredient ideas:

Potato and chorizo
Cauliflower and kale
Lentil and squash
Roast tomato and basil
Roast peppers and courgette
Chicken and mushroom

Curried parsnip and
  coconut milk
Carrot and coriander
Broccoli and Stilton
Pea and ham

Method:

Throw all the base ingredients except the stock into a large, heavy-bottomed pan. Sweat out on a low–medium heat until soft but not brown. Stir in your chopped main ingredient (e.g. parsnips or tomatoes) and cook for a couple of minutes in the base. Add any spices you fancy (this is where I'd add chilli and garlic, for example). Pour in your stock. Simmer for as long as you like (but minimum 20 minutes, especially if you've used root vegetables). When cooked, remove the bay leaf or thyme sprig, put in your hand blender (see page 89) and blitz until smooth. Check for salt and pepper, and add more stock if the soup is too thick. Chop a soft herb (like parsley, coriander or basil) and throw into the finished soup for colour and flavour. Serve.

If you are making a chunky soup, don't blend at the end.

If you are making a semi-chunky soup (like a creamy chicken soup with shreds of roast chicken, or pea and ham soup with chunks of ham), ladle out a third of the cooked soup, blend the remainder, then throw the removed third back in and stir.

If you are roasting some ingredients first, such as tomatoes and peppers, do that in the oven and throw into the soup as you would any uncooked main ingredient.

Allow to cool before refrigerating or freezing.

How to make a carbonara

I can only apologise in advance to Italians and purists for the garlic oil and removal of all egg whites (my Italian friends are insistent that three yolks and one white, is correct). But I am broadly albumen-averse and besides, I have a child who would countenance only four meal varieties for several years, and this was one of them – I am too scared to fix what isn't broken. Plus, it's incredibly easy, quick (around ten minutes) and absolutely delicious – and infinitely more authentic than those horrible gloopy, milky carbonaras you get in a pot at the supermarket.

127

Ingredients *(serves 2, greedily)*:

½ packet of dried spaghetti (linguine is also fine)

½ tablespoon garlic-infused olive oil (you can get it anywhere)

4 rashers of pancetta or smoked bacon (diced), or one of those packets of cubed pancetta from the fridge aisle of the supermarket

freshly ground black pepper

3 egg yolks (separate and freeze the whites for the next time you're making a meringue, or – heaven forfend – have an egg-white-omelette-eater visiting from America)

A large handful of grated Parmesan or pecorino

Method:

1. Place the spaghetti in a large pan of already boiling, slightly salted water (I would normally advise well-salted water for pasta, but the pancetta and Parmesan are both salty, so easier does it here). Cook according to the packet instructions, minus 1 minute.

2. Glug the garlic oil into a cold pan, add the pancetta, and place the cold pan on a medium heat. As it heats, the fat of the pancetta should render, i.e. release into the pan as clear oil. Grind in lots of black pepper. Fry the pancetta in this peppery, garlicky oil, browning it.

3. Beat the 3 egg yolks in a bowl, then add a handful of Parmesan or pecorino and mix together. Scoop a mug of pasta water from the spaghetti pan and set aside for a couple of minutes.

4. When the pancetta is brown and the pasta is a minute off being ready, move the spaghetti from the water with tongs and immediately place in the bacon pan, tossing in the oily mixture. Don't strain carefully as you go – some sloppy, starchy water is ideal to emulsify the sauce and stop the frying process. Turn off the heat.

5. Take the mug of slightly cooled pasta water and dash a little into the egg mixture to temper it (this will make it more liquid and stop the eggs becoming shocked into scrambling by the hot bacon and pasta). Scrape the egg yolk, cheese and water mixture into the spaghetti and toss well to coat.

6. Serve with more grated cheese and pepper. Does not freeze or reheat well (the eggs will scramble), so eat the lot in one sitting.

Vegetarians can make a very delicious version by substituting the pancetta with brown mushrooms and using vegetarian hard Italian cheese instead of Parmesan. When doing this variant, fry the mushrooms fully in a hot pan, allowing all the moisture to evaporate and the mushrooms to develop a golden surface. Do everything else as with the meaty carbonara, but add lots of black pepper to the egg mix (rather than at the frying stage) and finish the dish with a handful of chopped parsley.

Fashion

'Deciding who I was on any given day became a huge source of pleasure, freedom and creativity when being myself didn't even remotely appeal.'

I adore fashion and have since I was a little girl. My first legible Christmas list said: 'girls' ballet stuff', meaning something, anything feminine that hadn't previously been worn by my brothers and god knows who before them. Later, at primary school, when I was dressing myself in Madonna-alike clothes bought from the market and swapped back and forth with my friend Lynda, my love of fashion became an obsession that I knew would never tail off. My teenage party trick involved my mother holding up any fashion magazine and pointing randomly at a catwalk picture, so that I could identify the designer, model, makeup artist and hairdresser out loud (I had never even touched a designer item but I was determined to be ready). But as well as fashion, I also adore clothes, and this is an important distinction – then and now. Clothes are how we stay warm and modest, of course, but also how we communicate silently with the world, often how we make ourselves feel how we'd like to feel. Fashion is just an interest, a hobby, a culture and an industry. Clothes, whether trendy, vintage, flamboyant, minimalist, customised, recycled, conservative, classic, homemade or oblivious to anything going on outside their own wardrobe, encompass far, far more than that. Never purely functional, regardless of what anyone claims (the choice to not give them any thought is a conceit in itself), our clothes are, in my view, the outward expression of all our experiences and influences. Every single one of my memories – good, bad and terrible – begins with what I was wearing.

My style has evolved significantly over the years, in tandem with my finances, mental and physical state, childbearing status, social group and day job, but my way of shopping has remained much the same. I've always combined basics with fancier items bought second-hand and I'm asked as frequently about how to go about this as I am about foundation and sunscreen. I spent my early childhood in my brothers' cast-off jumpers, zip jeans and sweatshirts and my grandmother's jumble-sale finds. Their scruffiness wasn't really the issue (having little money was normal and not at all frowned upon – everyone was in much the same situation), but the lack of autonomy and femininity seemed hugely significant to me, the lone female in a highly unusual single-dad family set-up. In the absence of even a shred of paternal fashion sense, clothes were how I learned to express myself, often how I learned about other cultures, music genres,

133

how I celebrated being an outsider instead of struggling fruitlessly to blend in. Deciding who I was on any given day became a huge source of pleasure, freedom and creativity when being myself didn't even remotely appeal.

But although I still longed at the time for something feminine from Clockhouse at C&A (the pinnacle of designer fashion around my way), I can now see how much this early repurposing and recycling of hand-me-downs governed my teen and adult style in a wholly positive way.

I open my wardrobe now and see the influences so clearly. The clashing prints of the dressing-up box of fabric scraps and my mother's old clothes – my every-other-weekend access to femininity – remain in the form of leopard coats, floral dresses and spotty scarves, all of which I still wear unapologetically and delightedly. The pillars of my adult wardrobe are the same unfussy, masculine basics like jeans, crewnecks, duffle coats and donkey jackets acquired when my older brothers had outgrown them. These hang next to the occasional hyper-feminine frock like those my grandmother would buy me from the Peter Craig catalogue for 99p over twenty weeks, which made me feel happier and more confident, and gave me the sense of normalcy and belonging I craved. The clumpy black boots like those I lived in as a clubbing teenager, the odd ridiculously posh piece bought only after months of stalking happily for bargains, because managing finances carefully means my own children always know we'll have electricity and gas. I find dressing myself – and others, when they'll let me – the purest joy. Nothing makes me happier than an email from a friend or reader, asking where they might find the perfect work backpack or the best denim mini, and my husband can attest that I will not relax until I've found it. My clothes really, deeply matter to me and this long-term love affair has taught me a thing or three. I hope something here helps, or at the very least sparks some great memories for you.

The three-colour rule

While I'm not a fan of fashion rules generally, I make an exception for this one (used also in cinematography and interior design), because if you struggle to put together coherent outfits you feel great in, it can be a very helpful tool. The three-colour rule works on the principle that an outfit should contain no more than three colours (I would count any non-nude lipstick or eyeshadow, such as red, orange or hot pink, as part of the three), including blue denim but not including any black or white. For example:

> *Three colours + black:*
> - Camel coat
> - Blue jeans
> - Brown boots and bag
> - Black jumper
>
> *Three colours + white:*
> - Beige trench coat
> - Blue jeans
> - Red shoes and lipstick
> - White T-shirt
>
> *Three colours + black*
> - Black coat
> - Tan bag and shoes
> - Blue jeans
> - Cream jumper

A pattern or print counts as one of your three colours. However, I would then ensure that the other two colours in my trifecta were also present in the print, or simply use black and/or white against it. For example:

> - Brown, beige and black leopard-print skirt
> - White shirt
> - Black bag and shoes

> - Floral dress of orange, pink and red
> - Red shoes and lipstick
> - Black or red bag

Remember that three colours are the maximum – they're not obligatory. Two colours also looks fab (an all-black and camel outfit, for example). Four colours, though, are harder to pull off, so whenever in doubt, follow the rule and stop at three.

Does everyone need a perfect white shirt?

No. Every time I read this tired old cliché on a website or in a magazine, I assume space had to be filled in a hurry. Crisp, white shirts are sheer perfection on some people. Tom Ford looks better in a white shirt than anyone else I've met. Katharine Hepburn was the very embodiment of chic in her mannish white shirts. Marion Cotillard, Meghan Markle and Michelle Obama all look extraordinarily elegant when clad in sharply pressed white cotton poplin. In most white shirts, what I look like is a schoolgirl with a Saturday job at a carvery, dressed for the cack-handed serving of roasties with twin spoons. It is a lie that there is a white shirt to flatter everyone. It is an even bigger lie that white shirts suit everyone's style. On many of us, they look corporate, or uniformish, or buxom, matronly and boring. Don't tell a woman with big boobs that she'll feel great in a white shirt. I didn't even own one before my breast reduction and even now I do, I'm not always convinced.

Is there any coat that suits everyone?

Yes. A trench coat looks good on every body shape and size, without exception. Whether you are as straight as a board, or you curve like a slide in a water park, a trench will make you look great. Buy one size up for a mannish, Scandinavian vibe, or wear your regular size cinched in with the belt for a flattering, classic shape. I wear my trenches all of spring and much of autumn and they never fail to make me feel nice. The ultimate in versatile outerwear, they can be made sexy, casual, super smart, low key, cool or classic. And don't think trenches must be stone to look right (I love honey and navy, personally, but you can also buy them in reds, greens, greys and black), or that you have to go Burberry or bust – you can buy beautiful trenches on the high street. COS, Gap, Jigsaw and M&S tend to release stylish trench coats year after year.

Must the bag and shoes match?

No. I frequently match my bag and shoes but only because this is easy to do when you wear mostly neutral colours. But I certainly don't consider it essential. There is nothing wrong with black boots and a tan bag, or leopard shoes and a black bag, or brown shoes and a navy bag. Handbags, whether high street or high fashion, are more expensive than shoes. It's not at all feasible to own a bag in the same colour as every pair you buy, and besides, matching very distinctive shoes – satin stilettos, glittery trainers, neon pumps and so on – with an identical bag can look a bit laboured. Just let the shoes pull focus and sling on a black bag.

Which colours shouldn't be worn together?

I loathe colour rules. They seem so archaic, but also it seems to me that the most roundly accepted as unwearable are almost invariably the most stylish combinations. Take navy and black. Apparently not to be worn together but without a doubt, my favourite clothing colour scheme. So smart, so French and expensive-looking, the addition of navy gives more dimension and elegance to an all-black outfit and looks peerlessly chic. It also gets around the problem of matching up shades of black, which is much harder to do than one imagines. Speaking of mismatches, don't worry about white and cream – they're the best of friends (chunky cream jumper with white jeans in winter looks wonderful). Blue and green should never be seen? Such tosh. Navy blue and bottle-green are glorious worn together. Pink or orange worn with red is a modern and utterly fabulous clash. Yellow absolutely does go with blue, especially when a vivid or lemon yellow is teamed with faded blue jeans. The only combinations I personally avoid are red and brown, because I just don't love it myself; navy and red, because it feels like a British Airways uniform and, dare I say it, a bit flag-bedecked Brexiter screaming about his passport on a demo. And I don't do red and green because it feels too much to me like a Christmas-themed outfit. But these self-imposed rules are also influenced heavily by how awful I look in all red unless it's painted thickly on my mouth – they're nothing even approaching edicts everyone else should follow. If you love a brown bag with a red frock, or the red and navy full-on royal livery look, please do go for your life and feel fabulous. All that matters is you. And if ever you're in any doubt about colour combinations when planning an outfit, google a chart of traditional Scottish tartans

137

(that's plaid if you're American). Every conceivable colour clash exists somewhere in an unfailingly gorgeous clan tartan. The Scottish knew a thing or two about style (and Brexit. But I'll hush now).

Should I wear silver or gold jewellery?

As I type, gold jewellery is very much having a moment, but silver will be back soon enough. I tend to buy fine 'forever' jewellery in white gold or platinum and semi-fine (i.e. plated) jewellery in gold, but most people instinctively know which suits them best. If you don't, a good general rule of thumb is that if you have a cool skin tone (regardless of how pale or dark it is) with blueish veins, you probably look best in silver. If you have a warm skin tone and greenish veins, you probably look best in gold. If you have a neutral skin tone with both blueish and greenish veins, then you probably suit either gold or silver. If, like me, you fit into the last category (my veins look like the wiring in a UK plug) but can't decide, it's useful to determine what is your most important piece of jewellery, decide which metal suits that individual piece, then match any other important, pricey, worn-every-day staples to that. In my case, that's my engagement and wedding rings, and since I very much wanted vintage Art Deco rings, this automatically meant platinum. So my watch is white gold to match, as is my other pricey ring worn on my right hand. All these non-negotiable pieces are silver-toned. Everything else I wear is a free-for-all depending on mood (yellow gold tends to look quite classic and sophisticated, while silver lends itself to a sportier, edgier feel), and I like it that way.

Can I mix metals in jewellery and bags?

Lots of people feel very, very strongly that one should always match gold with gold, silver with silver, from the studs in your ears right down to the buckle on your belt and the brass snaffle on your loafer. Jewellery is such a personal thing that I can only tell you to follow your own taste. Speaking for myself, I mostly mix metals without a care. I regard gold and silver as neutrals that play perfectly nicely together and see no problem in wearing silver earrings with a gold necklace, silver watch and gold-chained bag – although I do think that mixed metals look better in multiples, for example in a stack of bracelets – two gold, one silver, maybe. Or swapping out one or two pieces for gold in an earful of silver piercings. That way, you won't have a single mismatched piece that looks as though it was mistakenly put on in the dark. Besides, different metals have different looks on different items. The only time I would make a point of matching metals is if the metallic features dominated an otherwise blank canvas of an outfit. For example, if I was wearing a plain outfit with a chunky belt buckle and big hoop earrings, I'd want them both in gold, because they'd be very prominent against an unforgiving backdrop. If you're still worried about mixing your metals, a good way to bring everything together is to add one item that includes both shades – I have a very handy pair of two-tone metal hoops that instantly make any mismatching metals look wholly intentional.

How to store and untangle jewellery

If you have neither the time nor patience to do a whole lot of polishing and untangling, you should organise and store your jewellery carefully. There are lots of lovely jewellery carriers and boxes around, but at home, I use cheap jewellery tray organisers, available from Muji and Amazon. They stack, meaning I can store silver and other easily tarnished items on the bottom, away from the open air, and have loads of little compartments for keeping earrings partnered and longer sections to allow each necklace to stretch its legs in its own bunk. Spread out like this, jewellery is super simple to select and throw on quickly and never tangles. Though if you do happen to get your chains in a twist, do as my grandmother Nance did, and sprinkle them with talcum powder before beginning to separate them with a needle. The whole thing becomes easier and less maddening.

Can one wear two prints at once?

Absolutely yes. In fact, I positively encourage it. A quick glance through my social media output will show that I'm a huge fan of mixing leopard with spots, paisley or even tartan. I think it looks fun and cool, and actually, it is a look that often requires the confidence of maturity to pull off (Iris Apfel is, of course, the ultimate example of this). My only tip – and it really is a tip, not a rule – is to make sure the darker of the two prints is on the larger bit of your body and the paler pattern on the smaller bits. For example, I might wear a pale leopard blouse with a dark paisley overcoat, or a dark floral frock with pale dotty socks. The bigger the area, the darker the print. It's more flattering on you and more soothing on the eye of the beholder.

Are posh handbags a good 'investment'?

No. Property is an investment. Stocks, shares, maybe art if one gets it right. What posh handbags are is beautiful, depending on your personal taste. Broadly speaking (and rare collectors' editions aside), there are only a few specific handbags that, when sold, will not see you out of pocket. The first is a classic handbag shape by Chanel. By 'classic', I mean one that Chanel makes season after season, year after year, like the Classic Flap (probably the best recognised, designed by Karl Lagerfeld in the 1980s), the 2:55 (by Coco Chanel in 1955) and the Wallet-On-Chain or WOC, which is not technically a handbag but, in practice, is. The same applies to Louis Vuitton canvas bags in classic shapes like the Speedy or Alma. These sorts of bags, when kept in good condition for a couple of years or more and retaining their dust bag, receipt and box (what's known as 'a full set') will likely sell for as much as, if not a little more, than you paid for them. But it's important to remember that this is primarily because Chanel and Louis Vuitton hike up their prices at least twice a year, and used bags simply benefit from a constantly rising market. The other types of bag that hold their value are the Hermès Kelly, Birkin and to a slightly lesser degree Constance handbags. Unlike the Chanels and the LVs, these don't just hold their value in a rising market, their value increases immediately and will typically cost more (sometimes even twice or three times as much, depending on condition and colourway) on the resale market than when bought new. This is because of the scarcity of these three styles only (which are handmade and cannot be mass produced to satisfy demand), which are not freely available in-store, but usually offered discriminately to loyal and selected Hermès customers after what can be a lengthy relationship and purchase history (there are exceptions, but there's no planning or accounting for them). People without the patience, time, money, access or desire to engage in this infamous dance with their sales associate simply pay a premium to jump the queue on the resale market. All of these bags cost thousands. Other designer handbags, while they can be every bit as classic, timeless and beautiful, will start to lose money from the moment you walk out of the shop. So my advice is always to buy a bag for love, never for money, and always look first at second-hand, where nearly new bags can cost half as much and any depreciation is someone else's problem.

The pouch system

If you have both the inclination and good fortune to own multiple handbags, as many of us do, you may find the pouch system makes for an easy and fast transition between them. I only keep four items in my handbags – my sunglasses and three small pouches containing many smaller items – and just swap them quickly in and out of bags when I've decided what I'm wearing that day. I began doing this a few years ago, having spent the previous two decades periodically and hurriedly emptying out a mountain of crap onto the bed and picking essentials from old receipts, fluff and bits of hair, when I should already have been en route to the station. This better way takes seconds, and means you can always find what you're looking for on the go. Which pouches you use isn't important; Muji and Superdrug do strong, durable, wipeable and very affordable transparent ones that will serve you well. But go as fancy or as basic as you like.

Pouch 1:
- Painkillers in case of period pain or headache
- Two cotton buds for any makeup smudges or weepy eyes
- Tissues
- Two emergency tampons
- Mints or gum for instant freshen-up
- Phone charger with folding plug
- Pen
- Lip balm
- Small hand sanitiser or anti-bacterial hand cream
- Small solid sun protection stick for unexpected spells outdoors
- USB stick
- Specs cleaning wipe
- Nail file

Pouch 2:
- Makeup, the works – but only because I tend to do my makeup in a quiet part of the train and frequently have to dress up for something more formal in the evening. If you get ready at home before leaving, then a powder compact and a lipstick should do it.

> • A travel perfume atomiser. Travalo makes excellent lipstick-sized perfume containers that refill from most regular perfume spray bottles, but Chanel, Frédéric Malle, Ormonde Jayne and others do great miniatures off the shelf. Jo Malone and Diptyque make small solid perfume compacts that also allow for travelling light.
>
> *Pouch 3:*
> • A coin purse with attached key chain, for debit cards, cash and keys.

How to buy great second-hand clothing

I accepted long ago that I'm an extravagant person. What I won't allow myself to be is a wasteful one. This is why I make sure that at least 50 per cent of all my clothing and accessories purchases are second-hand. Though 'make sure' implies that this is some worthy compromise requiring great self-discipline and sacrifice, and not the extremely fun and hugely satisfying hobby that it is. I have never in my life bought any new garment in a shop that made me feel better than the arrival of my black, Italian-made brogue boots, in terrific condition, for which I'd paid £100 while they were still selling online and in-store for £550. My black Max Mara wool and cashmere Crombie coat – available every winter for around £1,200, cost me £80 second-hand on eBay and is still going strong, almost a decade later. I don't own a pair of designer jeans that cost me more than a new pair from the Gap website. It is deeply gratifying to know that you are extending the life of an unwanted item, shopping more sustainably, saving a fortune and spending the same amount of money as you might on a poor-quality, less-comfortable fast-fashion item that may soon find its way into landfill. Things that are built for a long life should live one, and the much lower pricing of preloved clothing should incentivise our support for the slow-fashion movement. When you start buying second-hand, and buying extremely high-quality classics for the price of Dorothy Perkins, you will quickly realise that there's no going back.

Buy off season
The world and her husband are looking for a trench coat in spring, straw basket bags in summer, a wool coat in autumn and big boots in winter, because people are most likely to identify a gap in their wardrobe when they most urgently need to fill it. This drives up prices and decreases availability, so avoid the bunfight by planning ahead. At the end of each

season, I create a private Pinterest board of everything I've either been missing over the past couple of months, or which has come to the end of its natural life. Next season will be spent shopping for those items second-hand, at precisely the point where everyone else is clearing out their wardrobe for the change in weather (I've just bought a floor-length woollen coat at the beginning of spring, for example). The market becomes saturated with off-season clothes, driving down the price and giving you your pick of a large crop. I'm not much of a trend shopper, but if you like to be bang up to date, it helps to buy only classic items that won't be out of fashion next year this way – such as stripy tees, vintage denim and black coats. Then you can just accessorise them with more current bits later on.

Buy the wrong item from the right designer

Okay, this requires a bit of fashion knowledge but is such an important and useful tip that it's worth swotting up for. The best way of securing an infinitely wearable, very high-quality designer item for a fraction of its original cost is to shop for something that is famously made not by them, but by another designer. For example, if I say 'trench coat', your mind will rightly think 'Burberry and Aquascutum', because those are the designers best known for their trenches. What you probably won't think is 'Max Mara and A.P.C.', both of whom quietly make beautiful trench coats that will give you a very similar look and quality, but are much less frequently searched for and consequently cost much less in resale. Topshop were famous for their floral teadresses, which still fetch around £30–40 second-hand. But broaden your search to include Topshop's (also defunct) sister brand, Miss Selfridge, and you'll be in a much less crowded pool and pay maybe a tenner for essentially the same frock. Max Mara are famous for their wool, belted gown coats, but when I searched for an identical style by Acne Studios (more famous for their sweatshirts and boots), I uncovered the most beautiful, simple belted coat I've ever worn. Searching for an item seemingly at odds with a brand's popular signature look – flat shoes rather than stilettos from Manolo Blahnik, a Levi's sweatshirt rather than jeans, something low-key and minimalist like a black cashmere sweater from a maximalist designer like Versace, is far, far more likely to find you a very posh bargain than taking the obvious route. I have countless trophies from deploying this tactic. My second-hand navy cashmere Gucci peacoat (£280, never worn, tags still on while still being for sale on the Gucci

143

website for £2,200) found its way into my shopping cart because I actually wanted the near-identical style made famous by Yves Saint Laurent, which is owned by the same Kering Group as Gucci. So next time you see something you love on Instagram or in the pages of a fashion magazine, search for a similar style, not the same brand. Swerving the obvious pays dividends.

Don't be afraid of offers

Sellers want to sell their items, which is why so many eBay, Depop and Vestiaire listings allow for offers. Just their clicking the offer option upon listing shows that the seller is open to, and is expecting, some negotiation, so I would never not at least try. Vestiaire will not submit your offer if it's not at least 70 per cent of the listing price, which saves time, but eBay allows for any offer, which means you need to think more carefully about how you proceed, since both sites allow only three offers before you default back to the asking price. The first and most important thing you need to decide for yourself is how much you are really prepared to pay for an item. Which price would feel worthwhile to you, and at which price would losing out on the item cause you not to feel any regret? Then also consider the likely resale price if it doesn't work out. I recently bought some shoes that I loved enough to pay over the odds for, but since I hadn't tried them on, I knew I had to factor in how much someone would pay me if they turned out to be too big.

Avoid trends

The preloved market is not the ideal place to shop for trends. Very hot items will be scarce, as original owners will usually still be enjoying them. Those that do make their way onto resale sites, perhaps because they didn't suit or fit the owner or, as happens frequently, the owner is predicting the imminent death of a trend and wants to cash out before demand falls off a cliff, will likely be overpriced, sometimes even more expensive than they are or were in-store. The big bargains are in classics, basics and items that were either never super trendy, or those that were, but are now past their peak. My first Burberry trench (now £1,600 new) was bought for £70 on eBay at a time (2003) when trenches were seen as something a city trader or posh grandmother might wear. Nana chic has never put me off, so I snapped it up and wore it to death. When I came to sell it (because I'd found another that fitted me better), minimalist bloggers had made Burberry trenches trendy, and I earned back almost

144

five times what I'd paid. Timing is key, so sometimes it's worth hanging on to something a bit longer and waiting for the market to change.

Look across price points

I find the lure of designer clothes sold at premium high-street prices irresistible myself, but high-street labels, when sold second-hand, go for peanuts. I bought almost all of my kids' clothes on eBay, for example. The rapid physical development of small children means that many used items still look almost new when sold, and also that any money you spend on new clothes from shops will likely be wasted as your kids outgrow them. I couldn't stand the thought of spending money on a new jumper that may either be too small or too covered in spaghetti sauce to wear even a month later. Brands like GapKids, Next, Boden, OshKosh, H&M and Zara Kids are available by the truckload on eBay, Shopbop and Vinted (I personally prefer eBay because prices are set on the others), very often in large bundles – 'six girls' T-shirts, age 5–6', for example – and at very low cost. And when your child is too big for your purchases, you can sell them on and, spaghetti sauce notwithstanding, recoup your funds.

Don't be squeamish

While few people would take issue with a preloved bag or overcoat, many are resistant to wearing someone else's shoes and sweaters, so if you're made of sturdier stuff, the opportunities for bargains are even greater. Some of my best eBay and Vestiaire discounts have been for shoes. I just give them a little wipe down with Milton sterilising fluid before wearing, and if really needed, insert thin insoles to cover the old.

Embrace the rejects

Resale sites aren't just for second-hand clothing – they're a great place to buy factory seconds with often imperceptible defects. For years, I bought all my Fantasie and Freya lingerie brand new from factory shop sellers on eBay. A £40 bra might cost as little as £15 and arrive with tags still attached. I never once spotted what was wrong with any of them.

Don't forget denim

I practically never buy jeans anywhere but eBay. Preloved jeans look better than new and cost a tiny fraction of the price. My favourite boyfriend jeans, by Current Elliott, cost around £200 new, but rarely more than £40–50 on eBay (my favourite pair set me back a princely £25), and this way arrive perfectly worn in. I've bought pristine H&M jeans for a little over a fiver. If you know the style, brand and size you like, then you are bound to find a bargain. Even if you don't – and I'll admit it's tricky trying to work out if a pair of flat jeans photographed on a wooden floor, rather than professionally on a model, are right for you – the much lower price often makes a punt worthwhile. Especially since you can sell on again afterwards.

Bid an odd amount

If you're on an auction site, remember that most people will make their highest bid a nice, round number – £20, £50, £200 – so I always bid an odd amount, like £21.36. It's amazing how often it seals the deal. At this point I could suggest you use an online bidding app or service, to automatically swoop in at the last second to win you the auction, but I don't hold with them, personally. They do work and plenty of people do use them – I'm sure I've been beaten to many an item by them. It just seems to me to be against the whole ethos of second-hand shopping and takes the fun and goodwill out of something that gives me real joy. But each to their own.

Don't bid early

I never bid early unless I absolutely know I won't be around for the end of an auction. Mostly I join the auction in the last ten minutes – there's no use driving up the price prematurely.

Consider customs

Brexit has affected second-hand shopping hugely, because where I once was able to shop all of Europe as though on my doorstep, now any purchase will come with a customs charge that can easily take it from bargain to not quite worth the bother. It means I now rarely shop Paris-based Vestiaire Collective, for example, whereas it used to be my first port of call (I still use it frequently for assembling ideas, but rarely pull the trigger). Remember to consider any of these additional charges before bidding or buying, and if they're prohibitive (when applied to an already expensive item, for instance), then tick the UK-sellers-only option in your search results.

Stay onsite

Never, ever agree to leave the safety of eBay, Vestiaire or any other respectable selling platform in order to save money or 'make things easier'. When you walk off a platform, you walk away from your dispute management and financial redress privileges if the listing turns out to be inaccurate or dishonest. Any request by a vendor to complete a transaction off-platform should immediately sound alarm bells (my mind

'Brexit has affected second-hand shopping hugely ... now any purchase will come with a customs charge that can easily take it from bargain to not quite worth the bother.'

immediately goes to counterfeit goods). The only exception to this rule is when the eBay listing itself offers 'cash on collection' and you choose this as you check out in the normal way. Also, it is not uncommon when purchasing large items, like furniture, for the buyer to have to pay the seller's third-party courier company upon delivery, when the main item has been paid for separately on the selling platform.

File your coupons

All selling sites have occasional flash sales and promotional coupons and these can add yet more savings onto your total. I use them constantly to drive down already great prices. Mark them as 'not spam' in your email inbox so you never miss any.

Use PayPal

If you can use PayPal, do. I can think of at least five occasions where they've refunded a purchase in full when a seller has either lied or gone AWOL. Your credit card company may do this too, of course, but I like the relative customer anonymity, ease and speed of PayPal.

How to sell your clothes

I have sold so many of my clothes over the years, and I love it. It is deeply satisfying to take several ill-fitting, unloved or no longer worn items, pass them on to someone more appreciative, then pour the proceeds into one truly wanted item. I never make any big purchase without first wondering what I can sell to make a dent in the final price. It can be time-consuming, but when you're properly prepared, there's nothing more rewarding. Here are some best practices.

Choose the right platform

It's no longer a case of eBay or bust; there are now several options, depending on the value and target market of your item. I mostly sell on eBay, but items that will appeal to teens and twenty-somethings perform well on Depop. So for, say, a garment I haven't worn since the 1990s, which is now hugely cool to someone my son's age, I might list there instead. Children's clothes do especially well sold in bundles on Vinted and eBay. If an item is designer and perhaps more niche than is commonly sought on eBay, I could go for Vestiaire Collective, where shoppers are very well informed and fashion-savvy, but there I would need to weigh up the much higher seller commission against what could be a higher sale price. If I'm getting rid of items I think my friends will like, I'll pop them in a private Facebook group we all share for swapping and selling our clothes and accessories. For items of a lower value (but not fast fashion) that may not seem worth the admin, I may choose Thrift+, who send out a prepaid sack to fill, then sell on your clothes, passing either all or some of the proceeds to your chosen charity. Similarly, your local charity shop, depending on their specific needs and policies, will be very grateful for any clean clothes in good condition. They are not there to offload your mess, however; items not good enough for a charity shop should go in the textiles bank for recycling.

List on a Sunday

Sunday is when buyers have the most at-home time to browse and shop online, and when they are most likely to be near a device at an auction's end, so it makes sense to have your own auctions end then. Listing a seven-day item on Sunday afternoons will ensure it naturally ends at the best time (I generally aim for 5 p.m.-ish), but if you're not free, you can schedule your listing to start on a Sunday (or any other day and time). Sometimes there's a small fee for this, but a Sunday sale price will usually more than make up for it.

Get the right pictures

Good pictures sell items, while bad ones will rob you of a decent profit, so it's absolutely worth taking your time to do the following:

149

- Look out for free-fee days. Most auction and second-hand sale sites have promotional periods (often around holidays when people are most likely to clear out their wardrobes and reorganise) where they either reduce or scrap listing fees for sellers. This is to encourage selling activity, increase the onsite offering significantly and to recruit new sellers who may be dithering. It's the perfect time to start.
- Wash, de-lint and de-fuzz your item and ensure it's crease-free.
- Hang it on a decent hanger or, better still, dress it on a model and crop out their head for privacy. This gives buyers a much better idea of how the item will look on them, and reduces their purchasing risk.
- Place the item (either on the hanger or the model) against a plain background, like a blank wall. When items are presented simply and cleanly, buyers will assume they are from a clean home. Shooting in daytime, when natural light allows for accurate colour depiction, gives the best results, but if you can't clear the time, consider spending £20 on an artificial studio light.

- Hone in on detail, as far as the image allowance accommodates. If something is lined, or the pockets are interesting, or the tags are still attached, show the buyer. If there are any faults, make sure they are clearly visible. Turn over shoes to show wear (or lack of it) to the soles. Every detail shown upfront will save you lots of time and headaches later on. The last thing you want is an aggrieved buyer seeking a refund or opening a dispute against you when an item isn't as expected.

Be honest

Don't lie in your listing, ever. And never steal images from other stores or photo agencies. Copyrighted images will often see your listing removed, taking any active bids, and your sale, with it. More importantly, good feedback is what gives buyers the confidence to shop with you.

Be descriptive

After pictures, a proper description is your most powerful selling aid. It's surprising how few people really take the time to detail what's on offer. Include colour (it's often hard to tell from a photo), approximate measurements, retailer, original price where impressive and whether it fits true to size. Point out any flaws, and tell someone how fast you're able to post after auction. If something is authentic, explicitly state so (not using the word 'authentic' is how some fake sellers get around the rules, so make it clear you're not one of them). If you smoke, you really should say unless you are absolutely certain your item isn't tinged with its smell. I own one pair of Isabel Marant boots that I can neither wear nor sell on because they reek to high heaven of the previous owner's cigarettes. My feedback was no love letter. Be concise but thorough now and you'll save yourself heaps of time in answering basic and annoying questions during the listing.

Start low

Remember that something was making you precisely nothing while hanging in your wardrobe and start the price as low as you can bear. If listing on an auction site, pay attention to starting-bid suggestions made by the app – they are usually about right. It may seem counterintuitive, but starting an auction too high frequently results in a lower sale price. If you are inflexible (and you've every right to be), consider offering a Buy It Now price instead – there's usually an additional fee for this.

150

Don't try to make money on postage

Hiking up the delivery costs to increase profits is not only unfair, it's counterproductive. Consider combining postage to encourage buyers to shop your other items without paying for extra parcels. It consolidates your packing and admin and attracts more bids. Conversely, high shipping fees drive customers away.

Don't put off what you think will take ages

Most preloved and auction sites allow you to save listings as drafts until you're ready to go live, meaning you can prepare multiple listings one by one, over many days. And remember that you will definitely get faster as you go. You'll be banging out the orders in no time.

Send promptly

Try to get out your parcels soon after your buyers have paid (there's usually one annoying person who takes their time and misses the first drop at the post office, but you shouldn't make the rest wait for them). I always keep a stash of packing materials from previous online orders, so I can recycle on my own sales, and wrap any fragile or precious items in tissue, padded envelopes and so on. Even dropping a brief note into the parcel can benefit your feedback.

151

Leave feedback

If the platform allows for feedback, do leave it. Preloved sites work on politeness, honesty, cooperation and goodwill. Leaving positive comments for good buyers helps to keep things working as they should.

Are fashion influencers a good source of inspiration?

A very definite YES and a cautionary NO. Many women, having felt too poor, too ordinary, too fat, too short, too old, too everything for aspirational fashion shoots of models in magazines, can now find leagues of brilliantly stylish online influencers who may look and live much more as they do. It's really no wonder that a style video by a girl in her bedroom can be seen more times than a fashion billboard or front cover of *Elle*. If there is someone online who has great ideas on dressing that resonate with you and your style, and they have a way of communicating those in an inspiring, relatable or just plain entertaining way, then use the resource to your benefit. Pin any good outfits onto your Pinterest boards and refer back to them whenever you're unsure of what works.

The problem is that, unlike a photograph in a one-off fashion-magazine shoot, a fashion influencer presents an entire wardrobe, lifestyle and world, and – as can easily happen – becoming too influenced by the taste of another poses the danger of erasing any existing personal style altogether. I can't stress how important your own taste is – it's what gives you a signature aesthetic that no one will ever be able to capture as well. For example, a few years ago, I began reading minimalist Scandinavian interiors and style blogs. The women who wrote them looked so incredibly wonderful in every oversized car coat and detail-free blazer, but however much I admired them, and whenever I attempted to capture their exquisite style for myself, I just felt ... bland and boring. I am not a woman who can wear some lasercut trapeze dress and feel like myself – I'm going to have to throw on a posh earring or handbag, or a vivid orange lip, or a glittery sock, or an ever-so-slightly-flashy logo somewhere into the mix. I am too old to pretend that a wardrobe full of biscuity beige and mushroomy grey cashmere is who I really am, much as it's beyond chic on others. There were a few instances where I bought something that I didn't really love, simply because a complete stranger did. For a very brief while, I tried to be that woman and lost a sense of style that I'd always been so sure about.

And while I come to think of it:

Fashion habits that the internet will convince you are normal, but aren't

One-season purchases

One of the scarier monsters created by vlogger culture is luxury and designer clothing as fast fashion (and, now I think of it, fast fashion treated as something as disposable as a crisp packet). Items costing hundreds, even thousands, of pounds are hot one minute, old news the next. I recently saw a YouTube video in which a vlogger who had raved about a brand-new £1,500 designer bag just three videos before, declared she had already 'stopped reaching for it', sold it at a loss and moved on. And before anyone thinks I'm judging or blaming vloggers for that, I'm not. It's what happens when escapist, aspirational content becomes believable, influential and so relentlessly abundant that it skews how we view normal life (imagine if fashion magazines came out daily in an inexhaustible, ubiquitous supply; you'd start to feel weird about those, too).

People on both sides of the screen are complicit. I know from working in beauty that people would prefer to watch content about a new product than an older one that works better. Look at YouTube viewing figures for fashion – a video containing box after box and bag after bag of shiny new things, however unrelatable and unaffordable to most viewers, will typically fare far better, and see much higher viewing figures, than one on creative ways to style the existing items subscribers have previously seen. We demonstrably crave more and more content and newness; influencers show us what we want to see, and we, in turn, believe we must own it. Within months or even just a few weeks, the process refreshes and what would in the real world represent a once-in-a-lifetime purchase is as 'out' as this season's Zara frock. Bloggers can earn money from spending money on clothing, while viewers cannot. It is utterly dysfunctional and mad. I love fashion with quite literally my every fibre and understand completely the need for escapism and entertainment (and I know that there are content creators who manage to offer both brilliantly in a moderate and responsible way). But what I would want any viewer to remember daily is that just because a content creator has seemingly moved on from something you've only just bought, it doesn't mean that your item is no longer beautiful, or stylish, or useful or relevant in the world outside your window. It doesn't mean you need to update or renew at any point in the next few years. It just means someone is doing their job and feeding the beast.

153

Walk-in wardrobes

Here's the thing. Maybe I'm mixing in the wrong crowds, but no one I know has a walk-in wardrobe. Like most people, I have an (admittedly large) wardrobe in my bedroom. If it starts to look full, I know I either need to clear out and sell some things and/or that I've been feeling sad and am buying in order to feel better, which doesn't ultimately work. Having a huge walk-in wardrobe is no doubt very pleasing to those who own them, and yay for that. They look fabulous on YouTube and it's surely very gratifying for a clothes lover to look out at rows of colour-ordered sweaters stacked like macarons in identical shelving cells. I can see why it's exciting to have sixteen pairs of Christian Louboutin shoes, pointed toes poking from bespoke racks. I really do get it and enthusiastically applaud their owner's square footage. But it also represents a way of life that is not remotely achievable for the vast majority of people, and given that there are only a maximum of 365 days per year on which you can get dressed, I'm not sure it is all that helpful unless your job is to own clothes which, in an influencer's case, it literally is just that. Curating a wardrobe in which every item is loved, accessible and wearable is arguably more life-enhancing than piles and piles of stuff for stuff's sake – and I speak as someone who loves stuff. If my children ever decide to leave home (and, frankly, that's an increasingly tough one to call), I will not convert their bedrooms into clothing museums for myself. A home cinema or ball pool, perhaps.

Buying something every week

There was a time when, as a young teenager, I would catch the train to Cardiff every Saturday with my friends and use my pocket money to buy something like a lip balm in The Body Shop or a Value Meal in McDonald's. These are the only sorts of circumstances in which I would agree that weekly purchases are 'normal'. As an adult, it is not usual to open packages to yourself on a weekly or daily basis, as people online appear to. If you can afford to shop weekly and you love it, fabulous – enjoy. I love a self-gift. But know that weekly clothes shopping is not how anyone is reasonably expected to live in order to be fashionable (or, indeed, sustainable). Regular unboxings and shopping hauls are entertainment, frequently not paid for, and not remotely instructional for civilians.

Buying all the things you like

Bear with me here if this sounds completely mad to you, but it's important that we all remind ourselves that it is perfectly possible, even necessary, to see something, appreciate its beauty, think how lovely it will be for someone, then walk away without buying it. Beautiful things can give us joy without our having to own them. They can exist in the world without living in our houses. I worry we've all lost sight of this simple, previously obvious fact. Admire, don't acquire.

Buying lots of luxury items

A colleague once told me that she'd travelled with a fashion influencer who joylessly spent over £17,000 on high-fashion items before they'd even left the airport, barely cracking a smile for the remainder of the luxury work trip. Personally, I've never met anyone in the industry with this attitude and requisite cash to burn, but the story stayed with me as the most extreme demonstration of where such a strange culture can lead. The vast majority of people can't remotely afford to buy luxury items even if they desire them in the first place, which they frequently don't. But even those who want and can afford very posh things are likely to see them as a highly significant purchase requiring careful selection, planning and budgeting. I spent literally years choosing a watch and it took someone dying to prompt me to invest in an heirloom. For most people, a designer handbag is at best a thirtieth, fortieth or fiftieth birthday present, a big anniversary gift or landmark purchase, and all the lovelier for it. Acquiring expensive things on a regular basis is mostly confined to oligarchs and online influencers. By all means, enjoy vicariously, but never believe it's actually A Thing.

Is fast fashion always bad?

It really depends what we mean by the term 'fast' and whether we are, as is done frequently, conflating 'fast' with 'affordable'. The manufacturing of clothes is, by and large, an extremely wasteful business. And while it stands to reason that mass-market, high-street suppliers making millions of garments will likely create more waste than, say, a luxury designer manufacturing in small batches, it's also true that clothes worn for many years are less wasteful than those that are hot for one season, then discarded – regardless of how they were produced, how much they cost and from where they were bought. It strikes me as obscenely elitist and unjust to lay the blame for the environmental crisis on those whose budgets require them to shop cheaply, and not on luxury shoppers who may turn over a larger number of garments per year. ASOS doesn't have the monopoly on faddishness. Fashion can be fast – and therefore wasteful – at any price. More responsible choices resulting in less environmental impact can be made everywhere, from the high street to Sloane Street. Wherever you shop and whatever you can afford, choosing garments that suit your style and will look great way beyond a trend's lifespan is the most important thing.

155

How to develop a personal style

What is personal style? Read any interview with a fashion designer and they always give the same dull definition: confidence. I find this Route One explanation somewhat unhelpful to anyone who doesn't look like a model and have piles of cash at her disposal. It's easy to feel confident in a £500 dress draped over a perfectly proportioned figure. Most of us are more limited in our choices. To me, style is how you express yourself visually. It's a hundred tiny visual cues, each hinting at what you're about, how you feel about things and who you are as a person. Style to me is working with what you have – your body and personality – and complementing both to the best of your abilities and budget.

In life, I absolutely loathe fuss, so I'm unlikely to look and feel good with ornate detailing, big frills and lots of logos on my clothes. I'm forthright and straight, so I'm drawn to bold, neutral shades. I'm tomboyish so will rarely be seen in pastels, least of all baby pink. I don't believe in astrology, fate or ghosts, so anything floaty, hippy and bohemian jars with my personality to an almost comic degree. I'm far too sentimental a person to throw out trendy garments after three months, so I need lasting classics in quality fabrics. This need for self-awareness in developing style is one of the reasons it comes later in life for many of us. And that's just the way it should be. Adolescence is about trying on everything for size, experimenting to see what works on the self you're still getting to know. As we know ourselves better, we dress ourselves better. Only when you understand what makes you look the best you can, fitting comfily into your lifestyle and flattering your shape while allowing you to still feel like yourself only better, does that elusive 'confidence' come.

There are myriad online and real-life resources that can help us hone our dress sense. My private Pinterest boards are where I often loosely plan my look for the season ahead and build wishlists to fill any gaps in my wardrobe. If I'm considering a significant purchase, I'll turn to Pinterest to see all the ways in which others are wearing the same thing. I might consult YouTube for reviews on its quality and wear. But more useful still is an old-fashioned try-on session in my bedroom. Here we can put together outfits, assess what we're not wearing and why. Just pulling out your five most-worn garments and asking yourself what it is that prompts you to reach for them can be more insightful than days spent scrolling fashion posts on Instagram. Is it the colour you're drawn to? Maybe you've found your palette. Is it the defined shoulders? Perhaps this is your silhouette. Is it the feel of that sweater? Perhaps for you, it's all about the luxury, classic fabrics. Or is it wearing something very fashionable that makes you feel most fabulous? Then a handful of trend pieces may make your season. Pay attention to the clothes that make you happy – they are information-gatherers that will lead you to your personal style.

But don't obsess over the notion that authentic signature style comes entirely from the same moodboard, colour palette and aesthetic.

I take issue with the idea that we must be consistent to be ourselves. I think it's perfectly normal to have elements of your personal style that are at odds with one another and yet coexist happily in different outfits as your mood changes. For example, the vast majority of my day clothes are from a neutral colour palette, fairly minimalist in design, and classic. But for a special occasion, I wouldn't think of wearing the evening equivalent. Instead, I'm prone to cracking out prints, glitzy lamé and bold colour. Real people are contradictory and all the better for it. My friend Sam – tall, extremely glamorous and usually in bold-printed dresses or power tailoring – recently bought herself a pair of rainbow Crocs and, despite teasing her mercilessly, I had to concede they worked. The idea that personal style is about defining one narrow aesthetic that appeals exclusively is one that ignores what makes us all unique. Use your style as a tool, a filter through which you can pass – and block – unsuitable, unflattering purchases. But also know it is fine to be chameleon-like, fun to be a bit rock and roll one day, prim and pretty the next, interesting to be unpredictable. As long as your clothes are authentically you, then they automatically fit the brief.

How do you save money on online purchases?

I never buy anything without first checking to see if there's money to be saved on the list price. I do this via discount tracking and cashback sites. I use:

Karma – a computer or device plugin that monitors the price of items on your wishlist and informs you of any discount so you can buy at the right time. It works so brilliantly that I'm prepared to overlook how irritating a presence it is on my desktop.

Quidco – a cashback site. Whenever I know I'm going to pull the trigger on any item, I check to see if the retail site is listed on Quidco. If it is (and heaps are, including some resale sites like Vestiaire Collective), I click through from Quidco and complete my purchase. A percentage of that purchase price will be stored in my account as cashback, to be returned to me at the end of the year. It is absolutely worth your while.

My banking app – look at yours, as there's every chance your favourite stores are offering you either cashback or a discount if you visit their sites through the bank's app instead of via your browser. Brands like Apple, John Lewis, Nike and so on are frequently available this way.

Honey – a discount code site. In my experience, searching those voucher sites for discount codes is a total waste of time. They invariably come up as expired, invalid or not known at checkout. Instead, I use Honey, a plugin that automatically applies every existing discount code at checkout. It takes around thirty seconds and I frequently manage to snag 10–20 per cent off.

Multiple email addresses – lots of sites offer great discounts to new customers only, so using different email addresses increases the number of times one can take advantage of a code.

Best of all, every one of these money-saving methods (with the exception of banking apps and Quidco, which can't be used at one and the same time) can be used together. It's not at all unusual for me to capitalise on a price drop, discount code and cashback, all in a single transaction.

How to best store clothes

Forget those lovely wooden hangers; they're so chunky that you lose half your hanging space to accommodate them. Conversely, wire hangers, like those provided at the dry cleaners, are terrible. They make your garments' shoulders poke out horribly and sometimes even permanently. The ideal solution is a velveteen-covered thin hanger (available also with skirt and trouser clips) bought cheaply in bulk online from a shop outfitters or Amazon. The matte fabric coating stops any garment slippage and the thin, rounded hanger shape preserves the line of your clothes. Having one style of hanger for all of your clothes means they are all equally visible, and slide on the pole like a dream, for fast, efficient selection. Most knitwear, however, should be folded. Even the best hanger is in danger of misshaping a fine-gauge jumper. I have mine stacked in drawers lined with moth paper, the more precious pieces packed in large ziplock sandwich bags. Formal dresses and tailoring are stored in hanging bags, with a handwritten paper luggage tag tied around each bag's neck to identify the frock without unzipping (I also do this for identical-looking items like jeans or black trousers, so I can select at a glance). My bags live in open dustbags (the more expensive ones containing handbag shapers) in the top of the wardrobe – keeping them boxed can send them sticky or cause surface bubbling. Coats (my addiction) need a full length of wardrobe, otherwise the hems become too creased and ruin the line of your whole outfit. Blouses and cardigans should be buttoned at the top third (no need to do the rest) to maintain their shape. Roll any uncreasable items like Lycra, leggings and workout wear – it saves space and makes selection painless. Pyjama bottoms are placed inside their top prior to folding. T-shirts are also best folded and stacked. I worked at Gap for years, so I practically do this in my sleep, but if the skill eludes you, fold tees around a glossy magazine, then slide it out of the top when each is a perfect rectangle.

How to buy jeans that fit

I generally avoid the horror of the changing room if I can possibly help it, but finding the right new jeans (as opposed to a style you've been wearing for years and can confidently buy online) can take so many wrong turns and duff pairs that to order and try on sufficient quantities at home can involve dozens of styles and sizes and possibly a sizeable bank loan. So if you're unsure of size, and on which style might best flatter, it's worth biting the bullet and visiting a store – horrible fluorescent lighting and all. Most big stores, from high-street chains like H&M to high-end department stores like Selfridges, will have denim specialists who really know their cuts and washes, so make the most of them. They will have seen every bum shape and leg length and will know exactly which jeans look best on whom.

159

   Jeans look great on women of all sizes and shapes, with some details flattering every type of figure. By and large, a high rise – a longer distance between crotch seam and waistband – will hit you at the narrowest part of the waist and give a smoother, more flattering shape to your abdomen, keeping you nicely contained (I cannot relax if I'm spilling out of anything), and also gives the illusion of longer legs (high-waisted jeans with flat shoes make me look taller than mid-rise jeans and high heels). Unlike actual leg length and, to a degree, leg shape, a rise cannot be altered or tailored later, so get it right now and you're at least halfway there. Those with very short torsos and long legs to spare may wish to drop to a mid-rise. Few women – even those with the most banging bodies – look their best in a low rise. Who wants jeans that don't allow for period bloat or a long, boozy lunch?

   It's a myth that cropped trousers make legs look shorter. In fact, a flash of ankle usually makes short legs seem longer, and works for most footwear choices, either shoe or boot. For the most part, only the very tall can get away with bunched-up fabric at the shoes. The exception to this rule is flares, which should mostly cover the shoe to not look weird.

Consider colour

In theory, the darker the colour, the smarter the jean. The paler the denim, the more casual. My style is somewhere in the middle, so I mostly opt for indigo and other mid-blue. Dark navy rinse is elegant, slimming and can look dressy enough for even corporate wear. Faded jeans look utterly fab on some people, but I am very much not American in style and I am old enough to have lived through the Nineties once, so, for me, very washed-out denim is a hard pass unless I'm wearing cut-off shorts on holiday. True-black denim can look super smart, especially if, like me, you find most proper 'trousers' either unflattering or a bit 'office Christmas party', but bear in mind that a true black usually comes up smaller and you'll need to size up one. Classic black denim (that is, denim that is, in reality, dark grey) is a good way to break up an all-black outfit, adding a little dimension and tone, and really very stylish. With a little stretch, white or natural denim can be flattering, looks fab with chunky knitwear and boots and is deceptively easy to keep clean.

To stretch or not to stretch?

Each to her own, but after decades of enthusiastic research, I've concluded that 95–97 per cent cotton denim jeans, i.e. 'medium stretch', are the most flattering. Much less cotton than that and the denim can cling visibly to your cellulite and bag over time in the knees and bum. Any more than 97 per cent and you have yourself a rigid denim (you'll probably need to go up a size), which is perfectly cool if you're blessed with a figure that delights you, but I personally favour a little suction to the mum-belly and thighs, a little lift to the backside. Ignore the percentage of elastane, since this doesn't give the full picture. Elastane, polyester and/or nylon, Tencel and other fibres are frequently in the mix and, all together, will come to no more than 3–5 per cent of the final fabric makeup for the perfect jean denim, so just check the cotton count on the label and ignore the rest. Remember that the life expectancy of any jeans with elastane will shorten dramatically if you wash above forty degrees or tumble dry.

Think about pockets

Big pockets make for a smaller backside, small pockets make for a bigger-looking one – so choose according to your own bum fantasies. The reason

I loathe jeans without pockets is not that they make one's arse look large (I know that very big bums are now very much the thing), but because they make mine look flat. I also can't really accept pocketless denims – they really have no business calling themselves jeans at all. If you agree, look for larger pockets that are scaled up proportionally, i.e. the pockets are larger on a size-18 pair of jeans than on the size 8, and cover most of your bottom. Pockets that tilt slightly upwards at the outer corner make for a peachier shape still.

Zip or buttons?

I mostly prefer button flies, since they are usually attached to better-made, better-quality jeans (they're more expensive to manufacture). However, they will never have the stomach-suction powers of a zip, so if you're looking for a smooth, streamlined look, it's worth having a zippy pair in stock (my favourites are H&M Embrace – the only jeans I ever buy new).

Be realistic about shoes

I have jeans I wear with flats and jeans I wear with heels. The only jeans that work with either are those with both a slim leg and a ⅞ crop. A full-length jean that works with a stiletto is likely to bunch up around trainers and flat boots. Meanwhile, flares and bell bottoms look a bit rubbish with most flats except sneakers. If you wear lots of hi-tops and boots, you'll need denim that's either thin enough to tuck in, or a leg shape that's wide enough to glide over the top. Matchmake your jeans and shoes carefully.

Do they fit?

Here's a quite literally uncomfortable truth: the right-sized jeans feel half a size too small when new. They're not painful – they will do up with relative ease and you won't have to hold your breath. But they will feel a tiny bit more snug than you will want them, and than they will soon be. Stretch denim will usually 'give' about half a size within a wearing. A rigid denim (like classic 501s) may take a couple of wearings. Thereafter, they will tighten up again in the wash, but yield quite quickly again after dressing. Jeans that feel perfectly relaxed and comfy upon purchase will quickly feel too big, which is fine if you're buying loose boyfriend styles or pairs you plan to cinch in with a belt, but not ideal otherwise.

Who makes jeans for most shapes?

Good American
Don't let the involvement of a Kardashian (Khloe) stop you from checking out these most woman-friendly of jeans. High-waisted, bum-lifting, bump-smoothing and leg-lengthening jeans, in many washes and (dress) sizes from UK 4–30. Very helpfully, the website allows you to choose the size of model wearing the jeans in the photograph, and the prices, while not cheap (around £90), aren't as horrific as they could probably quite easily get away with. You can also find lots of them preloved on eBay.

Levi's
The original and still very often the best, Levi's make women's jeans from a size 0 up to a UK dress 24. Unlike most brands, they don't assume larger women don't come in the same array of heights as smaller ones, and offer three different leg lengths (sometimes more) across the brand. They also have an advantage over many excellent 'plus-sized' ranges, in having UK-based stores and website (the plus-sized selection on American sites is usually better, but returns can be a royal pain). The latter features larger models for a more realistic idea of how everything might look.

H&M
I'm a huge fan of H&M jeans, which are far better than they need to be for their low cost. They do skinny and high-waisted shapes especially well, shoot them on a diverse range of models and sell in (dress) sizes 4–26. Look out for the Premium Collection (better fabric, traceable manufacturing process and the most comfortable and flattering, sucky-inny 'Embrace' skinny jeans I've ever owned) and cool collaborations with denim giant Lee.

Gap
At around £34–50, Gap offers the best price–quality ratio in the business. The number of shapes and washes, both classic and seasonal, is vast but easily navigable online (alas, all stores have now been closed). Sizes go from a UK dress 2 up to 24.

Purchases that never work out well

Suede
What an absolute waste of everyone's time and money most suede is. The spoilt child of fabrics, it stains easily, picks up all the dye from

whatever else you're wearing, is ruined by the lightest drizzle, looks almost immediately grubby and costs the same as proper leather. I will never understand why people choose suede from the two. You'd be as well making clothing from spun sugar.

Clothes to slim into

No, no, no. A world of no. Do not pay hard-earned money for a garment to tell you you're fat every time you open your wardrobe. As much as dress sizes can feel like the enemy, they are here to help us. The right and most flattering size is the one that fits now, when you are here and wearing clothes in which to live your life. You don't deserve nice things when you're slimmer – you deserve them right now, in whichever body is kind enough to carry you around.

Clothes that need alteration

If you are a whizz on the sewing machine or content to hem with Wundaweb (needs must, on occasion, though only as a temporary measure), go right ahead and buy items on which you can work your magic. If, like me, you require a seamstress to take in dresses, let out waistbands and essentially do anything more than replace a fallen button, you should either act immediately after purchase or walk away from the cashwrap. Anything that hasn't been altered within the first fortnight of moving in is probably never going to be. If you really can't live without something, ask about alterations in-store, or visit your dry cleaner or repair shop on the way home.

163

Buying multiple colours

If you find a pair of trousers or a jumper that works brilliantly for you, that you're constantly washing and wearing, that makes you feel nice, then it's sensible to buy it in a second colour. Great. What rarely works, in my experience, is buying the same item in three or more colours, because however much you love the style, there will always be a couple of colours you instinctively gravitate towards, while swerving the other. The only exception to this rule is basic outfit-building blocks like T-shirts, socks, bras and vests, where it's useful to own white, black, nude, maybe navy. For anything else, two is plenty.

Items for another woman with another life

This is a huge one, and a lesson that took me many years to learn the hard way. Sure, I can look at a folky blouse or a statement necklace and appreciate it all I want, but is it for me, or is it for the kind of woman who wears gypsy blouses and statement necklaces? Why yes, those mules are beyond chic, but could I stomp through town at my desired speed without kicking them clean through a shop window? That sharp, shit-kicking blazer is making me swoon, but where would I wear it when I haven't worked in an office since 2004? While it now seems perfectly obvious that I am not bohemian Sienna Miller, or willowy Kristin Scott Thomas, or a corporate, athletic, super-sexy, preppy or eccentric type, for years there was some confusion and possibly aspiration that cost me dear. I am free to appreciate all of these looks without handing over my card.

Uncomfortable shoes

You won't wear them. And even if you do, you will look and feel crap in a way that will hinder your evening's enjoyment. And whatever the sales associate tells you, a too-small pair of shoes emphatically will not 'give' enough over time to make them fit.

164

The thing that's nearly like the thing you really want

That bag you're saving up for – that's the one you actually want, not the one that's in the same general area and affordable a couple of months earlier. Similarly, the dress you fell in love with, that you can't wait to come back into stock or turn up on a resale site, will still be on your mind as you wear an imitation or approximation of the real thing. Believe me, you will never, ever love a substitute as much as the desired original, however much you try to talk yourself into it, and ultimately, you'll be back to square one, having wasted the money you could have put towards the real thing. Stay focused, do not be derailed and be patient.

Mohair

Itchy, rash-inducing, boiling hot and prone to leaving long, irritating fibres in your eyelashes, lipstick and dinner, mohair is an utter pest of a material, cool though it undoubtedly looks. Against my better judgement, I once wore a mohair jumper to host an onstage event. Twenty minutes in, I was so itchy and red that I had to excuse myself while I removed it, then spent the remainder in a vest. It's so, so tempting to buy mohair, but truly, no good can come of it.

Items where it's good to save

Jeans

Buying very expensive designer jeans at full price is pointless for a number of reasons. Firstly, they always end up much cheaper in the sale and on sites like theoutnet.com. Secondly, once you know which ones you like, they are almost always available on eBay at high-street prices. Thirdly, high-street denim is brilliant. Weekday, & Other Stories, Gap, Arket and H&M all make terrific jeans that are as stylish as posh ones and make me feel every bit as good.

Knitwear

There is no fashion disaster more dispiriting than a moth attack on a spendy sweater. And provided there are no unique design features (logos, sleeve shape or specific slogan, for instance) and the fibres are natural, there is usually no telling the difference between a jumper from the high street and catwalk. So you might as well save your money. Uniqlo and M&S's cashmeres aren't just as good as their designer counterparts, they're often better. My chunky Reiss sweater is much softer than my Acne Studios equivalent, and I have a chunky, brightly coloured sweater from Zara that looks every bit as gorgeous, and feels every bit as itchy, as a similar one bought for six times its price at Ganni. Mohair is an equal-opportunities abuser.

T-shirts

Arket makes the best plain cotton, casual T-shirts and this is, in my view, simple fact. Not too short, not too long, neither too boxy nor too fitted. They wash like a dream and the heavyweight variety can be pulled on creaseless from the dryer. Everlane comes a close second. Neither are fast-fashion cheap (they're about £15 at time of writing), but nor are they the eye-watering prices charged by designers for an inferior product (£300 on something that will be ruined if you ever drip your pizza cheese? Are people mad?). The only expensive T-shirts ever to wow me are those by Sunspel, which are impossible to twist, exceptionally well cut and very fine-textured. At £50-odd I reserve them exclusively for when I'm wearing a T-shirt dressily, for example in a work environment, under a blazer.

Trainers

Many will disagree – and all power to them – but I personally believe that overall, the best trainers are made by sportswear companies – Adidas, Veja,

Nike, New Balance, Converse, Puma, Asics and the like. I have a strong aversion to most trainers made by fashion designers I'd normally covet, including Chanel, Saint Laurent, Gucci, Prada and so on. I'd no more buy Louis Vuitton trainers than I would a Puma handbag. To me, most posh trainers look anything but, and ironically, seem at least to me to be deeply uncool. And don't get me started on those £300 pre-distressed pairs that look as though they've been fished from a skip.

Leopard-print coats

Faux leopard coats, of which I have more than is decent, are not meant to be refined and elegant. They're meant to look a bit brassy, sexy and as though they've seen some scrapes – the essence of 1950s pub landlady in outerwear form. Think Christine Keeler, not Lady Astor. With very few exceptions, I feel about designer leopard coats how I feel about sweet potato fries instead of chips on a menu – some things are too precious, and too glorious, for gentrification.

Summer clothes

If I lived in Monte Carlo, then maybe I'd at least look at posh summer threads, but I don't and so cannot bring myself to pay heaps of money for thin fabrics I may or may not get much chance to wear. My holiday wardrobe consists almost exclusively of high-street and second-hand finds that won't make me cry when I spill my Ambre Solaire.

Workout wear

If spending an extra tenner on your leggings ensures they don't fall down with your kettlebell, then the premium's worthwhile. If the thought of wearing a lovely new spotty vest is what propels you out of bed and onto an exercise bike, then I get that too. But no one on earth actually needs to spend lots of money on clothes that, with the best will in the world, are soon drenched in sweat and threadbare at the crotch. What little activewear I have for what little activity I do is from Nike or Hush, which feels plenty fancy to me.

Items where it's good to spend

Winter coats

As a self-diagnosed outerwear addict, I have learned the hard way that cheap coats don't last. Manmade fibres quickly become shabby, the silhouette loses its shape, bobbling and pilling occurs. I definitely don't think a great-looking coat means designer, I'm saying that the difference between a £70 wool-mix coat and a £100 wool one is a good three winters. H&M Premium Collection, & Other Stories, Mango, M&S, Arket and (if you can stretch the budget a bit further) Jigsaw or Whistles all make fantastic, stylish coats that last (and are abundant on the preloved market).

Sunglasses

Your eyes and surrounding skin need protecting properly from the sun and those £5 street-market sunnies won't cut it. Good sunglasses work better and instantly elevate an outfit, making inexpensive summer clothes seem much more put together. I'm not talking about spending hundreds here. Arket has a small but perfectly curated selection of sunglasses at around the £40 mark, and for similar cash, there's the terrific Le Specs (sold on Net-a-Porter, Hush and elsewhere online). Ray-Bans are a bit more, but are usually cheaper at an airport, often go on sale and in any case are worth it. All that said, it's worth noting that designer sunglasses lose their value drastically at resale, so if you're a fan of Celine, Tom Ford and the like, start on Vestiaire Collective and eBay.

Boots

In the British climate, boots get worn a lot. I live in mine, wearing them to balance leather mini skirts, add bulk to skinny jeans, toughen up midi dresses and remove any trace of corporate from smart trousers. I want them to stay looking great for years, be easily repairable by a cobbler, and I'm absolutely not prepared to put up with several weeks or even days of blisters. In my experience, that means spending money on proper boots from a proper shoe brand, not from a high-street fashion retailer that displays shoes on hooks next to the earrings and iPhone cases. I'm pretty devoted to Grenson myself, while many of my friends live very comfortably in their Dr. Martens (they shred my feet and don't do half sizes), so trying on is crucial. Whichever you choose, investing in better quality pays dividends in longevity and comfort.

Belts

The PVC belts that come with a new skirt or trousers are as useless as the sponge applicators and brushes that come with makeup compacts. Spending a little money on real leather (or high-calibre vegan leather) belts – one in black, another in tan or brown – will pay for itself many times over. Good-quality belts, whether plain or ornate (personally, I'm mostly over name-logo belts, but whatever works for your style), will make inexpensive trousers and dresses look smarter instantly and improve with age. Choose your metal carefully and buy them in person – I've never once in my life bought a belt online that didn't require an exchange for a bigger or smaller size.

Scarves

I treat myself to a nice scarf every winter and it invariably plays a significant and refreshing role in my seasonal wardrobe. A great-quality scarf elevates an inexpensive outfit and introduces potentially transformative colour to a look, all without your having to buy much else or think too hard about it. A stripe, colourblock, pattern or different texture adds interest and some individuality to a look. Keeping two or three at hand offers almost endless options.

Bags

Just because I have bag issues myself, it certainly does not mean I think you or anyone else should too. My friend Nic is as baffled by my bag obsession as I am with her fixation on horses and slow cookers, and I like us as we are. But since pretty much every woman carries one regardless, I do think buying a bag made from real leather or high-quality vegan leather (which is plant-based, not plastic) makes all the difference to your outfit and general smartness. Black goes with everything, tan adds a lovely touch of Parisian chic, navy is a less obvious choice and all the better for it. You don't need to spend stacks unless that's what floats your boat, but spending £150 on a new bag will take you past a pretty definite quality marker, into brands like Whistles, All Saints, Jigsaw, Furla, Hush, Arket, & Other Stories, Toast and Reiss (as a general rule, I avoid obvious logos unless from classic houses that are unlikely ever to change their branding). If you're prepared to take the preloved route, you can get even more bag for your money. I recently bought a navy Enny bag exactly like the one my grandmother was given when she retired from the local Girl Guides Association, for £18 on eBay, and it's as good quality as my black equivalent from Celine. A good bag with minimal branding will last you years and usually get better with age, and is potentially the one item you'll wear every single day, with every outfit, and entrust with your worldly possessions, so why not make it lovely?

Everyday jewellery

I rarely remove my jewellery – I sleep, shower and bathe in the same few necklaces, earrings, rings and bangle, so I try to make each piece at least semi-fine (i.e. gold-plated or sterling silver) to withstand the wear and tear. I occasionally like big, statement costume pieces for fun, but will always get the most wear from a simple pair of real gold sleepers, a vermeil chain or platinum ring. Real metals and unfussy designs from a jeweller often cost roughly the same as designer nickel, and I would strongly suggest investing in the former – designer costume jewellery especially is often a colossal waste of money, especially if it contains crystals, pearls and other stones, which seem invariably to fall out. I also have a strong aversion to the inclusion of logos in precious jewellery specifically, but that's me.

Which colours suit everybody?

I've been obsessed with this question for years and have come to the satisfying conclusion that there are two colours that look unfailingly great on everyone. One is bold, one is classic, but both are failsafe. Bright cobalt blue instantly brightens all faces of all colours and ages and makes them look noticeably perky and in glowing good health. It is a magic but unique colour that, consequently, is not to everyone's taste or style (I love how it looks, but I rarely have cause to wear it, since I mostly dress in neutrals). The other colour is a no-brainer and gratifyingly easy in every respect: navy. Navy blue flatters all skin tones, with cool or warm undertones. Truly miraculous, it suits those with a classic, chic or conservative style, those who prefer to be more edgy and modern, the ultra-feminine and the tomboys. It works as well on babies as on children and adults, and suits any fabric, from denim and jersey to silk and tweed. It looks expensive and refined while being quietly rebellious for not being black. It is the only colour one can wear to both a wedding and a funeral without looking wrong at either. Navy is the best colour in the world. I will brook no ripostes.

How to shorten jeans

For at least a couple of decades, all my jeans needed shortening as standard, which is why I almost always waited for a rare trip to America before I bought new ones, since all the department stores there offer fast, neat alterations on purchasing (there are some stores here that offer this service – Selfridges is one). The advent of cropped jeans (those that are around ⅞ of regular jeans, not those capri pants that only really look good with full 1950s get up, including polka-dot head scarf and cat-eye sunglasses) meant that I could quite easily buy jeans at roughly the right length, but there's still the odd occasion where losing an inch or more is required. There are three ways to shorten jeans and two depend on the level of your sewing skills:

Wundaweb

Wundaweb is sticky webbing tape available at Robert Dyas, any haberdashers and Amazon. It sticks raw hemlines in place without stitches and is a brilliantly easy (with practice) way to shorten trousers and skirts. Wundaweb comes in a few pack types – for jeans, you'll need the web for heavier fabrics. To use, simply fold your hemline to the desired length and iron in the new fold. When that's cooled, slip a length of Wundaweb into the new hem so the web is concealed inside it. Cover the whole thing with a clean, damp cloth (I find a baby or cleansing muslin is ideal), then press firmly with an iron for ten or so seconds. Allow to cool thoroughly (about ten minutes) before you attempt to handle the fabric. Wundaweb is terrific in an emergency, but in my experience it will need to be reinforced with real stitches within a few months and/or multiple machine washes.

Neat hemlines

For a perfect hemline, do not simply cut down the jeans and turn up the hems. It is usual for jeans to be washed and finished as a complete garment by the manufacturer, meaning the hems will look the same as all the other seams around the pockets and waistband. Cutting off the ankle hems and shortening what's left means they'll never match again and will look a bit strange, so ask your local repair and alteration shop (there's at least one in every town, plus a dry cleaners with a seamstress) to cut off the hems, shorten the jeans, and then sew the original hemlines back on to match. They will know exactly what you mean and will usually do such an excellent job that no one will ever be able to tell they've been shortened. This costs around £20, which I think is pretty fair, but if you're handy with a sewing machine, you can save your cash and DIY.

Raw/distressed hemlines

The other way to shorten jeans is to create a raw hemline. This is particularly important when converting old jeans into denim shorts. For this, do not use a pair of scissors to cut to the required length. You will get way too clean a line and it will be near impossible to soften it after the fact, without sacrificing some length to forcibly fray it. Instead, fold the jeans vertically so the legs and each half of the waistband line up exactly. Keeping the jeans folded and cutting through both legs simultaneously, use sharp scissors to cut around two inches longer than required. Try on the jeans and make sure you know where you want the finished hem (too short a cut is irreversible). Remove and fold them in half again, adding a pin to act as a marker for the final length. Place on a kitchen chopping board. Take a serrated bread knife and cut through in a sawing motion. You shouldn't have to do this for long before the denim pulls away with a gentle tug, leaving behind a frayed hemline.

How to put holes in jeans and shorts

If you want your denim to appear aged and ragged, take some small nail scissors and make small horizontal nicks in the denim, wherever you want a hole to appear. Then, with a piece of sandpaper, rub each nick back and forth. The holes will become looser, the surrounding areas more worn and threadbare. If you don't have any sandpaper, a fine cheese grater works well.

How to buy maternity wear

Unless you are planning to become pregnant every year for the next ten, second-hand is absolutely the way to go; eBay is awash with high-quality maternity wear that's been worn for a total of six months, so start here then assess any wardrobe gaps later. It's tempting, particularly during a first pregnancy, to buy loads, as though one must replace one's entire wardrobe, but try to resist – I guarantee you'll end up wearing the same five or six simple pieces on rotation and the rest will go to waste. What is also easily done is forgetting your usual aesthetic entirely and thinking you must adopt a new one for pregnancy. I should know. With my now-seventeen-year-old in utero, I went to a very expensive maternity shop in Islington and spent money I definitely didn't have on a sweatshirt embellished with mirrored discs and another garment with pintucks that I can only describe as 'russet'. I blame hormones, childhood baggage and some resulting belief that I must 'do motherhood' as I imagined other, better women did – £300 I spent in there; £300 that I could have spent on a breast pump whose noise didn't drown out the telly.

Retaining your own identity in pregnancy is tricky enough, without having to dress like someone else too. I just don't know why brands assume all women suddenly become hyper-feminine, bohemian, infantile (bows and ditsy florals – why? I think we've established that I'm over the age of consent) or inexplicably drawn to Breton stripes post-conception – and I happen to adore Breton stripes. I assume it's the same mad reasoning that leads them to believe women over a size 16 crave flammable fabrics and butterfly prints. In fact, maternity clothes are most useful when they are simple, practical, comfortable and allow you to retain your usual style by acting as a relatively blank canvas over which you can layer existing wardrobe staples – cardigans, sunglasses, jewellery, scarves, bags and the like. I found stretchy cotton elastane or Lycra indispensable, since it supports heavy boobs and bump, lightening some of your load, and because it clings it doesn't cover all your body parts, tent-like, just to clear a hump in the middle.

These are the things I mostly lived in while the mirrors and russet sold on eBay at a loss:

Maternity tights

Even if you're not normally a tights person, opaque maternity tights can be extremely helpful in lightening your load. The stretchy belly cradles and contains your bump and a good elastane content supports weary, water-retaining legs. Spanx, Falke and all the usual maternity brands make them, but it's worth knowing that Primark sells some of the best on the market.

Maternity jeans

You can get away with wearing your usual jeans with a maternity extension panel for the first few months, but after that, some second-hand maternity jeans are a worthwhile investment for pregnancy and the months that follow it. They're essentially normal jeans with extra-stretchy cotton panels fitted to the sides, and a thick jersey band sewn around the top, and these all expand to accommodate a growing bump. My 7 For All Mankind maternity jeans (bought on eBay for £70) were worn every week for about four years – post-baby, they stretched comfortably around my larger waist, and the maternity panels were easily covered with tops and jumpers.

A formal dress

If you have a wedding or other formal event in the diary, it's worth having one good dress within reach. This is absolutely not worth buying new, since most formal maternity dresses on auction sites have similarly been worn only once or twice. I had a plain stretchy black Lycra frock from Isabella Oliver that I dressed up with jewellery and a ribbon belt for smart occasions and it made me feel comfortable and look deceptively effortful, and allowed for swift hoiking up for the average evening's twelve emergency wees.

Two belly bands

If you buy nothing else, get one of these in white and another in black. These are simple cotton Lycra hoops that look like boob tubes, only for the abdomen. They support your bump and, usefully, cover any widening gaps between your tops and bottoms. This allows you to keep wearing your old clothes – just match the band to the colour of your top for a barely perceptible transition. They're also terrific post-baby, for breastfeeding, since they cover up your bare belly while you nurse. They cost about a tenner.

Maternity bras

As mad as it may sound to the smaller-boobed, big-titted women will understand when I say that my biggest dread about pregnancy stemmed from the belief that all maternity bras were wireless. I had been in wires since I was twelve and felt horrible without them. So if you feel my former pain, let me tell you that discovering Anita underwired maternity bras changed my life. They lift and support as well as a regular bra, with no spiky underwires, and cups that drop down for feeding. I lived in them for a total of three years and they contributed hugely to my feeling more like myself. If wires are neither here nor there to you, your options are endless. Hot Milk make very good, well-structured feeding bras, Cosabella's are extremely comfortable and attractive, Fantasie nursing bras come in a proper and intelligent range of sizes and if you want sexy special-occasion feeding bras, Elle Macpherson is your girl (though hers is another maddening brand that thinks big boobs equal big back).

173

Two stretchy T-shirts

Long-sleeved for winter pregnancies, short for summer. I guarantee that if they're not on your back, they'll be in the wash. Go for a high elastane content for a supportive, sling-like effect on the bump and to stop any fabric stretching.

High-waisted stretchy skirt

Extremely useful for teaming with pre-pregnancy tops, a stretchy skirt is easy and versatile – pull it up to make a mini or down to form a pencil or midi skirt. Also very useful post-birth when feeding, since it prevents you from having to expose your tummy – just pull up to make it very high-waisted.

A cotton smock, trapeze or maxi dress

If you're pregnant at the height of summer (I have a September baby and can relate), you'll crave something light and gauzy that allows blissful air circulation around your downstairs. A loose-fitting dress is flattering, cool and often very useful post-baby, when you will almost certainly retain your larger abdomen for at least a couple of months, probably longer.

Flared jersey trousers

Very specifically, these should be jersey and elastane, have a wide waistband that can be pulled over or rolled under the baby bump, and be as suitable when worn in bed or lounging on the sofa as they are with trainers and a top on the go. Also very useful for if and when you're in hospital and want to wander down to the shop or lounge. Yoga and activewear shops are often the best places to buy them.

174

How to follow a dress code

Formal

This, even now, mostly means wearing the sort of long frock/gown one would wear to a red carpet awards ceremony if one ever actually had both cause and invitation to attend red carpet awards ceremonies. High heels are usual but by no means still obligatory, though shoes and bags do need to be smart and glamorous. Shorter dresses and trouser suits are allowed, of course, but the expectation for each would be raised. Essentially, they'd better be extra fabulous or sharp to pass code. This really is the top tier, so if you need to go formal only once in a blue moon, as most of us do, consider hiring something to save cash and wardrobe space. Men in bowties – either white or black (the invitation should tell you).

Semi-formal

Only a fraction more relaxed than above. Clothing should still be well considered and smart, but the main difference is that women will be free to choose the length of their skirts and men will wear a smart necktie, not a bow. Any suit worn by man or woman should be matching and in a man's case worn with a proper shirt rather than a jumper or polo shirt. Excessive jewellery, sequins, sparkly embellishments and the like aren't strictly on-code. Most traditional British weddings and garden parties are semi-formal, especially if they involve a daytime element.

Cocktail/cruise

A very nice party dress or very smart trouser/top get-up. Men in evening suits and tie (bow or modern necktie). Any colour goes; sparkles are encouraged; bold costume jewellery is never wrong. Again, high heels are no longer necessary, but make the shoes smart.

Corporate

Suits all round. For women, this can mean either a skirt or trouser suit, or a blazer worn over a tailored dress. Well-groomed hair; neat and subdued makeup, if worn. Simple, smart shoes – never trainers.

Wedding

Some weddings have a specific aesthetic, including for the guests. Weddings involving a different culture or religion to your own may involve an appropriate dress code and varying degrees of modesty, so don't be afraid to ask the couple for guidance, allowing them plenty of time before arrangements become more stressful. Some wedding invitations say 'evening wear', which is fair enough, others say 'all white', which is slightly unreasonable given the already steep cost of attending a wedding, not to mention deeply naff, but it's down to you to decide whether you want to make an allowance for someone's dream day (I'm inclined to go along with most things). A girlfriend of mine once received a wedding invitation with the strict dress code of 'cappuccino' (I'm not joking) and decided she and her skin tone had found their unexpected limit, but each to their own.

For a straightforward wedding, the code is a smart day-to-night outfit (dress or trousers) that isn't too revealing or ridiculously short. High heels are now wholly optional, but decent shoes are not. I personally wouldn't wear a white or cream outfit unless it was floral or otherwise patterned, or if the bride and I were very close and she had given me her blessing. I would also avoid the bridesmaids' colour if I knew it in advance. Americans don't traditionally wear hats at weddings. British people traditionally do and, I've noticed, have started doing so more again (certainly more than five years ago). I'm all for it, especially if the venue is spacious, for example a very large church or outside (for small venues, I do think variations on compact styles like a beret, cloche, boater or fedora look smarter and more modern than a fascinator). If you wear a larger hat, make sure it isn't so large as to obscure anyone's view, or if you really can't resist a whopper, sit at the back. Essentially: pay attention to what the couple want, look as nice as you can for their photos, without making any of it about you.

Funeral

Unless a family has made express wishes for people to dress brightly or casually, or in a specific colour symbolic to the deceased, I would strongly encourage everyone to wear black or dark navy and to make a proper effort. This means no wet hair, dirty shoes or last night's mascara. And nothing revealing, micro-short or overtly sexy – again, unless that is the explicitly stated theme of the day. (In 1991, I attended a friend's funeral followed by an absolutely scandalous wake at the Wag Club in Soho – indecorous clubwear was positively insisted upon.) At a regular funeral, your appearance should blend in with the congregation while showing that you respect both the dead and their loved ones enough to have taken some real time to look presentable. I'm shocked when I see people attend funerals having made less effort than if they were attending an important work meeting, birthday party or night out, because it seems to me that the honouring of an entire life should be by definition a bigger fuss. Even if it doesn't matter to you, it definitely will matter to someone having a harder time. Hats are optional, but I must say that I like the tradition, and usually wear a beret.

Modest

Modest clothing is very important in the weddings, funerals and other special events within many cultures – especially when an event is held in a place of worship. If you don't have any personal experience within a culture, make it your business to find out what is acceptable well in advance. Modest dressing is remarkably easy to do stylishly these days (trying to find a long-sleeved maxi dress was no mean feat five years ago), but there are dozens of variables specific to different values and occasions. For example, exposed shoulders are generally not acceptable in a cathedral, gurdwara or synagogue but are often fine later, at a reception. Covered arms and long dresses may be required all day, while head scarves may be obligatory during a ceremony, so know your stuff in order to not stand out or unintentionally cause offence.

Smart-casual/dress-down

Not full-on corporate garb, but also not the kind of Zoom-call loungewear one could conceivably wear for a jog. This is often as corporate-looking as the media industry gets. Broadly, smart-casual means smart shapes in casual fabrics. For example, well-fitting trousers made from jersey, corduroy or denim rather than suiting flannel or wool, and smart shirts and blouses in chambray, twill or jersey instead of cotton poplin or silk. What smart-casual is telling you is to relax and feel more comfortable, but not at the apparent expense of your professionalism or respect for colleagues, clients or fellow guests. I wouldn't wear trainers unless they were leather or leather-like, and spotless.

Casual

Comfy and practical but not scruffy and slobby. Jeans, trainers, T-shirts, unsweaty sweats – all are fine. You still need to look clean and presentable, but so you can otherwise relax.

Are expensive watches worth it?

It depends if they're worth it to you. 'Expensive' is a relative term and depends not only on your own personal budget, but on spending and priorities (I wear an expensive watch but also balk at what other people spend on cars and holidays). It is absolutely the case that one can buy a reliable, accurate, high-quality and stylish watch for a hundred pounds-odd, while also being true that the craftsmanship of a Swiss heirloom timepiece is second to none. You should buy what you can afford and what you love. However, my one strongly held belief about watches is that you should always buy one from a company that first and foremost makes watches, NOT a fashion brand with a side hustle in them. This rule applies at every price point, from high street to high luxury. I'd always buy a Casio over something from Accessorize, a Swatch over a Ted Baker watch, a Timex over a DKNY, an Oris before a Gucci, and a Rolex before a Chanel. Wherever a brand sits in the chain, the reputation of a dedicated watchmaker lives and dies with the quality of its watches. They don't make watches as some brand extension to flesh out a jeans or handbag empire. Despite being of comparable price to the real deal, fashion-brand watches are never as good, don't hold their value and are much less likely to be around to pass down to your grandkids.

And the same applies to boots . . .

Considerable experience has taught me that when you're looking for comfortable, hardwearing, long-living, beautifully constructed, repairable and fantastic-looking boots, you are almost always infinitely better off with a shoe brand that does nothing else (Grenson, Church's, Dr. Martens, Trickers, Kickers) than you are with a fashion clothing brand that happens also to make shoes. A pair of Reiss boots costs roughly the same as some Grensons, for example. Saint Laurent boots cost more than Church's. In both cases, the difference in quality and comfort is night and day.

How to make clothes look instantly more expensive

Swap the buttons – even lovely buttons are comparatively cheap and make unexceptional cardigans, blouses and blazers look luxurious.

Change the belt – the belt that came with your garment will almost certainly be rubbish.

Change the laces – I frequently swap out the laces in new shoes for a higher-quality or thicker version bought very cheaply online. An extra four quid can make shoes appear a good hundred quid more valuable.

De-lint it – fluff makes clothing look cheap and tatty. Always keep a lint roller on hand, especially if you have pets.

De-bobble it – pilling is normal on knitwear but makes any garment seem old and worn. Buy a cashmere comb, electric bobble-off device or, at a push, use a regular razor to very carefully stroke the fabric.

Steam it – I loathe ironing but even if you love it, all that pressure on the seams makes them shiny. Use a steamer instead – they're inexpensive, extremely easy and give a much sleeker, more polished finish. Put your garment on a hanger, hang from a doorframe or shower rail, and wear a protective glove (usually the carrying pouch of a hand steamer) to hold the fabric taut. A shirt takes three minutes.

The anti-capsule wardrobe

I know, I know. You will find a thousand videos and a million links relating to 'the capsule wardrobe'. You know exactly what they'll say you need – a blazer, a pair of ballet flats, a little black dress, perfect white T-shirt and Chanel-style flap bag. You know the drill and don't need my version. The truth is that I love neutral colours and happen to be a relatively minimalist dresser who actively loves a camel coat. But even I'd lose my mind if I dressed solely like this. It is simply not the case that everyone looks good in a tailored blazer, or a pair of slim black trousers (I've found one pair I love in four decades). I don't want my wardrobe to look the same as a friend's, or a blogger's, or a celebrity's. I want it to look like mine. Capsule wardrobes are a great starting point if you love wearing basics, but even if you do, my view is that they're no placeholder for personal style and individual character. So here are some unapproved, unessential items that I think you should consider alongside them:

A mad thing

I'm talking about something that doesn't relate to current trends, doesn't look like anything else you own – or, indeed, like much else in the shops, but that you deeply, truly love. I own a huge, chunky grey jumper emblazoned across the front with a graphic from The Beatles' *Yellow Submarine*. I bought it a few years ago in the sales, presumably because no one else knew what to do with it, and I've worn it to death. It makes me smile every time I see it, which automatically means it suits me and the rest of my wardrobe. It was never in fashion so it will never be out of fashion. An animation graphic doesn't go with anything, and so it goes with everything. I have another jumper that looks like Charlie Brown's. I do think that in the world of fashion, there is something to be said for a sense of humour and an occasionally laid-back approach instead of meticulous coordination.

179

A shaggable thing

I'm not suggesting you buy clothes to pull in – though if you do, knock yourself out – I'm saying that everyone should own something that makes them feel sexy in themselves. A silk shirt that dips in just the right place, a pair of jeans that give you a bum you feel like reaching around and groping yourself, a bra that pushes your boobs into the juiciest cleavage, some shoes that make you strut – whatever it is, a garment that screams sex to you will bring joy whenever you need a boost.

An edgy thing

This is an essential if, like me, you are instinctively a minimalist classicist who finds slavish minimalist classicism impossibly, and joylessly, dull. Neutral colours and iconic shapes are wonderful and endlessly useful, but without something to offset them, you look like a billion other women. An earring that looks like a simple gold sleeper but is, on closer inspection, a safety pin. A classic Mary Jane shoe only with a very pointy toe that would never pass school uniform code. Traditional loafers worn with glittery socks. A little black dress with slightly exaggerated shoulders, a traditional overcoat with a loose, oversized fit, a ladylike bag with a heavy chain strap, or a flash of neon in an unexpected place. Anything that might give a future mother-in-law pause can make an outfit look more interesting, considered, individual and modern.

Leopard print is a neutral

Let's get this straight – beige/brown/camel/black leopard print (i.e. the classic colourway as opposed to the coloured versions) is as neutral as plain black, navy, white and beige and can be worn by anyone of any age, anywhere but a funeral. Leopard's neutral status is unique in the animal kingdom – ponyskin, snakeskin, tiger, cow or cheetah prints, stylish though they are, are not neutrals and are more of a statement to be deployed judiciously.

How to walk in high heels

It is a fact of life that for the most part (with many exceptions, of course), shorter women typically fare better in heels than those with a higher centre of gravity. It is also a fact that in the 2020s, this no longer poses any sartorial challenge to anyone. We live in a time when there is simply no longer a need for someone who cannot walk in heels to attempt to walk in heels, just so they can drink in the beauty of their shoes. Flats are now cool, stylish, feminine and infinite in their variety and, besides, even an ugly flat looks better than a precarious, uncomfortable hobble in pretty heels. Practise around the house for several evenings – back straight, neck aligned, confident strides – but if it's still not happening, it probably never will and just be thankful you're not hobbling down the Strand at midnight, not a taxi in sight. Move on to flats and chalk heels down as something that just aren't for you, like cycling shorts aren't for me. If you fare better, fabulous. The most comfortable high heels are around 80mm and remember that anything involving a wedge, strap or platform will likely be a little more comfy than balancing on thin stilettos. Manolo Blahnik stilettos are the comfiest of all. While Christian Louboutins, for about the same money, are agonising. Your mileage may vary, of course, but my point is that it is not the heel height per se that causes discomfort – it's about how the surrounding shoe has been engineered to support it.

Should you match your bra and knickers?

You do you, but I'd sooner sweep the M25 than wear a black bra with white knickers. I just can't. It feels like wearing odd socks. There is an argument that one should match underwear not to itself, but to the garment it sits underneath, but I'm just not in the habit of wearing transparent trousers and skirts, so can't think of an occasion when it would apply. Every time I buy a new bra, I buy two pairs of matching knickers. I wear the bra for two days (unless it's a sports bra), the knickers for one, then the whole three-piece set goes in the wash. This way everything ages evenly.

How to buy a bra

I am obsessed with bras. Having carried around disproportionately huge boobs for three decades before finally undergoing a surgical reduction (absolutely not the desired or affordable choice for everyone, but I personally felt I'd paid my dues and my shoulders deserved a rest), I know a lot about underwear.

Much as I hate to quote an online troll, one of mine once declared, in a conversation about how I was certainly lying about my bra size, that 'it is impossible to be a size 8 and a G cup'. I repeat this pointless guff only because it demonstrates how widely misunderstood bra sizes are. In fact, the statement is the opposite of true. What is almost 'impossible' is for a size-8 dress to be a 34-inch band size, which is why I'm a 30 – cup size is neither here nor there. Even well-informed women constantly conflate band size (the ribcage) with cup size (the boob flesh) and consequently end up with the wrong bras, feeling nowhere near as nice in them as they should.

Here is what is true of almost every woman I have ever met, and probably those I haven't: your cups are too small and your band is too big. It is simply not possible for such a vast number of women, of all shapes and sizes, to be a 34B or a 36C. It's just not. Big boobs do not automatically mean a big band size. I know: I used to be a G-cup and had hurtled down the alphabet without ever once creeping past a 30 band. Conversely, small boobs don't mean a low number – it is perfectly possible to be a 38AA. Stop guessing your size based on preconceptions or prejudices you have about your body and those of others. Stop accepting the size that sounds about right in a culture where most talk of bra cups occurs in tabloid newspapers (it drives me mad when they say 'the model had implants to take her from a 32D to a 38FF' – not possible unless she also now has a silicone back). Instead, get fitted for a new bra in a proper lingerie boutique or department store, and prepare to feel and look so much better in your clothes – instantly.

Of course, we now like to shop online, would prefer not to schlep and seek easy solutions to common problems, and I daresay you could google some magic formula involving a tape measure and band-to-cup size equation, but trust me – these conversion tables are no longer fit for purpose. Boobs have grown exponentially in recent decades. There are now many more cup sizes than when the cup sizing system was conceived and developed. Different fabrics and sizes can also yield different results. So finding your bra size really is a question of trying lots on. I suggest heading into town for a fitting appointment at a specialist such as Bravissimo, Rigby & Peller, M&S, John Lewis or one of the many excellent specialist independent lingerie boutiques around the country, who are generally very generous with their time and expertise. If you're too shy or busy and budget allows, you can order heaps of bras online and make an afternoon of it at home, but you'll need to know how a great-fitting bra should look and feel. The following should help:

182

- If your boobs bulge out of the top of your bra, almost as though you have four separate boobs, but are neat at the armpit, you are at least one cup size too big for the bra you're wearing.
- If your boobs bulge at the top of your bra, and also bulge at the armpits, you need to increase by two cup sizes, possibly more.
- If your back band is riding up your back, making a concave arch, then your band size is too big – this effect often goes hand in hand with divots in the shoulders, as your tight straps work too hard to carry what your ill-fitting band should be supporting on its own.
- If your bra band is riding downwards, so that your boobs no longer reach the bottom of the cups, it is simply seeking a narrow point to sit comfortably, which is probably nearer your waist. Your band is too small. Your band should sit at the same level, front and back.
- If there are creases in the fabric of your cups, they are probably a bit too big, so go down one. They should be smooth.
- If your underwire is stabbing you in the armpit (a unique joy), then you are either wearing cups that are too small or have incorrectly machine washed or tumble dried your bras (this can be done safely – see pages 28–9) and damaged them, or both.

- If your underwire is stabbing you in the cleavage, you are either wearing cups that are too small, and/or you have boobs that are very close together and therefore better suited to a plunge or T-shirt-style bra than they are to a push-up or balconette. This is also true if the wide-apart straps on your push-up or balconette are constantly slipping down – make the switch to plunge.
- Ask a friend or your partner to pinch the bra band at the back and pull it outwards. If they are able to pull the band away more than 3–4cm from your body, the band is too big.
- If your bra becomes too loose over time and you haven't lost weight, you've been wearing your bra in too big a band size and wearing it on the tightest hook. All elastic gives over time, so buying a size that fits perfectly on the loosest hook gives you somewhere to go as the bra stretches.
- If your boobs are escaping out of the bottom of your bra, your cups are too small and your band is too big. Again.
- If your back band is coming away from your body, leaving a gap at the bottom of the bra between it and your torso, then again your cups are too damn small. They are almost always too damn small.

Where can you buy bras with small bands and big cups?

I'm convinced that the reason so many women believe big boobs equal big band sizes is because, for decades, bra companies treated these very different measurements as mutually exclusive. For years, I was forced to choose between bras that fitted my back or those that fitted my boobs and even, on more than one occasion, to make Frankenstein's bras by sewing straps from one onto the cups of another, or cutting slits into my cups to expand them. And that was before I could even dare think about attractive design. Things are different now, though fashion brands, both high street and posh, still seem to believe that everyone is a 32–36B or C. Fortunately, proper bra brands like Fantasie, Freya, Miss Mandalay, Bravissimo, M&S, Curvy Kate and Cosabella know the score and most of them offer either wired or unwired designs. Their commitment to supporting big-knockered women has changed many lives, including mine. They are invariably more expensive than fashion bras, but worth every penny.

Do I need wires?

This is a very personal and free choice. Most women will have an instinctive reaction one way or another to underwires and they will be right about themselves. Pre-breast reduction, I would never, ever have considered a non-wired bra (I literally slept in wires) and now I wear unwired bralettes almost exclusively (I keep a couple of pretty wired bras for special occasions only, as well as a wired sports bra, which is worn even less often). Your choice to wear or not wear wires is really down to how you feel in them, in terms of physical comfort and mental confidence, and what you're doing in them at the time. I'd argue that a sports bra is necessary for anyone planning to jiggle and bounce around lots, but follow your own preference for wires or none, and ignore any preaching by anyone else.

The neckline lie

Here's a lie women have been told for too long: V-necks are the ideal choice for big boobs, while polonecks and turtlenecks should be avoided. Absolutely not true. In fact, practically the opposite is true. V-necks have to be exactly the right depth to flatter big boobs – even a fraction too high a V (common) makes perfectly lovely tits flat and saggy and looks bloody awful. Conversely, polonecks can look fabulous and chic on women of all shapes and sizes, lengthening and slimming the neck. Just choose one that fits the neck snugly but not tightly, rather than a big, thick, sloppy cowl-neck-type affair (which I love, but they're harder to pull off and not as universally flattering). I wear polonecks often, particularly with chain necklaces and pendants worn over the top, for that cool 1970s mum vibe – shaggy perm and Lambert & Butler fag not included.

What women need but can't buy

Dear British High-street Retailers,

I am a forty-something woman with an upcoming award ceremony, three weddings, several important work engagements, a holiday in the unreliable British climate, another abroad, and some pottering about doing bugger all. I have spent decades browsing your wares, both online and in your bricks-and-mortar stores. My question for you is this: where, particularly in the past five years, have all the clothes gone?

Let's begin with sleeves, for these cast a shadow over my entire shopping experience. Despite your apparent belief that my life is one long high-school prom, I would always like to cover my arms, at least to just beyond the elbow. I would not like cap sleeves to highlight the fact that I've lifted one kettlebell in my life, nor a bandeau top that precludes me from wearing a bra. I don't want to pick up any more nice-seeming dresses, only to find the entire back of it missing. I am literally always going to be wearing a bra, whatever strip of wide elastic you so optimistically sew in to replace it. Like most women over thirty-five, who have either breastfed babies or done way too much reckless jiggling at underground raves (I know you're shocked), I like my boobs firmly encased, not increasing my dress size by two, and covering my belly like a stab vest.

Aaah, bellies. Mine is not taut, or flat, and I'm mostly okay about it. What I'm not okay about is your obsession with tops that finish exactly around its middle, which, when teamed with your persistently low-rise jeans, expose my protruding midriff for the first time since Madonna went nuclear and I cut up my Aertex hockey blouse. I'd like, ideally, a T-shirt or jumper to reach my hips, skimming breezily across my stomach as if to say 'nothing to see here', ideally with enough fabric to ruche so no one is quite sure where excess flesh ends and surplus cotton begins.

I say 'cotton', because you are quite mistaken in thinking that I'd like fabrics I can't safely wear near a naked flame. I want natural, soft cloth that stays the same size in a dryer, doesn't need dry cleaning, can be put on a radiator without emerging as tactile as a Ryvita, and still looks good on someone who hasn't ironed this decade. And my larger friends (middle-aged and therefore numerous) would like their fabrics to be the same as mine, not sourced for three pence a yard from the cash and carry, nor emblazoned with mimsy butterflies, ditsy florals or garish Aztec prints like pelmets from a static caravan circa 1992. When you do give them something more modern, they'd appreciate your not assuming any body confidence they do possess should manifest in dressing like a dancer at Spearmint Rhino. They're not ashamed, dowdy or inherently bubbly and outrageous. Please stop presuming that fat automatically equals tall with massive knockers and thin equals short with a flat chest. Larger women's lives and desires are the same as those of thin women. All of us want normal, nice, fashionable but unfaddy clothes with a design flourish here and there, that make our respective bodies look their best.

Although while we're at it, I'm a size 8 (except in & Other Stories, where I'm a size 10, Gap, where I'm a size 2, M&S, where I'm a 6 and Whistles, where I'm at least three different sizes – do please all meet up for coffee and chat) and also feel strongly disinclined to show as much flesh as the teenage models on ASOS. com. Contrary to your sales blurbs, for many of us 'bodycon' is less an irresistible selling point, more a helpful signal that we will spend our evenings draped in a coat, unable to nibble more than an olive. Likewise, many of us haven't shared your love of tight-waisted skating dresses since puberty, think 'cold shoulder' detailing makes us look a bit mad, and we're not sure we'll ever be old enough for bias-cut linen. What would better tempt us is a whole department of 'eating dresses' – flattering frocks, neat at the shoulders, sleeves and neck, but with enough fabric around the middle to invisibly accommodate a bottle of red and more than nineteen calories.

Not that thirty-, forty- and fifty-something women are all about socialising. We have busy jobs to do, families to care for, schedules to manage and bills to pay. Instead of 'occasionwear' seemingly aimed at black-tie beach parties we've neither hosted nor been invited to, ever, how about a plain dress that, with a quick slick of red lipstick and black liner or a fancier shoe, can be worn straight out to drinks from a boring work meeting? Speaking of shoes, our taste didn't vanish with our flexible foot tendons. We like the bright colours, quality leather, femininity and high design spec of stilettos, even though many of us would like to be able to run from a mugger after dark. Do put a little more effort into cheaper brogues, Oxfords, ballet flats and slides – in fact, go mad. Our feet are where we're up for anything – studs, neons, jewels, bonkers prints – safe in the knowledge that they'll fit almost everyone and inject some fun and personality into our outfits without going full top-to-toe Su Pollard.

So, once-beloved high-street retailers, when lamenting your declining profits, do consider putting into production this failsafe shopping list of garments that practically every woman over thirty, from size 6–30, would buy tomorrow: a flattering sweatshirt dress available in several colours for school runs, evenings with close friends, dog walking and trips to the supermarket. One perfect tunic dress like those made by Goat and Victoria Beckham only for less than a monthly mortgage repayment, which can be worn to any wedding, funeral or party, depending on accessories. A fancier, more fitted midi dress in a vintage print. A soft, navy, Paddington-style duffle coat with a hood. Pockets on everything. Sucky-in tights in different lengths as well as widths, which don't make us bloat and ache as though we've just flown long haul. Long-length T-shirts and sweatshirts that don't shrink, twist or bag. Slim-fit, washable cardigans that finish mid-hip and have buttons spaced close enough to avoid gape. Some jumpers that go in and out as our bodies do, and have a deep-enough V-neck to stop our tits looking massive and saggy. A couple of A-line skirts that hit the knee. A *Mad Men*-style pencil skirt with a sturdy control panel across the belly.

I am a forty-something woman who is wondering where all the high-street clothes have gone. My friends are all similarly perplexed. We are all in charge of our household budgets, all have some money, all love fashion and all want to look nice. So why, failing high-street retailers, do you so persistently ignore us? The lucrative answer to many of your problems is standing right in front of you, desperately searching for sleeves.

How not to make bad sale shopping decisions

1. Would you still covet this at full price? If the answer is no, don't buy it.
2. What will you not wear from your existing wardrobe in order to wear this on any given day? Do you like this more or less than the item it will replace in an outfit? If the answer is less, don't buy it.
3. Have you ever noticed that this is missing from your wardrobe? If you've never felt the need to own one or spotted an opportunity to wear one, don't buy it.
4. Can you think of a similar garment that's proved extremely useful? If you can't, don't buy it.
5. Is it a little bit like the item you really want but don't want to wait any longer to save for? You will never like this as much – don't buy it.
6. Does it require alteration, workouts or dieting for it to fit properly? If it does, don't buy it.
7. Regardless of sale price, what will the ultimate cost-per-wear likely be? If a special-occasion sale dress is £150 and will be worn only twice, then £75 each time you leave the house in it is actually extortionate. Don't buy it.

How to have a wardrobe clearout

The 2020 lockdown sparked not one, but a series of three big wardrobe clearouts for me. As it became clear that we were looking at months, rather than weeks, confined to our homes, what hung in our wardrobes began to look slightly daft. I had over a dozen party frocks, but little to wear for a daily walk in the park. My work-meeting clothes – high heels, pencil skirts, tights – were made redundant as my lower half disappeared from Zoom view. The garments that would comfort, warm and console me were sort of sprinkled around various drawers and cupboards – the also-rans and understudies, uncoordinated and unprepared to be drafted for service.

The cull was dramatic (I got rid of all but five pairs of high heels), but even now, in calmer times, it's best practice to undertake at least one critical analysis of your wardrobe each season. I generally do mine at the same time as the changeover between spring/summer and autumn/winter, but whenever you can clear an entire afternoon for the job is fine.

I should say now that I'm not about to go organisational guru, here. I'm not someone who endorses ruthlessness for its own sake. But having been raised by a hoarder in a house I was too ashamed to have any friends visit, I do feel very strongly that if you keep everything, you value nothing. Having piles and piles of clothes frequently makes it harder to choose a coherent outfit in a timely fashion. It means that really great pieces are underexposed, because they're jostling with mediocre ones for weartime. Too much stuff is confusing, wasteful of time, money and space, and bad for the environment. And so you don't need to be ruthless, but you do need to be honest and firm with yourself, for the greater good. Here's how:

Take two cheap clothing rails (they're a tenner at Argos, come apart for storage and are useful things to own anyway) and place them side by side. Take each item from your wardrobe and decide which one of the following four categories it falls into:

A. Worn in the past six months.
B. Not worn in the past six months.
C. Doesn't fit/don't like/haven't worn at all.
D. Legacy pieces.

Place A on one rail. Hang B and D on the other. Place C in a pile on the floor. Do this until your wardrobe is empty. Now ask yourself:

Why do the legacy pieces matter?

It's all very well going full Marie Kondo and bagging up anything you don't love now, but what if the memories of wearing a long-since-retired frock still spark considerable joy? Sure, there are clothes you haven't worn for years but there are also family photographs you may not have looked at recently either. They're no less precious to you. It is completely understandable to want to keep your wedding dress, or your baby's first bathrobe, or the blouse you wore when you graduated. But prioritise and limit yourself to those that really, truly matter. The skirt in which you passed your driving test when you were two sizes smaller probably doesn't, on balance. A discerning selection of sentimental items (five or six, max) is plenty and if there's storage space to put them all in a box instead of hanging in your everyday wardrobe, then that's ideal. Divide the rest into what can be sold, gifted or donated to charity, and give your memories a new life.

Why do you like the A rail?

We're keeping them all, for sure, but what is it about these pieces that has you reaching for them so often? Is it the cut, colour, fabric, comfort, trend? Really pay attention to their great qualities and think about any gaps in your favourites that might need filling. Maybe that jacket you love could be worn even more often if you had a good black skirt as well as your existing trousers. Maybe some loafers would give all your good trousers a whole different look. Make a list of items that would add even more wearing opportunities – this sort of targeted, thoughtful and slow shopping saves time, money and wasteful mistakes.

Are the B-list items inferior doubles?

Among the most common reasons women don't wear the clothes they have is that they have overshopped for things that are slightly inferior versions of things they already own and are happy with. For example, I have a second-hand denim APC shirt dress that I bought for £20 on eBay and love madly. I feel great in it; people often compliment me on it. So if I'm shopping, and feeling sad, weak, vulnerable or bored, a denim dress seems like a dependable and joy-bringing buy. Which is how I came to buy the lovely Warehouse denim dress. This is a darker denim, with aged gold buttons instead of poppers, and a slightly higher hemline. But make no mistake, it is STILL A DENIM SHIRT DRESS. There are only 365 days in a year. At absolute most, I may wish to wear a denim shirt dress of any kind every couple of weeks. That's just twenty-six wears per year. Why would I choose to ignore the APC dress I love, in order to wear the not-quite-as-great Warehouse version instead? I have a washing machine – I will just keep choosing the one I love. People do this all the time. If you have something at home that you already love, do not effectively take mistress garments to compete with it for your attention.

Are the unworn items off season?

If anything you haven't worn in six months has been unwearable for the past six months, put it in a box of things that aren't seasonal and should only come back out when fit for purpose and climate. These get a stay of execution.

Does the remaining B list have tags still attached?

These purchases were an error of judgement. Maybe a sad purchase, or a period purchase. We are none of us wholly immune (arse-skimming pinafore dress with cat-shaped bib detail, anyone? See Brighton Oxfam). But if you've left on the tags you are, on some level, hedging your bets and refusing to commit. You simply don't love them. Ask yourself why you bought them in the first place and keep this firmly in mind to avoid similar future errors. Leave on the tags to make the items more sellable on eBay or by a charity shop, and write them off as an expensive mistake.

Which of rail B are you unsure of?

There will be items on rail B that you'd forgotten about, or which you can't quite decide on. There will be some that you suspect may come back round, and any rashness now will lead to regret later on (I still think about the very pointy 1999 Gucci Mary Janes I sold eighteen months before major revivals of both Gucci and 1990s fashion. Donor's remorse is real). That's okay. We're not getting rid of them. We're putting them on death row, in clothing purgatory, if you will. They still have the right of appeal. Place the untagged, rail-B items in good condition into a plastic airtight box (I source mine from the Really Useful Company) and hide them wherever you have space – under the bed, on top of the wardrobe, up in the loft. Set a reminder on your phone for six months from now. If you miss or want to wear any of these items at any point in the next six months, get them down and enjoy. If you don't, then a full year has passed and it really is time to give them a new home.

Is the C pile in a sellable state?

It needs to go, but where? I ask you to think carefully about this because, to be blunt, people treat charity shops like landfill and skip away proudly as though they're being terribly helpful, while some poor volunteer is saddled with five bin bags of their unwashed trash. It's selfish, disingenuous and really rather patronising. Charity shop customers need clothes that are clean, unstained and in a state of good repair, just like everyone else. If you wouldn't hand over a couple of quid for each of your items, then don't expect others to either. Clothes that don't meet the acceptable threshold should be deposited in garment recycling bins locally. Clothes that do can be folded into bags and handed over to (never dumped outside) a charity shop, or passed on to friends. For more valuable items, you can either sell on Depop, Vinted or Vestiaire, or via eBay or Thrift+, both of whom allow you to donate a portion of your proceeds directly to charity.

Can you lose some undies?

Laddered tights need to go. Blood-stained knickers should be binned. Bras with escaping wires, socks whose partner is never coming back, pyjamas marked indelibly with bacon grease. You deserve better. Lose them all to the recycling bank.

191

What is the ideal outcome?

You should have lost enough clothing bulk to be able to slide your hangers across the pole and see fully what's next in the queue. Your folded T-shirts and jumpers should all be visible and easy to select from the stack. If you can separate them further – for example, the printed T-shirts in one pile, the plain in another; poloneck jumpers in one stack, crew necks in another – then all the better.

Items that are fashion immune

Times when you must ignore fashion:

Jeans

Who are these people with multiple jeans shapes that flatter their bodies equally? Most people have one, maybe two, shapes that make them look and feel great. It took me a few years of trying to realise that straight jeans – so beloved by, and effortlessly cool on, willowy fashion blogger types – make my thighs look positively distorted. Meanwhile, there's no use telling me that skinnies are too 2005, or that boyfriend jeans were a flash in the pan. They are best for my body shape and so those are the jeans I will wear. Similarly, my friend Kate looks like a goddess in flares, which flap in and out of fashion as the wind changes. Good jeans are essential and fads are beneath them.

The only time trends are useful in denim is when previously unavailable styles flood the shelves for a needlessly limited period. An example of this is high-waisted jeans, which are extremely flattering on those – small, large or medium – who don't own an abdomen like an ironing board. But could you get them between 1980 Brooke Shields and 2009 Jessica Simpson? Could you hell. See also now, when cropped and ⅞ jeans are everywhere and women of 5ft 4in and under can finally wear denims that fit. The moral is this: when denim trends don't suit you, ignore them, and don't fear a shape that's technically 'out'. When a trend does flatter, make hay while the sun shines and stock up, like a squirrel preparing for hibernation. Because soon they may be snatched away.

UGG boots

You're groaning, possibly, but hear me out. I've been on a journey with UGGs, and they've proven themselves irreplaceable, regardless of whether

or not *Grazia* currently approves. Because UGG boots are cosy, they are warm, they slip straight on without your having to find any socks in order to nip to the Co-op for an emergency Curly Wurly. They're also – and I stand firm on this – good looking when worn with a massive jumper, woolly hat and jeans (I'm sorry, but it's a look. It just is), especially if they're the mini UGGs that don't interfere with the silhouette or hemline. Would I wear UGGs on a day out where the rest of my outfit is more effortful? No. Do I always ensure I own a pair for when I essentially need an indoor slipper with an outdoor sole that doesn't embarrass me when I need to drop off a teenager, or take out the bins?* Yes, now and forever. (*I never take out the bins.)

Swimwear

Our respective boobs wish to be supported and comfortable, and we wish them to be flattered. No one should force a round peg into a triangular hole by donning a string bikini because a small-breasted influencer looks incredible in hers. Everyone looks sexiest and happiest in things that fit them properly, whatever the size, and in which they feel comfortable. Feeling confident in swimwear is hard enough without the added pressure of fashion.

Tights

Periodically, fashion journalists, designers and influencers will tell us that tights are done with, and everyone ignores them and pulls on theirs as always. Those who find tights uncomfortable, uncool or unattractive are absolutely free to carry on without them – I just wish they'd do it without showily shouting 'OH MY GOD, AREN'T YOU HOT?!?' at anyone they spot in black opaques, but this is apparently too much to ask (please don't do this. It's so rude). If you are a tight-hater, please know that not everyone feels nice bare-legged. Not everyone likes to show skin. Not everyone has a taut, smooth body they're happy to unleash, or invisible veins or soft, even-toned limbs with a golden gleam. Or maybe they just feel the cold. For many people, tights – whether sheer or opaque – are extremely useful wardrobe workhorses that should be as fashion immune as bras and pants.

Specs

I say this advisedly because there's no doubt that my glasses have grown exponentially over the years I've needed to wear them. I see photos of my first pair, circa 2008, and I can't believe my vision wasn't permanently obscured by the tiny letterbox frames. But I do think that had large frames been as widely available at the time as they are now (see jean shapes), I'd have gone giant from the off. Glasses should be about flattering your face and complementing your personality (a gregarious, fashion-focused type is not, for example, going to suit invisible metal frames). Typically, round and heart-shaped faces suit squared frames, square faces suit round, oval faces look good in either. If you don't instinctively know your face shape, stand facing a bathroom mirror and trace around your reflection with an eye pencil – it's easier to assess a featureless shape. When you know, take your time in choosing the right specs – there's a good chance you'll connect instantly with one pair, but do keep trying on the wrong ones to be sure. Listen to the expert opinion of your optician or her sales associate, but ultimately take the ones that look and feel good to you.

193

Handbags

When it comes to handbag designs, colours, leathers and so on, by all means follow fashion if you can afford to. But when choosing a fashionable style of bag, understand fully that while trends come and go, your preference will prevail whether or not you attempt to override it. I love how ladylike top-handle bags look on others, but I know that if I have to surrender an entire hand to carrying one, I will become murderous within the hour.

Similarly, satchels are so adorable and classic, but if those buckles are real and not concealing hidden magnets, then my patience for opening and closing the damn thing will expire at the cash till. I can appreciate that a single strap hanging from my shoulder looks chic over a winter coat, while knowing it will almost certainly slide off it relentlessly until the day I sadly sell it on. Don't even get me started on clutches – they're a mugging waiting to happen (at least you'll only stand to lose a slender Tampax and a Polo mint). Whether fashion wants me carrying a pouch, clutch, mini bucket, briefcase or hobo, I have learnt to my cost that what I want, nine times out of ten, is a roomy crossbody bag, probably in black, tan, brown or navy, and most others will quickly prove a distressing waste of money. If you need to carry a laptop and all but the kitchen sink, you're probably a tote girl. If you need things organised, you're not. If you carry lots and dash about, get a backpack. Whatever the season, decide realistically what you need to take with you, and where your tolerance for impracticality ends, then choose accordingly and do not stray – to hell with fashion.

Pants

Big pants for stomach security, boy shorts for full bum and bits concealment, leg-lengthening bikini briefs, or the joyous vulva aeration of French knickers = you know what type of knicker woman you are (the odd dirty weekend, effortful date night or other special occasion notwithstanding) and however everyone else is dressing their downstairs should not come into it. I speak as someone who didn't wear thongs even when they were standard issue for all women between eighteen and forty, and still doesn't own any now. I'd sooner have VPL than be picking a shoestring from my bumcrack whenever the coast is clear.

'I'd sooner have VPL than be picking a shoestring from my bumcrack whenever the coast is clear.'

Health
& Beauty

'*While people will no doubt have many fair concerns about the beauty industry, I have my own about the world of "wellness".*'

One of my formative early childhood memories is of waking up on the floor of a dermatologist's hospital treatment room, nurses gathered around me, my mother's shouting about the long wait finally halted by the shock of my fainting. A very small chunk of my buttock still sat in a plastic screw container, ready for biopsy, which is where I caught sight of it and apparently fell to the ground, hitting my head on an equipment trolley. I don't remember much else except that my mother shouted at me all the way out of the building and into the car park, and I cried a fair bit. It was traumatic, but since no one died on that occasion, it was the least depressing and stressful hospital visit of my life, and yet possibly the most influential. In the ensuing four decades, I have been very scared of hospitals and utterly obsessed with skin – possibly because I deduced that the proper care of the latter might allow me to avoid the former, and it did. Despite having inherited a difficult skin condition (ichthyosis) from my father, my early focus on treating and improving it, where my dad had never bothered, meant that I was discharged from dermatologists' care some time around age ten or eleven. My passion for skincare never waned, and resulted, quite accidentally, in my training as a makeup artist and a career in beauty journalism. Sadly, the hospital phobia barely improved either, and nor did the fainting upon entrance much. I will do almost anything to avoid them (including, very happily, safely and with the full support of the NHS, giving birth to both of my children at home). I don't ignore ailments, but I do try to mitigate their effects with a little DIY maintenance.

199

It was at one time very common for journalists who wrote about beauty to also be expected to cover matters pertaining to health, and from the get-go, I either resisted or flat-out refused. I understand completely why, for many, the bodies we live in are incredibly interesting and the ways in which they can reach peak physical health are perhaps the most important topics in life. And so I can only apologise when I say that my fascination with health extends only to the skin and the brain and beyond that, I find it quite thunderingly dull. And while people will no doubt have many fair concerns about the beauty industry, I have my own about the world of 'wellness', where, it seems to me, quite disordered eating is dressed up respectably as 'health' and not the perhaps more likely but ethically outmoded desire to be thin in a crop top. Entire food groups are cut out for 'health', with either scant or extremely vague and woolly science to support it. I know someone who eats only red meat and green vegetables, 365 days a year. His grocery shopping bill could fund a hospital's new cardiac wing, where he may very soon require a bed. I know a woman who believes her body to be 'intolerant' of all red and white foods. I know plenty more who will consume salt only if it's a Pinterest-pinnable shade of pink. One of my closest friends, a properly qualified, state-registered dietitian, spends his life attempting to undo health-threatening eating disorders acquired via Instagram in the pursuit of wellness. The virus has spread into beauty too, of course, with words like 'clean' and 'non-toxic' creeping onto the labels of products that, by stringent law, have long since been anything but. I am sent so many useless collagen skin supplements that I now keep them in a big box and invite any visitor of a Gwyneth Paltrow disposition to fill their boots before the expired capsules end up in the bin. Naturally, there are no doubt sage and credible wellness gurus as well as appropriately critical thinkers who follow them with genuine interest. But I swerve the whole thing. And so what follows is very much a case of me staying unambitiously in my lane and writing about what I myself – a practically minded, lay beauty expert with two grown kids, a hatred of exercise, a history of mental ill health and absolutely no medical expertise beyond Red Cross First Aid training – have lived through and learned from, what my readers ask me, and the advice they tell me has proved helpful. In almost every case, the following should be read on the implicit understanding that when things aren't right, one should always consult a proper doctor. They are very unlikely to remove any buttock.

The right order to apply skincare products

The layering of skincare is without question the thing that most confuses non-professional beauty people. So I'm going to strip back any waffle and ambiguity. Here's the basic routine I follow.

Morning

1. CLEANSE. Milk, cream or gel-to-milk cleanser removed with hot, wrung-out, terry towelling cloth (use a face wash in the shower if you prefer).
2. EXFOLIATE. Liquid exfoliant, i.e. AHA, BHA or PHA, swept over the entire face (including eyes) and neck with a washable cotton pad – throw in the laundry after each use. I do this maybe three mornings a week.
3. TREAT. Vitamin C serum, ideally including hyaluronic acid (standard) and niacinamide (not standard but definitely approaching it), massaged into the entire face, neck and around the eyes.
4. PROTECT. Eye cream, if you use it (I rarely do).
   Moisturiser.
   OR
   Moisturiser with SPF.
   OR
   Dedicated sunscreen.
   Pick one. If you go with the first, I would always follow with a high-protection tinted moisturiser or foundation, and even then, only if I wasn't planning to be outdoors much. For extended periods outside, use a sunscreen before makeup.
5. MAKEUP. Only if you choose to wear it, of course.
6. FRESHEN UP. Mist containing hyaluronic acid at any point during the day. Keep in or out of the fridge, as you prefer. Particularly pleasant if pregnant, menopausal, tired, flustered or dehydrated.

Evening

1. REMOVE MAKEUP. Balm cleanser removed with hot, wrung-out, terry towelling cloth. I use a balm that emulsifies on contact with warm water, then comes clean away with no greasy film left behind.
   OR
   Micellar water swept over with washable cotton pad.

OR

Microfibre makeup-removing cloth or disc (wet with warm water and wring out – no product required).

2. CLEANSE. (If you've been wearing makeup or SPF.)
Balm or milk cleanser removed with hot, wrung-out, terry towelling cloth.

OR

Face wash, if preferred.

3. TREAT. Prescription tretinoin or over-the-counter retinol serum (if used). Should contain hyaluronic acid as standard.

OR

General, multipurpose night serum.

4. PROTECT. (Optional unless dry.)
Night cream, pressed firmly in.

OR

Facial oil, pressed firmly in.

OR

Facial oil (if extremely dry in winter), then some night cream.

But do you actually need sunscreen?

Yes, you really do. It's tedious, isn't it? But you will be thankful when you don't have brown blotches of sun damage on your cheeks and are able to wear a V-neck without the slightest self-consciousness. The effect of UV rays on the appearance of skin is the lesser concern, of course. All of us would choose wrinkles and sunspots over cancers. But what I have learnt over the years is that the latter is just too abstract a concept to persuade most people to wear sunscreen, unless they're lying in equatorial heat and grudgingly accept that they may be at risk. It's akin to telling someone that a delicious pizza may one day cause them a heart attack. As vain as it may be, what does get people reaching for the SPF is the everyday, very real connection between inadequate sun protection and uneven skin tone, a crepey texture, premature wrinkling and sagging. Being outside requires UV-protective skincare. And I say 'being' not 'lying' very deliberately here, since SPF is not the preserve of lazy beach holidays in the strongest sunlight. In fact, the need for SPF is not linked to climate at all – it relates to the amount of time spent outdoors, regardless of temperature. If you are to be outside for extended periods – sitting in a beer garden, playing sports, walking the dog in the park, dining al fresco or tending to your garden – you need a dedicated sunscreen. If you are merely nipping out for a paper, or to collect your kids, or to drive to the supermarket, then in my view, the SPF in your moisturiser or makeup is likely sufficient. In any case, your sun protection should be an SPF of 30 or higher. This, I believe, is the most realistic advice and most achievable goal. There is another, increasingly noisy, school of thought that believes SPF to be bad and the cause of serious vitamin D deficiency, resulting in greater likelihood of ill health than exposure to the sun. There is a grain of validity to this, but in practice, it is nonsense. Vitamin D is essential to physical and mental health and our understanding of its wide benefits is increasing all the time. It is also true that, owing to our climate, practically everyone in the UK is deficient in this vital vitamin. It is also true that sunscreen prevents vitamin D absorption. However, this is easily managed. Some sun is absolutely a good thing – but one doesn't have to offer up one's undereyes to get it. In spring and summer, a short bout of summer sunlight (roughly speaking, two to eight minutes for Caucasian people, twenty-five to forty-five for people of colour) on exposed, unprotected arms while your face and neck are safely creamed, at around noon each day, should see us suitably topped up with vitamin D. In winter in the UK, there is little chance of getting enough even if one were to parade the beaches naked, so keep taking those D3 supplements (in conjunction with K2, ideally, to direct the resulting increased calcium levels appropriately).

203

Physical or chemical sunscreen?

For a start, let's rename them, because both commonly used terms are misleading. Everything, even natural sunscreens, is made up of chemicals. And neither type physically blocks the sun. So, let's call them instead 'mineral sunscreens', i.e. those made from zinc or titanium oxides that deflect and scatter UV rays, and 'synthetic sunscreens', i.e. those made from manmade ingredients that absorb and process UV rays (disarm them, if you will). There is no qualitative benefit of one over the other, in terms of sun protection, but your skin type and concerns may make one more suitable for you than the other.

Sensitive skin

By and large, it is fair to say that sensitive skins fare better with mineral sunscreens. I am not particularly sensitive-skinned myself, and even I find that numerous synthetic sunscreens make my face itch. Those with eczema, rosacea or generally delicate or intolerant skin are usually best to swerve them in favour of minerals. For the same reasons, I would generally choose mineral sunscreens for small children and babies.

Olive, brown and Black skin

There are certainly exceptions, but by and large, synthetic sunscreens are almost guaranteed not to leave an ashy, white, grey or lavender cast on deeper skin tones, whereas finding an invisible mineral sunscreen is a little more challenging, though achievable and worth seeking out if your deeper-toned skin is sensitive in temperament. Supergoop, Dr Sam Bunting, Coola, Versed, Dr Dennis Gross and Paula's Choice are just a few clear mineral sunscreen-makers that spring to mind, but a little research will yield many more.

Sensitive eyes

Synthetic sunscreens are, in my experience, far more likely than mineral versions to cause watering if they migrate to the eyes, which is easily done on a hot day. It's not a word of exaggeration to say that I've previously had to come off a motorway and into a service-station ladies' room for a face wash, after a wandering synthetic sunscreen was seriously affecting my ability to see the road. If you love the fine texture, ungreasiness and comparative invisibility of synthetics, you may wish to use those over the majority of your face, but first use a mineral sunscreen in the immediate eye area. At the time of writing, Skinceuticals, Clinique, Kiehl's, Ultrasun and Sarah Chapman all make mineral SPF eye creams.

Oily skin

Mineral and synthetic sunscreens come in formulae for all skintypes, but it's fair to say that the oily-skinned will find suitable synthetics in greater abundance, and many minerals a little on the richer side. Again, there are exceptions. Dermalogica, La Roche-Posay, Skinceuticals, Dr Sam Bunting and Coola all make terrific mineral sunscreens that feel untypically featherlight.

Melasma/chloasma

Some studies and dermatologists now believe that mineral sunscreens may better mitigate the sun's effect on melasma (often called chloasma in pregnancy), an acquired and often hormone-triggered skin condition that results in large brown patches on the face, which typically worsen in the summer months. As a sufferer myself, I can't say that I've noticed a huge difference either way (I will become blotchy no matter what, since heat also makes a contribution), but I still think the argument for deflecting rays off melasma with minerals, rather than absorbing them with synthetics, is commonsensical and compelling. And so I would always recommend that melasma sufferers try to find their perfect sunscreen in mineral form, or choose one that combines both mineral and synthetic filters (these are often my own favourites).

How to choose a foundation shade

When I first began working in the beauty industry, all foundations from major brands were pink in tone. The introduction of yellow-toned bases by Prescriptives and Shiseido, and later, Bobbi Brown and NARS, ensured there was a more flattering foundation for everyone, but still, it's only quite recently that brands have acknowledged a third category present in white, yellow, olive, brown and Black skins that ensures everyone can find their perfect match: neutral.

Not sure on which podium you stand? This should help.

Warm undertone

Warm skin tones have a yellowy, golden tinge. Warm-toned people will generally have greenish-toned veins visible in their forearms, backs of knees and temples (or wherever else veins show) and will usually find gold jewellery is more flattering against their face. If your skin tans easily, it is likely (but not certain) that you are warm-toned.

Cool undertone

Cool skins are pinkish in undertone. Their visible veins will typically have a bluer/more purple appearance. Silver-toned jewellery will usually be more flattering against their skin. Those prone to blushing and burning in the sun are usually cool-toned, but not always. It is a common myth that brown and Black skin is always warm-toned – over the course of my career, I've colour-matched countless cool-toned Black complexions, and I find that well over half of olive and South Asian complexions are neutral-toned. Similarly, it is not the case that very white skins are always cool-toned.

Neutral undertone

Neutral skin tones are neither pink nor yellow, but a fairly even balance of both undertones. Possessors may previously have found most foundations too pink or too yellow. Neutral-toned people will typically have a mix

205

of greenish and bluish veins (or a shade somewhere between the two) peeking through the skin and will suit gold and silver jewellery equally.

Remember that if you have a skin condition that affects your skin tone – for example, rosacea (pink) or melasma (yellowish brown) – you are still matching a foundation to the base undertone beneath those irregularities. At the same time, if you have melasma, it is often worth going up a shade to bridge the discrepancy between your dark patches and underlying skin colour. This helps considerably in disguising the condition.

Picking a shade

So now you have your undertone. Visit a makeup counter – I really do strongly recommend this, since there is no online service that adequately replicates an in-person colour-matching. The best brands for colour-matching are MAC and Bobbi Brown (it is a simple fact that American-owned brands cater most comprehensively for all skin colours and tones). If you can get an on-counter artist to help you, then all the better, but in any case, be sure you're happy before parting with your cash.

Select three or four shades of foundation that do not contain SPF (which can temporarily look different on application). All four should be in your undertone and look near enough to your own shade. Ask for a cotton bud or have one from home at the ready.

Paint all four shades in parallel stripes down your makeup-free cheek. Not on your hand (usually darker), or your neck (usually lighter), or anywhere else – foundation needs to be matched to the skin where you will wear it.

When all the shades are lined up on your cheek, stand back from the mirror and squint. The stripe that becomes invisible is your shade. If one becomes almost indiscernible, go up or down one shade. If all are very visible, your undertone needs checking and is probably off.

A short note on formula

Packaging will usually give you a visual cue on what to expect from a foundation's finish. Typically, a matte or frosted glass bottle indicates a matte-finish foundation (I instinctively avoid these, when it comes to my own personal use), while a classic glass bottle normally indicates that the finish will be satiny and perhaps more dewy. A pearlised tube will almost certainly contain glowy, light-reflecting makeup. A cream or balm foundation will better suit dry complexions; cushion formulas are usually very thin, and lend themselves to oilier types. Liquids are pretty versatile for all. Don't get too hung up on heavy-handed signposting about the inclusion of hydrating hyaluronic acid, since it's very much (and quite rightly) a standard baseline in almost all foundations nowadays – it's about as boastworthy as a jug of tap water on a restaurant table. Whichever foundation type you choose, always bear in mind that any foundation containing a significant SPF (over 15) will typically not look great upon application but will improve noticeably in about fifteen to twenty minutes. This is entirely normal and no cause for concern, but do allow time for it to settle before committing to buying. It's also worth taking a quick selfie with the flash switched on, to see how it photographs.

How to remove a splinter

If I could monetise my splinter-removal skills, I'd long since have made it my full-time profession. My husband and children deliberately save their splinters until I'm home because, truly, there is nothing more satisfying to me than a full, clean and painless extraction.

1. Take a small alcohol wipe and swipe over the splinter very lightly (so as not to push it further into the skin).
2. Using a clean needle (I keep sterile medical-grade ones at home, but any sewing needle or fine pin will work, provided it is very clean), slide the sharp end under the very top layer of skin. Flick upwards slightly to break open the layer. There should never be bleeding, as we are dealing only with dead surface skin.
3. Take sharp, clean tweezers (Rubis make the best) to grip the uppermost end of the splinter. Grasp as much as possible, to minimise the likelihood of breakage. With one swift, upward movement, tweeze out the interloper.
4. Examine the area to ensure there's no debris that could become embedded.
5. Sweep over the alcohol wipe again.

Do not attempt any of the above on the face or neck.

207

'The hunt for an NHS dentist is only marginally more straightforward than the procurement of a Gutenberg Bible.'

How to find an NHS dentist

The hunt for an NHS dentist is only marginally more straightforward than the procurement of a Gutenberg Bible. Most dental surgeries are at quota for NHS patients and will accept private patients only, so if the cost of treatment without the NHS subsidy (remember it's still not free if you're a working adult and not pregnant or post-partum) is unmanageable, or if you want to share the same practice as your children, then you'll need to put in the graft to secure NHS places on a surgery's books.

First, go to the NHS website (nhs.uk) and enter 'find a dentist' into the search bar. Here, you can access a list of all your local dental surgeries, which, at least in theory, take on NHS patients. Print off their contact details and get on the phone. Starting with any that come with a trusted personal recommendation, you will need to ring each practice individually and ask very politely whether they are currently accepting NHS patients. If they're not, ask about a waiting list and enquire as to its length. Tell them if you have children and mention their ages. Make it clear that you are seeking a regular, long-term dentist rather than an emergency one as a one-off. That said, if you really do need to see a dentist quickly, ask if it's worth coming in as a private patient, then moving over to NHS when a space becomes available (some surgeries will do this before accepting outside patients). If somewhere is local, pop in and be friendly, polite and patient. It's never a bad idea to book in with the hygienist (about £30–40 for a deep clean) at a practice and asking while in the chair.

What is of critical importance is that, having managed to become an NHS patient, one diligently books and attends regular checkups. Once-in-a-blue-moon-visitors will fall foul of routine book clearouts, where staff will reasonably decide a dormant patient's place would be best reassigned to someone who will better make use of it. A scale and polish with the hygienist every six months plus six-monthly checkups with the dentist is best practice and should keep your precious teeth out of danger.

How to wash makeup brushes

I have spent a good twenty years looking inside the makeup bags of women outside the industry, and one thing never fails to amaze me: people will spend fortunes on their makeup, then apply it all with bad brushes in need of an urgent wash. Clean makeup brushes are better for your skin (and your handbag), are more hygienic and give a smoother finish to

209

your face. I wash my brushes regularly, but I'm not neurotic about it. I wash brushes used for 'wet' products (foundation, concealer and cream eyeshadow) once a week, and those employed for powder products (eyeshadow, blusher, face powder and the like) every two to three weeks. If I was prone to acne and breakouts, I'd wash the lot once a week. My technique is thorough but quick.

1. Get a makeup brush cleaning mat, a plastic mitt with a bobbly surface to cause gentle friction that costs about a fiver from Amazon or Superdrug. If you don't want to buy one, don Marigolds and grab an old plastic hairbrush (a Tangle Teezer type works well).
2. Lie an old towel or tea towel on the countertop, folding it in half to protect the surface from any staining.
3. Divide your brushes into synthetic – the usually smooth, shiny bristles deployed for creams and liquids, and natural – the fluffy, more hair-like (genuine or faux) brushes used more commonly for powdery products.
4. Saturate the synthetics under a comfortably hot tap, squirting a dot of Fairy Liquid or similar into the cleaning mat or clean, upturned hairbrush, and gently move the wet brush in circular motions into the detergent. The makeup will bleed quickly from the brush in a disgusting but satisfying manner. Rinse well under the running tap. Repeat the detergent process if particularly filthy.
5. For the natural brushes, follow the same process, substituting the Fairy Liquid for any hair shampoo that doesn't describe itself as 'moisturising'. This needn't be anything special – the old advice of using only baby shampoo is no longer relevant, since pretty much all shampoos nowadays are gentler than they were. I like using anti-dandruff shampoos, since they contain an anti-fungal and anti-bacterial, but it's not important.
6. Each time you finish washing a brush, set it down on its side, resting fully on the folded towel. Do not place in a cup or mug, since the downstream of residual water causes glue to loosen and wooden handles to swell, and can easily ruin your brush.
7. Leave on the towel overnight, stroking the fatter, denser brushes over a dry patch of towel here and there to speed things up. If in a rush to get your brushes back to work, you can help them along with a blast of a hairdryer on a hot temperature setting.

Which makeup brushes do I need?

I'm fanatical about good brushes, but this doesn't mean I think we all need some vast battalion of beauty tools to put on an everyday face. I especially don't think you need to buy a full set, any more than I'd suggest you buy an entire music system from the same brand. Different producers excel in different areas and my own brush kit is an uncoordinated mishmash of the best from all of them. These basics will cover a lot of ground:

A synthetic foundation brush

Not the flat paddle type that paints on makeup, but the fat, round type that buffs it in. My own ride-or-die version is Bobbi Brown's Full Coverage Face Brush, but IT Cosmetics, Zoeva and Real Techniques all make similar models. Use for foundation and cream bronzer and blusher.

A concealer buffer

A mini version of the above for blending in corrector and concealer. My favourites are by Beauty Pie, Zoeva and Pat McGrath.

A medium-sized powder brush

For applying face powder and powder bronzer. Don't get one of those enormous tabletop things you see in the shops, which are too crude and clumsy to follow the contours of the face. The bristles should be soft, flexible and fine enough to reach the recesses of your outer nose and sweep powder from under your eye without poking it. I use the NARS Yachiyo Brush (which I carry in my handbag) or Bobbi Brown Sheer Powder Brush, but also like the Zoeva 106.

Blusher brush (only if you wear powder blush)

A rounded, 'natural' hair brush that's fatter than people think it needs to be. You know those little ones that come free in your blusher compact? It should be around eight times bigger than that if you want a seamless glow, not tiger stripes. My weapon of choice is by Charlotte Tilbury, but Laura Mercier, MAC and MyKitCo all make good ones.

Eyeshadow blending brush

A fat, fluffy eye brush about as wide as the tip of your index finger. This is for laying down colour all over the lid and blending out shadows for a smoky finish or to soften hard lines. My Holy Grail is a MAC 217, but I also frequently carry Real Techniques eye brushes, since they are cheap and require little care.

Eyeshadow pencil brush

A small detailing brush for applying undereye colour (cream or powder), artfully smudging eyeliner and applying dense colour to parts of the lid before smoothing out with the blending brush. My favourites for the role are the MAC 219, Charlotte Tilbury Eye Smudger Brush, Zoeva's 231 or 223 and NARS 14.

Brow brush

To groom brows and unclog clumpy lashes, I use an old mascara spoolie (brush) with any traces of mascara washed off with washing-up liquid, but an old toothbrush works fine too.

What I don't use

Lip brushes (life is short), makeup sponges (useful to have, but overrun with germs if not cleaned daily), fan brushes (I have never heard a compelling argument for their existence).

How to deal with jetlag

I never really understood what people meant by 'jetlag' until I first visited Australia. I think I assumed it was some extreme sort of fatigue, until my first night in Melbourne, when my consciousness left my body and looked down on it, sitting in a beer garden, for several hours, unable to reinhabit its physical form. If I hadn't been in such familiar and trusted company, I'd have thought I'd been drugged. True jetlag is awful and debilitating. Days are spent in this surreal, detached, sometimes hallucinogenic state, neither asleep nor awake, jumpy yet exhausted. This is not mere tiredness – it's what happens when your body loses its rhythm and is struggling to get back on track. It worsens with age, so a coping strategy must be devised. It took me a handful more long-haul trips to get the hang of it.

If travelling east, go to bed an hour early two days before flying, then two hours early the day before. After landing, keep adding an hour this way until you are back at your regular time (so if there's a six-hour time difference, this will take you four days into your trip or holiday to become fully regulated). When travelling west, you do the exact opposite and push your bedtime backwards – an hour late two days before the trip, two hours late the day before – and continue this pattern, adding an hour a night, until back to normal. I realise this sounds high-maintenance and something of a buzzkill when you'd like to hit the ground running and maximise enjoyment of your holiday. If you feel you can't manage the pattern, remember these key rules on arrival at your destination: don't sleep in the day, and get some sunlight when you wake up every morning. Exposure to natural light is pivotal in resetting your body clock.

How to avoid cystitis

If I thought anyone would publish it, I'd write four volumes on cystitis, a lifelong irritant, and for five long years the bane of my life. There was a period in my thirties where I got cystitis at least every fortnight. I ended up in A&E twice with a resulting kidney infection and took twelve courses of antibiotics in one year. When I became resistant to one of only two drugs that shifted it, I thought I was done for. So if you are anywhere close to this, or even just an occasional sufferer of UTIs, I feel your pain and wince. If every moment of sexual pleasure is later paid for with a scorching pain that reduces you to tears, please accept this hug through the pages. I proffer an imaginary hot water bottle. I can't and shouldn't tell you why you're suffering – you must get properly tested by your GP, insisting on a referral to a specialist if you're a habitual sufferer. But here are the basics that helped me, and the advanced steps that cured me completely. I haven't had a single bout in almost three years.

213

1. Always go for a pee immediately after sex. Even a fifteen-minute post-match cuddle can be too long. Hop out briefly and flush your system.
2. Drink gallons of water. I am rarely thirsty and consequently useless at this. But it is absolutely essential to force yourself.
3. Do not drink cranberry juice to treat an attack. It's as much use as a chocolate fireguard. This is a suggestion made by people who don't suffer from cystitis but who once read it in a magazine, and I dismiss it out of hand. Any specialist will tell you that sugary drinks and juices are more likely to aggravate UTIs than alleviate them.
4. Wipe front to back. I doubt any adult needs to be told this, but it's worth restating where cystitis is concerned.
5. Use unfragranced soap in the bath and shower. My urethra seemingly only has to sense the squeezing of a fruity shower gel to be triggered into total meltdown. Use the mildest, blandest wash or soap you can find (skincare company Gallinée makes an excellent one that was formulated by gynaecologists for exactly this purpose).

6. Take probiotics. I take OptiBac For Women and their 'intimate flora', which is a bit Barbara Cartland, but needs must. They definitely help.

7. Only use tampons on your heaviest days. Yes, I know, I know. Different hole, shouldn't make a difference. But absorbing all moisture makes a bout much more likely. When your period is finishing, switch to period pants or sanitary towels.

8. Wear cotton underwear. Look, I don't personally find this makes a difference for me (all undies have a cotton panel in the important place anyway), but I know that plenty of fellow sufferers find natural fibres better than manmade, so consider swapping out.

9. If you can persuade your GP to give you a referral, or you can afford a private consultation, do see an endocrinologist. After five years of trying to find out what was wrong with me, and having become depressed at the lack of interest and answers, I visited a hormone specialist. I had an underactive thyroid, suboptimal levels of progesterone and the worst case of vitamin-D deficiency the specialist had ever seen. I was given appropriate treatment for all three and, since that first prescription, I haven't experienced a single UTI. I dread to think how many women – and men – are currently crying on the loo and have no choice but to continue to do so. It was the best money I've ever spent.

214

How to prevent ingrown hairs

Ingrown hairs are common in shaved and waxed legs and bikini lines. Always ensure your razor blades are extremely sharp to minimise irritation. Exfoliating the site of ingrown hairs is crucial, but always before shaving, never after. For example, a pre-shave body scrub in the shower can be wonderful and result in smooth, silky limbs. The same scrub after shaving will more likely cause redness, bumps and more ingrowns. For existing ingrown hairs, saturate a cotton pad or bud with exfoliating face toner containing alpha and beta hydroxy acids, and sweep over the site.

Retinol best practice

The rise of retinoids – the umbrella term for over-the-counter retinol, the gentler (and less potent) retinyl palmitate, and prescription tretinoin – has been dizzying. I confess I'm somewhat surprised by their enormous popularity nowadays – not because they aren't brilliant (there truly is no skincare ingredient more effective in treating some signs of ageing, like wrinkles, enlarged pores, uneven skin tone and sagging), but because they can be not all that pleasant to use. I myself have a love/hate relationship with retinoids, having used them on and off for over a decade. I love what retinoids do to my pores (they smooth them dramatically), how they curtail my milia (tiny white lumps around my eyes) and how they all but magic away my pigmentation (along with vitamin-C products, retinol and tretinoin saw off quite an extreme case of hormone-triggered melasma, i.e. large brown patches on my face that appeared when I took a specific brand of contraceptive pill, and worsened significantly when I had children). Their effect on my teenagers' spots has also been miraculous. But what I don't love so much is actually using them. For many of us, retinol and the increasingly popular tretinoin (from a doctor only) leave our skins dry and less comfortable than less active skincare ingredients. Short term, there can and likely will be irritation. So rather than just chucking some retinol into your shopping cart and pledging to see what all the fuss is about, I would strongly recommend you make a plan, bearing these elements in mind:

Choosing a product

Over-the-counter retinol or prescription tretinoin? It is not true that retinol doesn't yield such good results as tretinoin – what the latter does is work faster and more directly. There are many additional pros to 'tret' if prescribed responsibly. These include: a dermatologist's input on dosage, stage-gating (more of that later), periodical check-ins as treatment progresses, an increased likelihood (purely in my experience with readers) of committed and diligent usage by the patient, thus increasing the likelihood of success. On the cons list are a financial commitment (usually a direct debit of at least three months to a specialist dermatological services company) and less luxurious formulations than those available in stores. Over-the-counter retinols give consumers a chance to dip their toes in the water, perhaps with a brand they already enjoy using, at a price point that feels comfortable and with formulas that, in my view, typically feel a bit nicer.

There is no right or wrong answer, but my advice would usually be to start with an over-the-counter retinol and finish the bottle, then either repurchase a stronger one or move over to tretinoin. The third option is retinyl palmitate. This is a good retinoid insofar as it is usually much gentler and more user-friendly, but I only really recommend it to the very sensitive-skinned, and even for those cases, a dermatologist can usually devise a good plan with prescription tret.

Percentages

There is a worrying obsession in modern beauty with percentages of active ingredients, in this case, of retinoids. I understand it and there is some validity in believing that higher doses will yield more noticeable results, but apart from the fact that low-dose retinols can be very beneficial, all this very much depends on whether the notoriously tricky retinoid continues functioning effectively throughout its application. In other words, a 0.03 per cent retinol that remains stable (active) until the end of the tube is better than a higher 0.1 per cent retinol that does not.

It is a generalisation, but big, mainstream beauty companies wary of litigation will typically focus more on product stability and on low incidences of skin irritation. They commonly will not declare the concentration of retinol in a product, but will usually sell one that stays intact. When they don't disclose, you can generally rely on it being on the lower end, somewhere between 0.01 and 0.03 per cent retinol – which, by the way, can still do plenty. Cult skincare brands tend to be more specific, in which case, I would start on the low side and gradually work up.

216

Plan your starting point

There's a good reason why retinol sales soared during the 2020/21 pandemic. Do not embark on your retinol or tretinoin – or even retinyl palmitate – adventure when you need your skin to look great in the next three weeks, or when you'll be spending significant periods of time outdoors. It is extremely common for skin to look and feel worse for a good fortnight, before it starts improving noticeably. It is common for makeup to go on less well than usual. It's common to experience flakiness. All this is entirely normal but not ideal if you have a special event or holiday planned. If you're a bride preparing for her own wedding, I would personally not start anything new with less than two months to go.

Stage-gating

This is the industry term for easing yourself into retinoid use. If it is your first time, it's wise to increase use gradually over a week or two. If using an over-the-counter retinol, stagger its introduction like this:

Week one: apply retinol product after nighttime cleansing, twice, three days apart.

Week two: apply retinol after nighttime cleansing, every other night.
Week three: apply retinol product every night after cleansing.

If using prescription tret, ignore the above and do exactly as your doctor says. It will already have been factored into your dosage and treatment plan.

Lay off the actives

It is perfectly fine to combine long-term retinoid use with other active skincare like acid exfoliants, and antioxidants like vitamin C. I use all three most days (the former before bed, the rest in the morning). But in the beginning, while your skin is becoming accustomed to any retinoid, give it space by temporarily pausing the others. When you are through the common (but not guaranteed) period of mild irritation – usually a fortnight or so – you can reintroduce your other active skincare products. Remember that hyaluronic acid can and should be used at any time, in any quantity, with anything else, so you can continue that as normal. Ditto other traditional humectants or emollients, such as glycerin, almond, olive and avocado oils, which will probably all be especially welcome as your retinoid-reacting skin craves comfort.

217

Retinol is not a moisturiser

If you are dry-skinned by nature, or experiencing the common short-term dryness associated with new retinoid use, I cannot stress enough that you must not seek to replace that moisture with your retinoid cream. It is tempting to add an extra pump of cream to parched skin, but you mustn't. You will merely be adding too much retinoid and increasing the chances of irritation and dryness. Instead, apply your proper dose, wait a few minutes, then apply a richer yet bland moisturiser. If unaccustomed to retinoids, you could reverse this and apply the moisturiser first.

Watch your eyes and neck

Your skin may take to retinoids like a duck to water, but don't be surprised if some parts of your face never acclimatise. I'm a seasoned retinol and tret user and my neck still becomes very sore and itchy if I veer below the chin. My eyes are more accepting, but only to a point, so I generally apply some bland moisturiser around my eyes before layering tret lightly over the top, thus providing the delicate skin with a buffer – a fireguard, if you will. I don't expect this ever to change, so be careful about 'pushing through' if your face does the same.

Move on up

When you have finished up the same over-the-counter retinol once or twice, and if you are seeing a plateau effect, consider moving up the 'retinol ladder' by switching to a product with a higher concentration. Many specialist skincare brands will have the percentage printed on the bottle. A natural progression during a course would be 0.01 per cent, 0.03 per cent, then 0.06 per cent, ending in 1.0 per cent.

SPF

You simply must wear SPF by day when using retinoids by night. It does not matter if you didn't apply it last night, or if it doesn't seem sunny. It does not matter if you are someone who tans easily. None of this makes any difference. When you sign up to any retinoid, you sign up to daily sunscreen of at least factor 30.

Be patient but realistic

Retinoids must be used regularly to be effective. After any stage-gating, nightly application is optimal and important if you'd like consistent improvements. Give it a good six months, perhaps even nine, before taking a view on whether you'd like to continue. But also do know at that point that retinoids are absolutely not for everyone. It is nonsense when people say otherwise. Some people see little effect from their use (even after increasing the concentration), some see results but the side-effects never diminish sufficiently to make them worthwhile. You can have wonderful skin without retinol, and people who refute this don't know what they're talking about.

Take a break

There is research to support the idea that, much like interval training in the gym, skin can be jolted into action after a break from active products, so don't assume retinoids are for ever or never. Some people like to take the summer off, others do three months on, a month off, all year round. Others find it easier to do it nightly long-term than to remember a new routine. Whatever works. You may find your skin has a less irritated reaction to subsequent courses than to the first. But don't panic. Irritation is not required for retinoids to work. Some people experience no side-effects at all from the start. They're just lucky.

How to deal with night anxiety

Given that not just whole books but whole sections of bookshops are devoted to dealing with anxiety, it would be folly to try to deal with it comprehensively here. But there are some things to consider, when staring at the ceiling, stomach washing-machining into the small hours, that might ease the path to a better night's sleep. They certainly help me. Anxiety can often be kept at bay for a time with activity and distraction, which is perhaps why, having lain in wait so patiently, it can flood in so devastatingly the minute the bedside light is switched off.

Whatever the cause of your anxiety, when the churning commences it's first worth considering this. There's an overwhelming likelihood that the problem, decision, person or situation that's causing your anxiety is not, in fact, causing your anxiety. Not this minute. This minute, what's causing your anxiety is thinking about that problem, person or thing. So, just stop thinking about the thing, right? No, that would be supremely irritating advice. Instead, just recognise that in the moment, the thing you think is making you anxious is probably not present. Of course, there are exceptions – the person lying next to you, the leaky ceiling above your head – but more often than not your thoughts are conjuring the threat, summoning it into the space, making it feel real and immediate. But it's not. Let's say what's worrying you is an unpaid final demand. It's a perfectly valid thing to be concerned about. But not at one in the morning. Because, however oppressive the thought of that bill is now, I guarantee you the pest who works on account defaults at your energy company isn't at their desk, drumming their fingers, waiting for your payment. They're sound asleep, as you should be. The boss whose performance review you're dreading? Away with the fairies. The medical test results you don't want to read? On a dormant computer in a dark surgery. Nothing about your situation will change tonight. The threat isn't with you as you lie awake and watch the numbers tick round. Just your thoughts about it. It feels like it's there, because the fight-or-flight reaction to those thoughts is pumping adrenaline around your body just as sure as if you'd turned mid-road to see a bus thundering towards you. Now, that would be a genuinely immediate threat. But adrenaline is just chemicals and most of the time those feelings, those chemicals, don't actually mean you have to throw yourself to safety this second or perish. If your thoughts had meandered in a different direction – let's say you hadn't heard the boiler clanking, which made you think about your gas supply, which made you think about your red bill – you wouldn't be worrying about it now. You'd be thinking about something else. And yet everything else in the world would still be the same. The bill would still be awaiting payment. So again, it's not the bill that's keeping you awake, it's you thinking about it. And once you acknowledge that, once you acknowledge that nothing needs doing this minute – or indeed *could* be done this minute, even if you wanted to – it can become a little easier to give yourself a few hours at least to park the worry and allow yourself the much healthier option of a bit of kip.

How to check your boobs

Having lost both my grandmother and mother to primarily women's cancers, I'd be the last person to suggest you should listen to me, and not a doctor, on breast-check best practice. Which is precisely why I'm going to tell you what the brilliant GP Dr Zoe Williams taught me at a special event held by Estée Lauder Companies (who, at the time of writing, have raised over $108 million globally for breast cancer research, education and services). Zoe's way is simple, thorough and easy to remember – though I still get a monthly SMS reminder from the brilliant breast cancer education charity Coppa Feel (sign up to this great service at coppafeel.org).

Whenever you check, it's important to remember, especially in the beginning, that you're not examining your breasts for cancer. You're fully acquainting yourself with them, so that you know their 'normal' lumpiness. This process helps you to identify anything that shouldn't be there in the future.

1. Stand in front of a mirror. Take off your bra and any clothes so you can see your breasts in their entirety. Look straight ahead and examine the shape, size, contour lines, skin texture and colour of your boobs. Compare them one to the other (remembering that almost no one has identical breasts). Do they look the same as usual, or are there any changes? Is there any unusual redness, puckering, flaking, dimpling or orange-peel appearance? Turn to the side and look again.

2. Look closely at your nipples and areola. Are they more sore than usual? (I never check during my period as I find this skews my perspective.) Are they newly puckered outwards or tethered inwards? Is there any discharge, colour change or a different skin texture?

3. Repeat steps 1 and 2, only this time with your hands behind your head, then with your hands on your hips. Engaging these different muscles gives you a different visual perspective on your boobs. Ask yourself all the same questions as before.

4. Choose somewhere comfy for the feeling bit. I like the bath, but anywhere works, whether bed, shower, office chair or sofa in front of *Countryfile*. Imagine using a lawn mower to mow those satisfying stripes into the grass – up, down, up, down – only your boobs are two lawns and the mower is your three flattened middle fingers. Press the fingers towards the ribcage on the opposite breast and move them gradually down in stripes, making little circles at each point to feel the surrounding tissue, then back up again. You may find it easier to do this with the other arm back, out of the way.

5. Now, using the same technique, mow the lawn between your breasts and your neck – all along the chest plate and collarbone. Repeat in both armpits and the surrounding areas. Up, down, up, down, making little circles with each move. Alternating the pressure helps you to examine both deep tissue (firmer pressure) and skin (lighter).

6. If you feel a lump, some thickening, a change of appearance or colour, swelling, pain, discharge or anything else that is different for you, call your doctor's surgery at once. Try not to panic. I've twice had cause to attend an emergency mammogram (my GP practice, like many these days, has a zero-dithering policy towards anything breast-related) and on both occasions there was nothing the matter and I was sent home relieved. Had there been something, my breast examination would have helped me get better, faster.

221

How to drink

I have an odd relationship with alcohol. My father was certainly an alcoholic, but a calm and functioning one who drank large quantities of wine and whisky on a daily basis without ever missing work, becoming aggressive or even noticeably drunk. My dad's behaviour meant I never made the connection between excessive alcohol intake and danger, but at the same time, I did associate it with sadness and ennui, a feeling that has never quite left me. I spent my young life never liking the taste of booze but loving its effects, and my older one loving the taste but hating the effects. I no longer enjoy being drunk and I hate feeling hungover.

This is absolutely not to say that I'm anywhere close to a time when I'll skip wine at a long lunch with girlfriends, or forgo a celebratory flute of champagne, or the occasional illicit West End cocktail, but a combination of age, a global pandemic and an increasing weariness around very drunk people has meant I now find myself saying no more often than yes. The pointers that follow are my personal guidelines, adopted over time, that allow me to have a happy relationship with alcohol, i.e. a fun time without any associated dread. Naturally, if you love the occasional piss-up and feel no ill effects on your life, then ignore my rules and get stuck in. Zero judgement. But for anyone who has spent many a Morning After mentally replaying the tape and cringing, or having to apologise for some drunken act, or feeling anxious and sad as a matter of course, these may prove useful.

Leave your phone in your pocket

In my twenties, I once texted my new boyfriend when drunk aboard a river boat, to tell him how much and how thoroughly I loved and desired him. This in itself could have been high risk (not to mention unnecessary, since he was about twelve feet away from me), but he had already stated his intention to marry me, which surely meant that he wouldn't be appalled or embarrassed by my own emotional nakedness. Sadly, the same could not be said for my boss at the time, to whom I actually sent the text, and who immediately replied (also from feet away) to explain that this was all a bit much to take in. Years before that, I'd texted my brother from a party to say I'd read a book on narcissism and sociopathy and had concluded that a relative of ours was a certifiable case. You can imagine which of the two received my text. Dignity prevents me from offering more examples, so just trust me when I say that texting anyone when drunk is almost unfailingly a terrible idea, and posting on social media an even worse one. The scope for cheek-burning shame later on is massive. Even if not drunk per se, we are all less inhibited when we drink and there is consequently no need whatsoever to put in writing things that we would never even say when sober. It's also too easy to mess up the delivery – sending to the wrong person, posting publicly when you intended to message privately, and so on – that delaying until tomorrow is the best policy. The only messages one should send are to close loved ones to relay important information, such as your ETA or safe arrival home. Check the recipient's name twice before sending.

Don't mix

Never, ever mix wine colours unless drinking very moderately with dinner, and in the full confidence you can leave it there. Similarly, don't mix spirits unless a single cocktail will be enough. Wine and spirits can be mixed, but only in two very distinct stages with no return. For example, one can begin with a gin or vodka and tonic, then switch to wine with dinner, or one can enjoy a glass of wine, then move on to vodka or gin for a safer pace (see 'Avoid white' below). But when the decision has been made, it cannot be reversed. Anything more varied than either tactic spells certain doom.

Avoid white

Having done decades of research on myself, and by observing others, I must conclude that white wine is evil. I love it; a cold glass on a sunny day is one of life's great joys, but nothing makes people more drunk, hungover, mortifying and mortified than too much white wine. Champagne has its own issues, of course, but bafflingly is way more manageable than non-fizzy white. Too much red will send you sleepy, stained and forgetful, but white will send you mad. White wine drunkenness will see you calling your ex and crying, adding something extortionate and ugly to your shopping cart, flirting with or snogging someone you loathe, or saying something horrid to a beloved friend before puking on your knees in the loo. One glass is bliss, three glasses are ruinous. If there's no alternative you like, order a spritzer and at least match every ounce with another of soda water. It slows the tide a bit.

Consider your words

This is the hardest part, and why so many of us feel so lousy the next day – on top of the physical effects, which worsen as we age. If you've had a drink and wonder if you should mention something you've avoided up until now, you shouldn't. If you have always kept someone's secret but now seems safe and constructive to tell it, it isn't. If you've been doubtful in the past, but are certain now, you're wrong to be. Stop. Hush. I know people who've been told by those they love that their children aren't very nice. I've been told by someone who adores me that I desperately need to enlarge my kitchen and shrink my nose when I'd previously never given a second's thought to either, but certainly have done periodically since. I daren't even recall the stupid things I've said myself, because I fear I'd never recover. Think about what you're saying. Being blind drunk is not a prerequisite for unintentionally uninhibited mischief making – it takes only a couple of drinks, so consider your words slowly and carefully before saying them, and avoid going past the point of being capable of that. The bolstering effects of alcohol are only ever useful if you and another single person have been mutually attracted for ages and are paralysed by shyness and fear. That can work very well. Everything else is a catastrophe in waiting.

Make room for a pitcher

Order tap water and separate glasses, and refill with every round. Drink it either by alternating sips (a faff, I agree) or alternating drinks (easy – no one notices).

Always have an exit plan

You must know how you are getting home. Always know when the last train leaves and set yourself a cut-off. If there's a chance you won't catch it, you must have either a sober lift, or the means to pay for a pre-booked cab or licensed street taxi. Never head for home without a plan in motion – fumbling about with your phone in the street is frequently disastrous.

Beware cocktails

So fun, so colourful, so completely delicious. The problem with cocktails is that they lie. When sitting on a bar stool drinking Martinis, one feels completely marvellous and as though this pace could continue all night without incident. It's only when attempts are made to reach a standing position and travel to the ladies' that one realises one's brain and legs are actually now wholly estranged.

Acknowledge The Moment

There's a feeling one gets, usually during a visit to the ladies' room, away from the main event. It's a sudden lightheadedness, when giddy cheer is replaced momentarily by self-awareness and the realisation that one is a bit drunk. It frequently occurs when one locks the lavatory door and is left alone and silent under horrible lighting, or when glancing in the mirror during a hand wash and realising something has shifted a smidge. It happens to us all. This fleeting moment is a crossroads. Old me would whack on some lipstick and get away from it as fast as possible to rejoin the party. New me is grateful for the warning and stops drinking for an hour. I don't go home if I'm around people I love being with. I continue to have fun, laugh and enjoy myself – more so since I know I'm in control and tomorrow won't be hideous – but I drink long, soft drinks and happily

224

bring myself back from the brink of no return. An hour or so later, I can generally order a vodka and feel normal.

Pass the A&E test

Police officers in films ask drivers to walk in a straight line to prove they're not drunk. I have my own personal threshold: if something were to happen to someone in my party, such as an unlucky fall resulting in a broken ankle, could I still summon the wherewithal to get them safely to hospital, fill out the appropriate paperwork, answer any questions and converse lucidly with medical personnel delivering care and important advice? Likewise, and more importantly, could I get home to do the same for my kids? For me, the answer needs to be yes or I feel immediately uneasy and stop drinking. It's not that I think I'll need to do any of the above, more that this hypothesis represents the line that my personality isn't happy to cross. Staying on the right side of it makes me feel much more comfortable and in control.

Water, water, water

As soon as you arrive home, drink a pint of water. Clean your teeth, however drunk you feel. Consider it an investment in the bearability of your hangover. Removing makeup may prove a bridge too far, but if you can manage it, you'll applaud yourself tomorrow when you wake up without grey, dehydrated skin and watering eyes. If you're a puker, place a towel on your pillowcase, because that's always comfortingly regressive, and a large bowl next to your bed. I find they increase the chances of not needing them, and provide enough reassurance to sleep.

My thoughts on Botox

If a product or treatment is safe, I'm all for defying nature if I want to, whether that's by using a posh vitamin-C serum on my sunspots, popping the contraceptive pill, dyeing my hair, or injecting away a frown line. And so twice a year, I visit a doctor in order to receive Botox injections. It goes around my eyes, in the 'number eleven' frown lines between them, and sometimes under my chin to stop my neck sagging downwards when I smile. These visits are as much a part of my self-care routine as haircuts and appointments with the dental hygienist, and I genuinely look forward to getting jabbed.

Decades since its introduction, we know that when properly administered, Botox is perfectly safe. It is, however, still woefully unregulated and women seem more cavalier about it than ever, nipping into hair salons, chiropodists and opticians for top-ups, even attending 'Botox parties' to pick at a vol-au-vent while waiting to be shot in the forehead with botulism. Here's how to Botox responsibly.

Manage your expectations

It's true that no serum, cream, facial treatment, gadget or massage can produce the same lasting results as a toxin injection. But at the same time, no toxin injection can do for the skin what thorough, diligent, good-quality skincare can. Botox weakens muscles, artificially softening lines. It has no effect on pores, acne, rosacea, clarity, pigmentation, scarring or anything non-structural. Botox doesn't improve the condition of anyone's skin – proper skincare does. The two are not remotely interchangeable. So next time you see someone with marvellous, unretouched skin on social media, don't dismiss her as merely having had Botox, which has no more to do with good skin than lines and wrinkles do. It's like saying someone's silk sheets are made beautiful by a mattress. In reality, what she has is either marvellous genes or (more likely) a diligent approach to good skincare.

226

Find a practitioner

You will know someone who has Botox. Do they look good? Are they happy with the service and outcome? There is nothing more reliable than personal recommendation. My own preference is to see a registered doctor rather than another aesthetic practitioner, which is absolutely not to say that there aren't terrific injectors trained in other professions. A doctor just gives me greater peace of mind. It's also worth checking resources like Alice Hart-Davis's TheTweakmentsGuide.com to see who's local. When you have one, find the practitioner's clinic's Instagram account or, at the very least, their website, and spend a decent amount of time looking at their gallery of case studies. Does their aesthetic chime with yours? What are their qualifications and registrations with professional bodies? These should be displayed conspicuously on their website and are easily checkable against associations such as the British College for Aesthetic Medicine, the General Medical Council and so on.

Be prepared to spend

Not all expensive Botox is good, but all very cheap Botox is bad. That is a fact. To buy the correctly licensed chemicals, keep a sanitary office, use proper equipment and pay comprehensive liability insurance costs responsible practitioners significant sums and this will be reflected in the consumer price. If your Botox is costing £50, many corners will have to have been cut to potentially disastrous effect. It is simply too cheap to be possible. As with so many things, it is unfair that there is a financial divide when it comes to good and bad injectables, but we are talking about your face – it deserves better than a bargain hunt. If you are not using a registered doctor, consider going with a company that has lots of cash and infrastructure and too much to lose in not doing things properly – chains such as Superdrug Skin Renew and SK:N, for example.

Have a consultation

However desperate you are to get jabbed on your first visit, this is only sometimes possible. Most responsible practitioners will treat new patients only after a consultation, and this should always be with the person who delivers the treatment, never a salesperson or assistant. If your practitioner advises you not to have something, listen and trust them. If they say yes to everything, then try to add yet more procedures on top, be wary. A good practitioner wants you and their work to look great, regardless of whether that yields less profit.

Prep and aftercare

There really isn't much. You are perfectly fine to attend the clinic with your makeup on if dashing from work. I mostly don't wear much, as I can't resist using makeup to mimic symmetry and I'd rather the doctor saw the slightly wonky reality than be misled. You will be offered anaesthetic cream, but the process is so quick and painless that I never bother, so consider your pain threshold. For twenty-four hours afterwards, don't be too firm with your skin. Leave it be. Use skincare that doesn't require firm massaging, keeping your touch light. If you like swimming, don't wear swimming goggles. I don't personally bruise, but it's not uncommon. Bruises will typically be of the faintly yellow variety, rather than a bright blue shiner, and are usually easily concealed with makeup. But if you bruise like a peach, warn your doctor.

At the end of your treatment, ask your doctor when you should return and book in the next appointment. You can always cancel later if it becomes inconvenient or undesirable, but it's sensible to have an appointment in the diary at the sweet spot where your treatment will be wearing off (my Botox lasts about six months) but hasn't completely vanished, sending your doctor back to square one. What you mustn't do is pop in frequently for top-ups, as this, I believe, is where people start to lose sight of how they normally look and what constitutes too much. They lose their frame of reference.

How to create the perfect ponytail

For my entire adult life, I deployed the ponytail only when painting walls, cleaning loos or feeling so full of some virus that I simply no longer cared. For anything more, I wore my hair down to look more elegant and disguise my bumpy head. Then the brilliant hair stylist Zoe Irwin taught me exactly where a ponytail should go to make the very best of one's skull and bone structure and it was revelatory. The perfect ponytail lands where an imaginary curved line from the chin to the back of the head – following along the jaw, skimming the outer ear – would naturally lead. This spot is in the centre of the back of your head, around a centimetre above the line of your eyebrow arch. On most straight, curly or coiled white, Black and Asian hair, this is helpfully at the point where your vertical parting dead-ends at the crown, and any parting in the hair becomes horizontal. Putting a ponytail here gives an extremely elegant shape to the neck and head, and, if firmly wrapped in your hair elastic (always hold the ponytail tightly as you wrap and don't let go until it's secure), lifts the face and eyes at exactly the right level to be flattering. Truly, the effect is remarkable and you'll never go back.

How to find your parting

Straight hair: With a wide-toothed comb or brush, scrape damp hair backwards. When it's all off your face, use your hand to push from the back of your hair forwards. Your natural parting is where the hair parts.
Curly or coiled hair: Using a wide-toothed comb, detangle and loosen wet hair. Tip your head forwards and use your fingers to rake hair forwards. Tip your head back upright and release your fingers. Where your parting falls is where it naturally lives.

How to create a side parting

Side partings are great for creating a soft, sweepy section of hair that is especially flattering on non-symmetrical faces (that's most of us) and fine, flat hair types, whether curly, coiled or straight. It's also a great way to add volume – just flip to the other side when your roots droop. In general, Black hair and thick, curly Asian or Caucasian hair has more stability and is consequently more helpful in creating a side parting – a tailcomb steered through the roots and smoothed either side will see it stay. Naturally straight Asian and Caucasian hair can flop about a bit and needs some help with the hairdryer – in which case, point the dryer downwards and sweep the hair with a brush in the opposite direction, as though you plan to part the other side of the one intended. A little product like mousse at the roots gives some grip. When dry, use a tailcomb to tunnel through the roots and smooth either side of the new parting. Do a little backcombing if you'd like some extra stability. Regardless of hair type, the most flattering side parting falls at the arch of the eyebrow. A deep side parting (not as flattering, but cool and striking) falls at the outer edge of the brow.

How to cut your own fringe

229

I know that by the time this book has travelled from laptop to bookshop, the following advice will be too little, too late. While we were busy fretting about the big and important stuff, Covid was also plaguing our hair. It turns out that cutting hair into something resembling a wearable hairstyle is really very hard. I've always been in awe of hairdressers and knew better than to imagine we could just acquire their skills when they were shut for business. I will only pick up the scissors in extremis to trim a friend's fringe, which I can now do pretty well. The key is to know your limits. Your job here is to restore vision and to tide someone over only until they can get to a hairdresser for a proper job, so go very easy and attempt nothing fancy.

Always start with clean, dry hair. Never, ever cut when wet or even damp – the hair will jump up when it dries and, in my experience, people are more likely to keep cutting wet hair to straighten out any unevenness, which is much less likely to show on dry hair. Clip back the rest of the hair, leaving the dry fringe isolated and loose. Comb through, and with the comb, gather the entire fringe into a single, flat, 2.5–cm section at the very centre of the forehead. Clamp it between two flat fingers at the bottom of the section, approximately 1cm from the hair's tips (you can use one of those plastic freezer-bag-sealing clips instead of fingers, if you prefer). Take the sharpest scissors you own and cut up into the 1cm section of tips, stopping at the fingers. Do not cut across, only upwards. When you've snipped the entire section, release your fingers and comb through to assess the length, snipping away any single hairs you may have missed (there will be some). If it's still too long (always preferable to too short), repeat the process, nudging fingers up only half a centimetre at a time, before combing through and checking. The same technique applies for kids.

How to treat a minor burn

Here's what's going to happen: you're going to put your just-grilled or burned finger under the running cold tap, to quell the immediate, urgent pain, and then a couple of minutes later, you're going to get bored. Your finger feels too cold now. It's uncomfortable and wasteful of water. You may think you'd prefer to sit down and watch telly, telling yourself you're probably fine now anyway. It's just a minor, household burn. Maybe you'll grab some peas from the freezer, or take a mug of cold water to the sofa and place your fingers inside it, like legs dangling lazily in a paddling pool. These may be your instincts, and you'd be foolish to act on them. You must stay put. Ten full minutes makes all the difference, taking the heat right out of the burn, cutting down dramatically on recovery time and that niggling sting that otherwise goes on for hours. Ten minutes. Not a second less.

Thoughts on insomnia

I remember the first time I absolutely could not get to sleep. I was six years old and sleeping over above a South Wales pub owned by the parents of some school friends. The twins and their little sister had gone to bed at 6.30 p.m., about three hours before my usual bedtime. I lay silently in a sleeping bag on their bedroom floor, eyes like saucers, wondering how I could possibly be expected to sleep when it was still light outside. As they all breathed deeply and rhythmically, I swore I could see Strawberry Shortcake and Care Bears twitch and move on their wall posters. The radiator clicked and I tried to Name That Tune. I could hear adults debating, laughing and singing downstairs in the bar. I longed to creep down and hide under a table with dogs lapping shandy from ashtrays. I felt trapped, lonely and what seemed to be interminably sleepless.

'My relationship with insomnia has outlasted my relationship with my parents, my first marriage and, in all probability, my career.'

It seems odd when I think, now, that my relationship with insomnia has outlasted my relationship with my parents, my first marriage and, in all probability, my career. For years I cheerfully attributed my sleeplessness to being a night owl. It's certainly true that I've always stayed up late – everyone in my family did. I loved my bed and yet I was always the last one to pass out from giggle exhaustion at sleepovers, always the last to flake at parties. I'll admit it's a handy skill when you're a raver, a new mother, or a writer on deadline trying to cram an entire book into an otherwise unchanged work and family timetable (I'm writing this sentence at 4.17 a.m.). But there comes a time – usually around now – when one must accept there's a deeper problem, and that there's something rather sad and lonely about insomnia in everyday life. The wider world is on a sensible schedule. Quite simply, I need to sleep more. I, and my insomnia, have become rather tired.

And yet decades after my first brush with sleeplessness, I'm still here, sleeping loved ones all around me while I listen to strangers in the dark. There are no longer babies in my house, no chorus of colicky wails to make wakefulness seem purposeful, or just part of a shared, empathetic experience among parents and neighbours. There's a local man with Tourette's syndrome who walks past the house at pretty much bang on midnight each night, shouting and ticking as he goes. When he doesn't, I fret that he's been mugged, or fallen ill, and that keeps me awake. Then there are shrieking students on their way home – invariably a girl who's had way too much to drink, crying loudly about some perceived slight from her clueless but belligerent boyfriend, also bladdered and making zero sense. There's usually a late-night taxi to collect someone, and I wonder if someone on my street is having an affair, as though life is a bad ITV1 drama. Sometime later, the posh hippy neighbours get home and insist on noodling around on unidentifiable stringed instruments, like the Levellers on barbiturates. I want to call the police, to shout at them to shut up, but at the same time feel faintly relieved to know I'm not the only person in Brighton still wide awake.

When the street has settled, I cycle aimlessly through social media apps, hoping someone, somewhere else, is still up. I have a little tribe of insomniacs who gather on late-night Facebook like local teens around a chip-shop Space Invaders. We often tell one another to go to bed in the hope it might be catching. There's a sort of desperate camaraderie, a verbal backslap to anyone not there, as though tonight they must've got lucky and zonked out. Then there's the American posse, just leaving their work as I'm obsessively calculating and adjusting the number of sleep-hours until mine begins. When page refreshes no longer bear fruit, and I've assessed every garment 'New In' at Whistles, Arket and Net-a-Porter, I listen to podcasts (TV is impossible – I share a bed). *This American Life* works well, albeit suddenly and only semi-unconsciously, just minutes before the end, when one has already invested fifty minutes in the story and characters. Sometimes I watch men carving tablets of soap on YouTube. Making myself very cold also seems to help. Standing in the back garden in my dressing gown until my hands feel frostbitten, then climbing back into bed to slowly warm up – with or without an electric blanket – has a soporific effect and I drift off. Some bedtime demarcation is essential – a deep cleanse and firm facial massage with a good oil, perhaps a bath too, all seem to talk my synapses down from the ledge. I've tried tea, no tea, exercise, rest, telly and no telly before bed, earlier nights, later nights, phone left downstairs, lavender eye masks, blue-light filters, pillow sprays and a 'calming' app that made me want to stab the narrator in both eyes. Melatonin will do the job – my friend Jamie, a fellow member of the insomniac club, sent me some. But it seems less than ideal to make it my regular nightcap. Often, the least-stressful tactic is to decide I'm not going to sleep, only to rest quietly, and that at least takes off some of the pressure.

And so on my brain whirs, into the early hours. I mull over my numerous mistakes and regrets, remember my dead friends and relatives. I think about my supermarket order, whether it needs amending, if I've missed the slot I wanted, how annoying it is that they discontinued their apricot oat bars. I wonder WTF my son has done with his expensive school blazer. I think of things I'd like to write, sentences I'd like to use, and sometimes write the lion's share of a column squinting at the Notes app, sure in the knowledge that by tomorrow, someone will have shaken the Etch A Sketch in my brain. I'll be exhausted, forgetful and resentful at having to wake up early and try to do some work. But I do it nonetheless. Because this is my life, I tell myself, as I pick out a dress and paint on a brave face. This is who I am. I'm just a night owl.

How to prevent and treat milia

Milium cysts (known collectively and commonly as milia) are those little white lumps that appear commonly around the eyes, on the cheeks and elsewhere. Made of protein and skin cells, they are harmless, not normally uncomfortable, but annoying nonetheless, and people frequently want rid of them. But first, prevention is better than cure, so it's good to have a solid skincare routine in place:

1. Always remove your makeup before bed.
   I know it's boring. I know you're exhausted, comfy and think it's probably fine just this once. And it is, but know this: properly cleansed skin not only looks much better than slept-in makeup, sweat and SPF within just a few days, it also helps prevent milia forming by clearing sweat ducts and pores.
2. Always exfoliate.
   I use liquid exfoliants all around the eye area, as this is where any flakiness looks worst under makeup. It's also a good way to stave off the formation of milia, as it sloughs away dead skin. Even if you're not an acid-exfoliant user, you should take your hot flannel around your eyes when performing your twice-daily cleanse. The cloth's mildly abrasive surface will buff away flakes – just move in circular motions, never dragging.
3. Massage in your skincare properly.
   Your skincare products need to be absorbed well into the skin, which can be more difficult around the eyes, where milia often develop. If your regular moisturiser isn't readily slurped up, you'll need a thinner, more absorbent eye cream. If you're dry or very dry of skin, you will probably find that your usual day and night creams work just fine all over. Whatever your skin type, work any serums, lotions or creams well into your face before applying makeup or heading to bed.
4. Use retinol.
   See 'Retinol best practice, page 214' for more on why it can be so beneficial to many skins. Retinoids can be extremely helpful in preventing milia – the number on my own face reduces to near nothing when I use tretinoin or retinol.
5. Take care of yourself.
   Being sleep-deprived, a smoker, a poor eater or a user of harsh skincare (using too many peels, for example) are all thought to exacerbate milia production.

How to remove milia

Do. Not. Squeeze.

Milia are too big and too hard to magically pop out of the pore with a little external pressure. All you'll do is cause irritation, redness and potential scarring. The lump will almost always work its way gradually to the surface over time (this will happen sooner with gentle but regular exfoliation), at which point it will be covered in such a thin shield of skin that some gentle agitation with a finger wrapped in a warm, wet face cloth should set it free. A professional beauty therapist can remove most milia very easily by inserting a sterile needle into the upper layers of the skin, then navigating the lump up through the newly created hole. I do this myself but only after having been shown professionally on many occasions, and I absolutely don't recommend that you give it a bash (it's extremely easy to go too far, especially around the eyes). Don't book a facial until you've determined that your therapist will include milia removal in the treatment protocol (the 'routine' performed), if that's important to you (it is to me), as it's by no means guaranteed. Alternatively, a skin clinic will usually be prepared to remove multiple milia for less money than you might imagine, so call and ask for options.

235

How to stop bleached blonde hair going green

Any blonde, particularly but not only the bottled kind, knows that swimming gives pale hair a greenish tinge. This isn't permanent – it's just chlorine, copper and magnesium clinging to the hair shaft and temporarily discolouring it. You can prevent this by never getting into the pool with dry hair, otherwise you're just asking it to drink up the green. Instead, saturate your hair first in clean water, then add a barrier. You could use any hair oil but you'd be wasting money unduly. Just coat the wet hair in any colourless oil (coconut, for example), tie hair in a topknot, cover with a cap and dive in.

How to fake tan your back

I got this excellent tip a while back from *Strictly Come Dancing* tanner to the stars Jules Von Hep. Pop a tanning mitt onto a wooden spoon and secure with a rubber band. Use the spoon to reach around and apply the product to your back.

How to cover dark undereye circles

If people take nothing else from this book, I'd love them to take this, since no matter how often I answer elsewhere, 'Which eye cream gets rid of dark circles?' remains the most-asked question in my professional life. The answer is none. An over-the-counter cream will not change the colour of your skin and nor should it. Any noticeable fixes to uneven skin tone will be cosmetic and temporary. The best three ways of achieving this are via corrector, concealer and light-reflecting particles in either your skincare or makeup, or both.

Please let us start with corrector, as we'd all do well to. Corrector is not concealer. The two are completely distinct products but the very best of friends that bunk one atop the other. Corrector cancels out the opposing tones in dark circles and is consequently never the colour of your skin. For white skin and grey-blue circles, correctors are usually a sickly salmon pink. For brown skin with greenish-brown circles, they're a peachier tone, and for Black skin with greyish-brown circles, an orangey one. In all cases, think of corrector as the sucky-inny shapewear that does the grunt work so the frock on top has to do nothing more than feel comfy and look pretty.

236

Concealer is the frock. This is the product that does need to match and flatter your skin. So either on a bare face or after your foundation, if you're wearing it, pat your corrector along the undereye. Wait a few moments, then pat or buff on a thin amount of concealer over the top. This two-step process is not for everyone. It's an extra thirty seconds in a demanding day and an additional £10–20 product, I do realise. Which is why it's completely fine to wear only concealer. Just know that it will never brighten dark circles as effectively, no matter how much you pile on (and perversely, applying heaps of concealer starts to look grey in itself).

While we're on the subject, bags are not circles. 'Undereye bags' are pockets of slackened skin, either hereditary or a natural part of the ageing process, and aren't necessarily dark. 'Dark circles' describe only the brownish/bluish/greyish crescents beneath the eyes that occur when we're tired, ill, run-down or – as is often the case – they simply run in the family. That said, what they do have in common is that no eye cream will shift either. Eye bags can be temporarily tightened and lifted with topical products but not, in my view, in any lasting way without either a needle or scalpel. Dark circles can be brightened temporarily with eye creams and covered beautifully with corrector and concealer, using the method above. But they will not change colour from the outside in, whatever the packaging may tell you.

Should I go grey?

The answer is dependent on just two things: what you want and what you can afford. Nothing and no one else should have a say, or even an opinion. I'm going grey. It started about seven years ago, with a single, bright white hair nestling in my fringe. As I'm not some sitcom archetype; I didn't scream, wail or fall into an existential crisis. It didn't bother me very much at all. Still, being a brunette had been part of the signature look I'd enjoyed my whole life, and so for a while I changed my hairstyle to conceal the greys, moving my parting, spraying on temporary touch-up for work. But in recent times, and despite being positively delighted to be in my forties, I became less enamoured with my salt-and-pepper look.

If, as your years advance, your hair undergoes a comprehensive change and naturally falls like some pearlescent satin nightgown, then I positively envy you. Mine did not. A colony of whites had now sprouted around my temples while the rest of my hair stubbornly resisted transition. I couldn't dye it back to its former colour (I'm allergic to the PPD and PTD present in all 100-per-cent grey-covering dark dyes – believe me, I've done over ten solid years of intense research on this and consulted with hair companies at the highest level on how this should change and it hasn't), and so I was presented with two choices: let nature have its way or bleach my hair white and tint it temporarily with silver, platinum or ice-cream shades of pink, green or lavender, none of which I'm allergic to. I certainly didn't relish the maintenance of the latter but nor did I particularly like the look of the former on me personally, and so I donned the gown of no return and went permanently grey overnight. My job allows for no painful growing-out period hidden under hats, and even if I were a vet, bus driver or CEO, I'd honestly have no desire to embark on it. I somehow feel more in control having made a drastic and sudden change on my own terms, steering into the skid, if you will. My real colour will just have to play catch-up when it's ready.

Despite spending my life defending the very concept of beauty to complete strangers, even I was shocked at the reaction to my plan when I mentioned it online. Both social acquaintances and women I'd never met

237

were horrified that I or anyone else would choose not to let nature take its course and apparently felt completely comfortable telling me point-blank to step away from the bleach. While some women felt I'd look 'too old', many others felt personally offended and let down by my decision, telling me repeatedly that I should 'grow old gracefully', an expression more likely to send me hurtling down a path towards extreme facelifts and a cryogenic chamber. A brief internet search yielded thousands of articles and posts calling for women to stop dyeing their hair at once, as though this was less about a simple choice of hair colour and more about moral weakness and a pitiful ignorance of the ways of the patriarchy – a maddeningly patronising implication as sexist as the problem it purports to oppose. I feel no more obliged to go grey naturally than I do to stop painting my nails or shaving my legs. I am as authentically myself with red lipstick and false lashes as I am barefaced in pyjamas with egg yolk down my chin.

If you want to save a load of time, expense and chemicals by opting out of the dyeing cycle, and feel a sense of liberation, then I enthusiastically applaud that choice. I'm as likely to gawp in admiration at a grey-, white- or silver-haired woman as I am at any other. Likewise, I don't care if your hair is dyed red, blonde, green, purple; is fake, real, short, long, curly, coiled or chemically straightened; is badly or well looked after. None of it affects my life and nor should it inform how I present myself to the world. The prescriptive judgement of how women should look and any qualitative value placed on their choices is exactly what we should be fighting against. It wasn't our game to begin with. Let's not play it and, for goodness' sake, let's get out of each other's hair.

Is hair self-cleaning?

You will, at least once in your life, meet someone who tells you proudly that they no longer wash their hair.

In my experience (which is extensive, since these people always seem especially keen to tell me), they will say the hair is self-cleaning (true in a very limited sense) and claim that shampoo deposits chemicals that prove toxic to the human body (not true), harsh ingredients that will strip hair and detergents that will harm the environment (decreasingly true and very easily avoided now that sulphate-free shampoos are available everywhere). They will sometimes tell you that people of colour don't shampoo their hair and manage perfectly well with only conditioner, which is both massively racist and a straightforward lie. They will frequently claim that after an initial period of rancidness, their hair has never felt or styled better, which is fine as long as they don't expect me to touch it.

Here's what is true of hair's ability to self-clean: for some people with very specific hair types (mostly dry or coarse), the increased levels of natural oils in unwashed hair will create a softer, more manageable feeling. For the rest of us, it will most likely not. Fine and flat hair, for example, will typically respond very badly to shampoo-dodging, becoming greasy and lank. More importantly, scalps are emphatically not self-cleaning, and avoiding shampoo will quickly cause a build-up of greasy dead skin, which at best will cause itchiness and irritation, and at worst affect the hair's ability to emerge from it (think about your bathroom shower head when clogged with limescale, and those pitiful shoots of water that spit haphazardly out of random holes). Even if someone believes the old wives' tale that the build-up of natural oils in hair will, after a month, obviate the need for shampoo, they'd do well to remember that those natural oils will carry rather than remove smells. Their magic hair cannot override the whiff of a barbecue, or proof itself against the fumes of sizzling bacon.

Hair is only 'self-cleaning' insofar as the skin is technically self-cleaning and the vulva is technically self-cleaning – who on earth would consider not washing those? If you want hair more as nature intended, cut down on blow-drying, straightening and other heat styling. But shampoo is our friend, and a polite gesture to those around us. If you'd like to avoid detergent, look for sulphate-free shampoos, and if you'd like to avoid packaging, buy a solid bar. There are now plenty of good ones.

239

How to look in the mirror

I feel very privileged to spend so much time gazing into the faces of women around the country. I love every moment except those when, with absolute inevitability, they tell me they have 'huge pores' and I have to squint to make them out. Women are lousy at looking in the mirror. They are too critical, too blind to see the beauty. Quicker to spot perceived flaws than virtues. While it's no wonder when we so often see ourselves described negatively, I wish we were encouraged to view ourselves as the vast majority of real people do. When someone glances in your direction, the best they will think, oh so fleetingly, is 'she looks nice', then be on

'Tattooing is not for everyone ... if you're likely to be hurt by the narrow-minded, think before you ink.'

their way. At worst, they will think nothing. Absolutely nothing. And that, in its own way, is wonderful.

How to get a tattoo

I have eight tattoos and I love them. Three on my wrists, another behind my ear, a much larger one – a swallow – on my back, and large arrangements of botanicals and bees on both arms. I have another planned for this summer and I daresay there will be more. I have no opinion on whether you should have even one, but the odds are that you've at least considered joining me and the some 40 per cent of British people with skin inkings. Before you take the plunge, there are some things you should know.

Firstly, you should be someone who is able to rise above the comments easily. The untattooed feel unfathomably furious about the decisions strangers and loved ones make for their own bodies, and remarkably free and easy in registering their revulsion in a way they simply wouldn't over a haircut, dress or flat bum. I've heard plenty of disparaging comments about tattoos over the years, but I actively enjoy the fact that some people don't get it. Tattooing is not for everyone, too painful for some (though I've had worse bikini waxes and lip threadings, in all honesty), not at all appealing to others, and that suits most of us just fine, but if you're likely to be hurt by the narrow-minded, think before you ink.

241

1. Download the Pinterest app and start searching either by theme, e.g. 'rose tattoos', or placement, e.g. 'shoulder tattoos'. Add in terms such as 'small', 'colour', 'black and white', 'feminine' or 'traditional sailor' to narrow the search. You can do the same on Instagram using hashtags. Keep a folder on Pinterest, Instagram or in your phone's photo album, so you can refer back, adding and deleting as appropriate.
2. Avoid band names unless your commitment to them has been lifelong. Don't get a partner or spouse's name (or, frankly, even go out with someone who expects you to). Remember that tattoo removal is much more painful and expensive than tattooing, takes ages and almost always leaves a trace.
3. Follow as many artists on Instagram as are named on your picks and scroll through their many designs. Contact your favourite and make an appointment. Expect to wait – good tattoo artists are frequently booked for many weeks or even months in advance. It's a good sign.

4. Give your chosen artists an advance idea of what you'd like in terms of design, theme, size and placement. Send all your visual references, saying which elements appeal. Don't expect an artist to copy wholesale a design you send them. It's insulting to a tattooist, unethical to the original artist and a wasted opportunity for you. A good artist will interpret your idea, adapting it to create options that will be unique to you. Never just point at something in a book as though choosing a burger from a takeaway menu – unless you don't mind having the same as a thousand other tourists.

5. Get an idea of pricing to avoid any nasty surprises on the day. Similarly to Botox, while it doesn't necessarily follow that expensive tattoos are always good, it is reliably true that cheap tattoos are crap. Talented artists making custom designs in sanitary conditions cost money. This is your body, and for ever. It is no time to make cutbacks.

6. Be well hydrated and rested on the day of your appointment. Take an ibuprofen if you think you'll need it. Be patient but honest and clear as the artist lays stencils on your skin. This is your last chance to get things absolutely right before the design is made permanent.

7. Try to relax. Tattooing is more painful when muscles are tense.

8. Impose a cool-off period. There's a huge adrenaline rush after getting a tattoo, where one can feel so euphoric that one immediately craves the next. I've felt this every single time. Understand what's happening and take yourself home to calm down without booking your next appointment. Tattoos need time, consideration and proper planning. You'll remember that tomorrow.

How to care for a new tattoo

1. Remove the cellophane wrapping as soon as you arrive home (it is there purely to protect others from your plasma and blood contamination) and rinse the tattoo under clear, tepid water. Very gently pat dry – never rub.

2. Apply a light coating of bland, fragrance-free moisturiser, such as Simple or CeraVe, or a nappy ointment like Bepanthen. This keeps the skin well lubricated to avoid cracking and uneven scabbing. Don't bother buying expensive tattoo creams at the studio.

3. Repeat the rinsing and moisturising routine, performing it three or four times a day. Don't apply a thick layer of moisturiser – skin should just be lubricated, not wet or greased.

4. Avoid bathing for ten days and shower (after the first twenty-four hours) instead. If you must bathe, keep the tattoo dry. Soaking it can delay healing or give a patchy finish to the healed tattoo. When showering, just let the clean water wash over the ink – don't use soap or shower gel.
5. Don't cover the tattoo with a plaster, dressing or bandage. The greater its exposure to the air, the faster and more evenly it will heal.
6. Don't pick any scabbing, ever. You will ruin your tattoo. Steer clear of body scrubs and loofah sponges for a couple of months. Just keep the tattoo lubricated and let nature take its course.
7. Remember that tattoos get brighter when they're healed. They will usually look more vibrant a couple of weeks after inking.

Should you squeeze a spot?

I think we all know perfectly well when we need to squeeze a spot and when we really shouldn't. The issue is whether we ignore our better judgement and start meddling regardless. A spot is ripe for squeezing when it has a visible whitish head. Sometimes there is no head but the uncomfortable sensation of pressure against the surface of the skin is so great that we can't be convinced of a spot's unripeness and in we go. Tempting though this is, it rarely ends well – namely with swelling, redness and perhaps even a spatter of blood that can result easily in a scab and possibly even a scar.

This is best practice:

Spot ripe for squeezing
1. Cleanse face, removing all makeup, SPF and so on. Use a hot cloth to remove the cleanser.
2. Take an extraction tool (available on Amazon or any beauty supply site for under a fiver) and wash it thoroughly under running water with soap.
3. Use the looped end of the tool and lasso it around the entire spot. Very gently apply a little pressure to the loop, pressing it lightly into the surrounding skin to increase pressure on the spot's head (if you don't have an extraction tool, wrap a little torn tissue around clean fingers and use your opposing ring fingers to act as substitutes – do not use index or middle fingers. They are stronger and it's easy to go too far).

243

4. The spot should now pop. Apply a lighter pressure to ensure the head is fully released, then leave well alone. Do not keep expressing clear liquid after the head has been expelled. Continuing to flog an already dead horse will damage your skin and probably cause bleeding.
5. Sweep a cotton pad saturated in beta hydroxy acid (BHA) around the area.
6. Leave a few moments and apply other skincare as normal.

Spot unripe for squeezing

1. You probably know it's not ready and you're going to try anyway. I know this, so I'm going to tell you to follow the above steps 1 and 2.
2. Place the looped end of the tool and lasso it around the entire spot. Press very gently only once. If a head does not appear, stop.
3. Use a cotton bud to apply a BHA spot gel (available in any decent chemist – look for salicylic acid on the ingredients list) to the immediate area. Repeat this every four hours. Some peeling over the next day or two is normal.
4. Apply other skincare as normal, avoiding the area.
5. This will often result in the spot either disappearing altogether, or rising up to the skin's surface. If this happens, you can follow the steps for a ripe, squeezable spot.

How to get pierced without an allergic irritation

In recent years, it's become mainstream to wear multiple piercings – and not just in lobes. Nose studs, brow rings, piercings in the helix (upper ear), daith (the nobbly bit, halfway up), tragus (between the daith and lobe), conch (the ear's recess) and other visible locations can now be seen on bank managers, executives, stay-at-home parents and clergy. As the owner of six ear piercings myself, I'm all for it, but piercing must be done properly to be a pleasure. And when I say 'properly', I mean by a person whose profession is piercing by hand. I loathe piercing guns. Decades of speaking to friends and readers has left me in no doubt of the fact that those 'allergic to nickel and piercings' – that is, those prone to sticky, sore, gunky and oozing ears (and I was one of them) – have usually been pierced with a gun in a jewellery or clothes shop. My advice is always to allow existing piercings to close and heal, before starting from scratch at a piercing shop, where the heavily pierced experts invariably believe passionately in their art and do the job with greater thought, design and care, using hand-held needles that give neater holes, which heal fully and cleanly. At the end of this very different process, it is extremely common to discover that there was no metal allergy at all – only crap piercing.

I spent my adolescence with such horribly weeping ears (having been twice pierced by a gun in a jeweller's), that I ultimately let them close up to save myself the discomfort and hassle. I became convinced that, Princess and the Pea-like, my delicate skin could only barely tolerate solid gold. Then, following plastic surgery on my ears in adulthood, I was re-pierced with a needle by a heavily tattooed professional at Metal Morphosis in London (any council-licensed dedicated piercing shop is fine) and can now wear any old market tat without so much as an itch. Nickel, plastic, silver, vintage, cheap-as-chips high street or designer costume – my ears will wear anything with no complaint. I've sent many friends and readers down the same path with life-changing results. Proper needle piercings simply heal better, more cleanly and permanently in a way that gun piercings, for many of us, don't. Which isn't to say you should shove in any old tin from the start. The smartest and safest option is to buy the boring titanium studs, bars and balls from your piercing shop. They're cheap (from about £3) and putting up with them for just six to eight weeks is an unstylish investment in a lifetime of fancy earring-wearing thereafter. While they're healing with the correct jewellery, leave piercings well alone. I just leave mine untouched to wash in the shower, then shove my ears under the warm tap when cleaning my teeth before bed. If you prefer, you can use sterile saline for contact lenses, but there's usually no need. Don't fiddle.

Tiny acts for good mental health

I've always maintained that whatever huge event crashes into my life uninvited – whether depression, death, redundancy, illness, divorce or other trauma – it will be the little things that cumulatively make me feel better in the long run, not grand gestures made for their own sake. 'Never make life-changing decisions at life-changing times' has been my steadfast rule and despite enjoying a happy family life these past years, I've lately found this to be as pertinent as ever. There have been occasions when the world around me has felt too unfamiliar for comfort, when things have seemed so hostile, scary, chaotic and mean-spirited that I need tiny,

'When free time is so scant, there's simply no point feigning enthusiasm for tier-two engagements.'

outwardly meaningless things to help me feel human. While the big stuff in my life has mercifully remained constant, I've made some tiny tweaks and promises to myself that have proved so transformative, I've decided to make them permanent. My aim is not to write anyone else's prescription, but to encourage you to draw up your own action points, so tiny as to feel neither effortful nor pressurising.

Avoid rolling news

I've seen the headline, I've familiarised myself with the facts. I know how many people are dying and what appalling acts are being committed. Inevitably, all stories reach the point where literally nothing is developing but my anxiety. After the 2020 US presidential election, I made the decision not to watch rolling news for more than thirty minutes at a time, and became much calmer as a result. A slice of toast and an episode of *Broad City* was a much better way of looking after my mental health.

Stop showering

No, not in the manner of the no-shampoo brigade. I mean that simply exchanging a couple of morning showers per week for long evening baths can prove extremely mood-enhancing. I lock the door, pour in some bubbles, put on an old *You're Wrong About* or *Savage Love* podcast, and relax. It's part of my ongoing effort to turn the functional into the pleasurable, to reclaim my life from my schedule of responsibilities, to slow the hell down. Keeping clean has become the highlight of my day.

247

Don't accept invitations you'll resent

In my forties, I have finally accepted that I don't have enough time to see the people I really love, never mind those I don't, and that it's much more polite, thoughtful and realistic to turn down any invitation I will, at some point, long to cancel. I have a close set of friends I need to see every couple of months and a partner I love being alone with. When free time is so scant, there's simply no point feigning enthusiasm for tier-two engagements, only to spend the next six weeks unfairly resenting the commitment to attend.

Charge your phone in a different room

A couple of years ago, I made the, er, radical decision to keep only one iPhone charger permanently plugged into a bedside socket. This has changed my life hugely, in that it means I plug in my phone when my long working day is over and my evening of eating, chatting and telly watching can begin, uninterrupted by the buzzing, pinging, flashing of constant updates. I adore my phone, I can't live without it, but my decision to put it aside for a few hours a day has immeasurably improved my life, simply by allowing my poor, overworked synapses to put their feet up with a Horlicks.

Accepting what you can and can't control

The significant things I can control: the way I vote, my engagement with issues that matter, my charitable contributions, my parenting, my role in my friendships, my behaviour towards strangers. I can't do anything directly about war, terrorism, cyberstalking, the dark web, internet conspiracy theorists, nor the fact that people are fighting like cat and dog on social media because someone has had the audacity to express an opinion that isn't shared by every reader. It is simply not the medium for rational, calm and empathetic debate and my contribution will further nothing and change no minds. All any of us can do is live as much as possible offline, clean up our own side of the street, examine our own behaviours and look out for others where we're able. This has been the hardest lesson to learn. But it's a shift in attitude I've had to embrace for the sake of preserving sanity.

248

Where should you give birth?

Ideally where you will give birth is wherever you want to give birth – screaming down the walls of your own home, lying on an operating table, on all fours in a birthing pool, huffing on a tube linked to a huge canister of delicious gas, sitting up comfortably in a hospital bed, while an epidural drips into your lower back and your partner reads you this month's edition of *Viz*. In practice, though, you will give birth where the baby decides you'll be giving birth. Sometimes, wonderfully, these two things match. Often, they don't. As someone for whom things went only halfway to plan the first time (home birth, an agonising tear so awful that I wince to recall it), then blissfully to plan the next (home birth under an hour, barely a stitch), let me emphasise in the strongest terms: it is just one day. ONE DAY that you will barely remember beyond the arrival of your baby at the end of it. One day that your child will definitely not remember. One day that will soon be eclipsed by the gigantic demands of the daily job at hand and one day that you just have to get through in one piece – and that, while remarkable and undeniably heroic, says precisely

'In practice, though, you will give birth where the baby decides you'll be giving birth.'

nothing about your quality as a mother. Women who refuse all drugs and whack out a baby in minutes in a garden paddling pool and women who elect to undergo a caesarean from the moment they spot a blue line in the plastic window – both groups are comprised of exceptionally brilliant mothers, perfectly fine mothers and really bloody substandard mothers. It is just one day. No one tells you this. And by the time you understand it in your bones, hair and fingernails, it's too late to go back and relax.

How to grieve

Ever more frequently, those around me are experiencing what one might class as the major bereavements. Both my parents are dead, so sometimes friends ask me when their own pain might end, how long it took me to grieve, when they might again feel even a little bit okay. I am very touched when they do, since my relationships with my respective parents were odd and difficult and my feelings about them unusually conflicted. It takes an emotionally intelligent person to understand that this rarely, if ever, translates to a detached bereavement. So I desperately want to trade their understanding for my insight and experience, but the truth is, I've still no idea what grief really means.

Because here's the thing about bereavement. Like motherhood, you're meant to just know what to do without anyone telling you how. In the days and weeks following my father's death (and he really did die. I didn't lose him, he didn't 'pass'. His heart stopped beating and he died), people constantly told me to make sure I 'grieved properly'. I nodded and thanked them for their kind wishes. I told them I was coping when, in reality, I was entirely at sea, not understanding how to behave, what process I should be embarking on. It felt too embarrassing, almost disrespectful to my dad's memory, to say, 'I don't know what the hell I'm meant to be doing, here.' Good friends bought me Joan Didion's (very brilliant, I know) books and they read like foreign texts. I read bereavement websites but, in my chaotic state, felt wholly unable to relate.

I sincerely hope you've never lost someone you love, but as someone who has, and who comes from a family where no one really talks, and who dealt in particular with my father's death extremely badly, allow me to tell you what I learned during the two years in which I genuinely felt I'd gone insane. When people prescribe a grieving period, they are coming from a good place. They mean 'feel sad, allow this to dominate your thoughts and feelings for as long as is necessary'. It's a thing to say, to feel you're being supportive at the most terrible time in someone's life. But having heard it repeatedly myself, I will never prescribe grief to my own friends. Because apart from that sounding like a platitude from the same category as 'time heals', 'kids adapt' and, worst of all, 'everything happens for a reason', it's not something over which anyone has any say. Grief is not a choice, a project to manage or a course of medication to take. It just happens while you're unable to form a single sensible thought.

With the benefit of hindsight, I know that grief is a feeling, not an expression. You don't have to wail to show you care, or weep to make others feel comfortable that everything is in order. Despite the neat psychological theory, there are no stages to go through in predictable order – denial, anger, blah blah. Frankly, the whole thing is a bloody mess. You may say nothing, as I did for a long time. You may feel like punching walls, or people who've deigned to ask you for a favour during your personal apocalypse (this also happened). You may feel so completely 'nothing' that you'd fail to register if they walloped you back. You may want to eat everything, or nothing, sleep too much or hardly ever. You might want to meticulously paint on a brave face with makeup, or fester in a dressing gown and your own filth. You might be in a constant state of confusion over how the world can make sense when your parent is dead, about who on earth you are if not someone's daughter. You'll feel under constant attack from all the questions you never asked, the things you never got around to saying. You will probably feel guilt over not having seen them enough, whether you went home once a year or visited thrice-weekly without fail. You may well feel all of these things repeatedly, in one dizzying cycle of anguish.

251

Grief is when pain is visceral like a stab, not dull like toothache. It's acute agony, not chronic sadness. It's the period before the wound becomes a scar. And however long that takes, however much of a mind bend it most certainly will be, I can promise this much: it ends. Like a storm, grief is real and terrifying, but mercifully ephemeral. It trashes everything in its way, but leaves behind a stillness, some space for you to rearrange the pieces in a new formation. It can take months or years to do its worst (I was lucky – I got emergency therapy and felt human within eighteen months), and afterwards, you will permanently feel a little sadder than you did when the person you loved was alive. You will be more aware of your own mortality, of how – should life follow its correct course – your children will one day feel similar anguish. But within the hangover of grief, you will still be able to experience the joy of a great joke, of a kind gesture, of an excellent meal or Sunday morning in bed. Your laughs will be real and raucous, your precious moments unadulterated, even enhanced by a sense of increased gratitude.

Piece by piece, you will gradually arrive at a point where your late parent's cooking can be acknowledged as an abomination, where you and your siblings can criticise his drinking, or her lateness, or their atrocious handling of a school bullying incident. If your family is anything like mine, you'll come to accept that your relationship was complicated, sometimes distant, and understand that those deaths are every bit as harrowing as those within close, picture-perfect families. You'll remember the shock when they smacked you on the bum for singing anti-Nottingham Forest FC songs, and the horror of the times they failed to show up. As well as the good stuff, you'll remember that they had bandy legs or shocking dandruff, the same occasionally bad breath as anyone else. To lose reverence for the dead, to let go of the need to cling on to their many achievements, will be comforting because it's familiar and real, and it takes you right back to when he or she was alive, flaws and all. And while you'd give anything to experience their shortcomings again, to just remember them makes life a whole lot more bearable.

252

And if a dear friend you care about loses their parent first? I wish I had the answers, but I don't. But having been there, I suggest saying, 'This is horrible, this is complete and utter shit, this is the absolute pits of the pits', and never, ever look on the bright side of an utterly ghastly situation. Take round a pizza, leaving it on the doorstep if they can't bring themselves to answer the bell. Don't believe their stoic crap about being fine, but don't force them to discuss it either. Tell them you love them, tolerate their imperfect behaviour or intense neediness. Be patient when they want to talk of a dead person constantly and are not at their most dazzling on a night out. Accept their temporary madness with kindness, and check in often, even if only via text. And make time to see all the people you love, while you still can.

'Like a storm, grief is real and terrifying, but mercifully ephemeral. It trashes everything in its way, but leaves behind a stillness.'

'I wouldn't dream of jumping on the Dry January bandwagon at the very time when a comforting glass of wine is not so much a vice as a medical imperative.'

How to beat the January blues

The January blues, the post-Christmas slump, Blue Monday (the third in January), acute post-bank holiday depression syndrome – all are common, medically recognised terms for beginning-of-the-year sadness, depression, irritability, apathy and lethargy. Seasonal affective disorder (of which I am not a sufferer) peaks in January, as do, according to the Samaritans, UK suicide rates. While I am mercifully in the less serious category, I'm not at all surprised that some people feel they simply can't cope.

I've always felt extremely grim at the dawn of the new year. My low-level depression begins with hauling the naked, skeletal Christmas tree into the street, to be cleared away with soggy, torn wrapping paper and other detritus of good times past, and doesn't much improve until February. There's some comfort in knowing I'm far from alone. The post-holiday period is when David Bowie and Carrie Fisher died, a time when we're all poorer and heavier than before, with an interminable wait ahead of us before payday. We're crawling out of bed in darkness and returning to work before we're ready, and I for one invariably feel overwhelmed by huge projects I've yet to start, the pressure to achieve goals within a neat twelve-month timeframe, and anxiety around what might happen to the world in the year ahead. New year's resolutions – commitments made at a time when I am at my least healthy mentally – are a non-starter. I've long since given up the pretence of joining a gym I know full well I'll never visit, and despite not being a heavy drinker, I wouldn't dream of jumping on the Dry January bandwagon at the very time when a comforting glass of wine is not so much a vice as a medical imperative.

255

If you tend to feel fabulously gung-ho and ready to slay the new year, go forth and enjoy your good luck. But if you are more usually in the grips of a festive comedown that leaves you feeling despondent, weepy and left behind, I'm with you, each and every January. This is how I've learned to cope:

Don't begin hung over

Perhaps my one and only concession to superstition is never getting legless on New Year's Eve. I know, it's nauseating, but I promise my aim is not to feel smug or superior, but to be without an unshakable sense of foreboding the next day. To me, there is something symbolically dreadful about waking up on January 1st wearing last year's makeup, feeling sick to the stomach and smelling of wine. I will gladly toast in the new year, but always remain sober enough to get up, put on a face and get out on a dog walk the next morning. It feels like a positive and auspicious start.

Keep ambitions small

Quitting booze, dairy or cigarettes, changing career, learning a new language or starting a new business – all are admirable and exciting if you feel up to the challenge. But I know that small victories from realistic, lower-stake endeavours can make you feel just as good without the threat of failure. Going out of your way to do a small favour for someone appreciative – a stranger or loved one – imparts an immediate sense of wellbeing, as does the completion of minor domestic tasks. Thinking 'I'm going to clear out an entire clothes drawer, sew on three buttons that have needed doing since forever, and take some paperbacks to the Sue Ryder shop' is still setting a worthwhile goal, and will ultimately impart similar feelings of pleasure and accomplishment as something bigger. Whatever your equivalent, keep the task manageable and the moment right – one depressed girlfriend emptied out her entire loft during a mood upswing, then crashed and ended up staring at the mess, too tearful and overwhelmed even to clear a path back to her own sofa.

Be sociable

Few people can afford to go out lots in January, and it can be extremely tempting to hunker down until it's over, but financial (and physical) lockdown and poor weather can cause feelings of isolation and loneliness to creep up on us. Rather than cram my pre-Christmas schedule, I prefer to diarise January get-togethers when everyone needs them most, pandemics notwithstanding. Cheap dates like pizza evenings in front of the telly, group dog walks and coffee, a weekend matinee at the pictures – all help our wellbeing and keep the social machinery well oiled.

Book leave

I know, I know – it seems wasteful and greedy to book time off when you've just had a load, but psychologists believe that one of the most effective ways of handling the January slump is to book a small amount of time off (even if just one day) after a short period back at work. I've done exactly this for the past few years and the effect it's had on my back-to-school nerves is unprecedented. Knowing I'm in for just one week before taking a day out again – even if it means making up the time and money in previous or future months – has allowed me to ease into the new year without the familiar dread and exhaustion.

Be grateful

An important act all year round, but most useful at this time. It's never a bad idea to acknowledge that you have a warm house when others are enduring January on the streets, that you have a job to dread returning to, and loved ones you can still call in a crisis. A friend once gave me the idea of writing down everything good that had happened in the previous year, and pinning it on the kitchen wall. It forced me to see how surprisingly full and varied my year had been, despite having spent the beginning of it feeling depressed and pessimistic, and to acknowledge that this year would almost certainly level out in much the same way.

Economise creatively

I find the need to economise one of January's more satisfying challenges, because it forces me to be creative and disciplined. I like to batch-cook a huge vat of delicious soup from whatever I can find leftover in the fridge and cupboards (see: 'How to make almost any soup, page 126'), then feel smug at the astonishingly low penny and calorie counts per portion (if the latter is important to you, you can type your recipe into MyFitnessPal for these calculations, sharing them for the benefit of other users to feel extra virtuous). Another deeply gratifying and important exercise in cash control is to see if you can go a whole day a week without spending a single penny – walking everywhere, packing your own lunch, making your own coffee and living off existing supplies (if your commute renders this impossible, try using only cash – it makes for more mindful spending). Unless desperate for something practical, I usually pledge not to buy a single item in the January sales, and to my amazement, it invariably makes me feel happier than a new frock or shoes would have.

257

Move

The Instagram gym bunnies may be dispiriting if, like me, you loathe most exercise. But they have a point. It is an unequivocal fact that moving briskly for twenty minutes per day lifts one's mood and spirits. A needless sprint up the stairs, a premature disembarkation from the bus, a quick session at the local trampoline park (it's way more enjoyable and relaxing than you might imagine), an energetic dance session in your kitchen, a touch of Pilates or yoga on your living room floor (there are billions of classes on YouTube) – all are instantly uplifting and a cinch to do. Supplementing them with a more substantial weekly workout, ideally outside, provides extra endorphins and an important hit of vitamin D – levels are usually at their lowest in winter.

It is absolutely fine to hate January to March. It is absolutely not a bad omen for the year ahead, merely a sign that your brain and emotions won't adhere to someone else's schedule. When spring comes, you'll have the same shot as anyone else at achieving your goals. What you are experiencing now is real, justified and extremely common, and you need to be kind to yourself and get through it. It will pass.

How to get an abortion

If you are against abortion in principle, you should probably skip past this section. You are perfectly entitled to believe in whatever it is you believe in, to feel however it is you feel, provided your feelings don't impact on the freedoms of others. In soap operas and science lessons, women get pregnant and just have their babies, however unwanted. In real life, people make mistakes and civilised societies give them options. Your doctor will not shout at you, and if you're a British citizen, you will not have to beg, borrow or steal to pay for a safe termination. Yes, it's undesirable, will be uncomfortable and can be traumatic; no, you will not necessarily regret it for the rest of your life (the same should be taught of divorce).

258

On a personal level, I know that women can have abortions they don't regret because I'm one of them. I had a termination at nineteen years old, with the help of the Brook Advisory Service and my GP. I hadn't been raped, I wasn't suicidal, my life was not at risk in the physiological sense. My pregnancy occurred through foolishness, the irresponsibility of quite a messed-up teenager alone in London. But as stupid and reckless as I was in getting pregnant, what I did afterwards was one of the most responsible and considered decisions of my entire life. Instead of feeling guilty for the state of my young life back then, I feel proud that I chose to put it into some kind of order before subjecting an innocent human to my complete and utter inability to mother – either practically or emotionally – at that time. I'm relieved to have made a correct decision that gave me, and later on my children, the opportunity for a happy, stable and productive life. I feel certain I did the right thing, and grateful to live in a country where I was treated with kindness and respect at every step. I didn't feel terrible afterwards, only shaken, crampy and a whole lot wiser. I cried, I would have preferred it not to have happened, but I was, and am, just fine.

I think very rarely about it, in all honesty. My experience is pretty common throughout my social group, but I'm certainly not disputing that some women are more adversely affected by their decision to terminate a pregnancy. But feeling sad and conflicted about a past abortion is not the same as guilt, and feeling guilty over an abortion is not the same as regretting one. And none of these emotions are any justification for making women feel worse by lecturing them or, heaven forbid, standing outside a medical clinic and harassing them on an already shitty day.

Besides, making abortion illegal and punitive doesn't stop it happening, not for a minute. The abortion rate is roughly the same in countries where it is 'unavailable' as it is in countries where it's available. Banning terminations does not prevent significant numbers of women from having an abortion – it just makes obtaining a safe one extremely expensive, difficult and even more emotionally charged. In Britain (though not in the wider UK), our laws are progressive, if always under threat. Procedures and best practices are in place for women of all ages to access the health services they need and be treated by calm, qualified professionals allowed to deliver their services in comparative peace. If you find yourself in need of them, there are a few things to consider:

Call for help

The first step is to contact the British Pregnancy Advisory Service (BPAS) – who act on behalf of the NHS – or your GP, family planning clinic, Brook Advisory Centre or, if you prefer, a private clinic. Unless you are seeking an abortion for urgent medical reasons, you will be given an appointment at a later date. They will talk you through your options and help you complete the necessary paperwork and obtain doctors' signatures.

Act quickly

Terminations are legal in Britain until twenty-four weeks gestation, but very few take place this late. If you know you are pregnant (it's always worth keeping a record of your cycle, whether marking day one in your diary or using a tracking app), are sure about your decision, and are able to move swiftly, it is very much worth doing so. Very many early terminations that have missed the cut-off for the 'Morning After Pill', can now take place 'medically', i.e. in the privacy, comfort and security of your own home, via prescribed medication. This removes all manner of aspects of the experience that can make an already unwanted day grimmer. For example, you won't have to travel (NHS medication can be sent to your home address), or arrange for someone to collect you (more on that below), deal with any unwelcome demonstrators and leafleters outside the clinic, be among strangers, or spend time in a clinical setting when most craving the familiarity of your own bed. However, all this depends on knowing your situation early (at-home terminations mostly need to take place before ten weeks gestation). Medical terminations still take place regularly after ten weeks, but will usually require a visit to a clinic and a follow-up appointment.

What to expect from a medical termination

After giving the appropriate consent, you will usually be given a tablet called mifepristone to take orally. This will end the pregnancy. A day or so later, you will take another medication, misoprostol, which is a synthetic form of prostaglandin. This is inserted as a pessary into the vagina, and effectively causes a miscarriage. You will probably be required to repeat the medication a few hours later, but always listen carefully to your dispensing medic's individual advice. If you're at home, you should make yourself comfortable. If you're at a clinic, you will usually be permitted to leave as soon as you've taken your first medication. Side-effects from the procedure vary and can range from normal period-pain-type sensations to more extreme cramping, diarrhoea, nausea and headaches, but they don't usually persist for more than a day or two. You will certainly bleed, passing heavier blood and clots than a period. You may feel okay, but it's nonetheless important you take the time to rest as best you can, and allow your body and mind to recuperate. However you feel about your decision – and any feeling is perfectly valid – a termination is a significant event for your body and probably your mind too, so allow yourself to properly recover.

It's important to note that any medication carries risk and can sometimes fail. If the medical abortion does not work (there's over a 90 per cent chance it will), or you have second thoughts, a pregnancy cannot safely continue after it has been administered, and a surgical abortion will need to take place.

What to expect from a surgical termination

All abortions were surgical when I had mine and although I would have very much preferred the option of a medical termination, whether in a clinic or at home in my own bed, I will say that it was not, for me, traumatic. Surgical abortions are still necessary in many cases and while there are always risks associated with any procedure, you should not be frightened. Most terminations carried out this way now take place under local anaesthetic or sedation, but sometimes general anaesthetic is required in more complex cases or when a termination takes place past fifteen weeks gestation. A surgical termination will be either by 'vacuum aspiration' (suction) under local anaesthetic or sedation for pregnancies between ten and fifteen weeks gestation, or if the pregnancy is further on, by dilation and evacuation procedure carried out under general anaesthetic. For the former, you will usually go home soon afterwards; in the latter case, you may (though not always) be kept in hospital overnight.

Should you take someone to an abortion?

Honestly, the short answer is yes. I attended my abortion alone. It was not by choice, but I thought it would be okay since I'm a fairly private and self-sufficient person. In fact, it was really not very nice to wake up alone and explain (falsely, so they'd let me go) that my lift was waiting outside because there was nowhere handy to park. A trusted and non-judgemental friend, relative or partner to sit at your side, then accompany you home and fill a hot water bottle, chat, make some soup, hug or watch a film with you will make a difficult day easier and a memory better, regardless of how capable you know yourself to be. Just because we can do things alone, doesn't mean we should, or that we deserve to.

What should you have ready?

Provided you've been given no other medication or advice to the contrary, it's a good idea to have ibuprofen to hand, for any cramping. You will bleed, so have plenty of sanitary towels (rather than tampons, cups and period pants) both at the clinic and back at home. Have something convenient to eat so you don't need to exert yourself to cook. Most of all, have a clear diary for the following day at least. Finally, have future contraception. Clinics will usually insist you have a plan before leaving. Put it into action, whether by laying in a supply of pills and condoms, or making an appointment to get a coil or cap fitted, or an injection administered, at a date in the near future.

261

How to breastfeed

From the time a woman conceives, she is inundated with information on the imperative to breastfeed. Every baby magazine, every medical professional, every midwife and NCT group tells mums – quite rightly – that breast is best and that six months of feeding your baby represents the healthiest start. We get it. The problem lies in how, in practice, we do it. Breastfeeding is not always 'easy' for women and babies. In fact, it was very difficult for the vast majority of my friends, many of whom felt so guilty and under pressure to breastfeed that their first months with their beloved child were tinged with anxiety, shame and great sorrow. In my experience, women don't need any convincing that breast is best. They are more likely to need convincing that they are still good mothers if, at six, eight, or even twenty weeks in, they stop spending every waking hour electronically pumping milk, crying and feeling like a failure, and reach for the formula and bottle.

In fact, the biggest problem with breastfeeding is not persuading anyone to do it, but properly teaching them how. Breastfeeding is a skill. It doesn't come naturally and blissfully to all women the moment they're handed a lovely baby, and yet this is what's often expected. Breastfeeds with my eldest child were so fraught that he'd spend most of the time screaming in frustration. Desperate to fulfil what I saw as my responsibility to breastfeed, I went to Sure Start groups, the La Leche League, three midwives, a celebrity lactation consultant who spent almost her full hour telling me my baby was merely traumatised by his decidedly unscary five-hour home birth, then the rest of the time counting her £150 payment. We were wrongly diagnosed with tongue-tie (this seems to be the stock lazy answer whenever anyone has no idea what the hell is going wrong but wants to give a desperate mother something she can cling to), colic, cranial problems, insufficient milk, too much milk – everything but the actual problem. Round and round we went, in a depressing cycle of guilt, pumping, bottle-feeding breastmilk, more guilt. I spent way more time on feeding admin than I did on enjoying my baby. I was heartbroken.

Meanwhile, all the well-meaning professionals patted me on the back and said, 'You're doing really well! Don't give up!' Except, a) I really wasn't, and b) I really should have. What I wanted and needed was a strict, clever nana type to tell me exactly what was going on and how to fix it, or, failing that, why I should throw in the towel and get my life back (I lasted six miserable months). This wisdom is exactly what I got from godlike feeding guru Clare Byam Cook (Clarebyam-cook.co.uk) when I had my second baby, who diagnosed overactive letdown (where milk is expelled too fast and furiously, like when one stands on a hosepipe) within about two minutes of meeting me and fixed the problem that very day (with a week of breast shields, which everyone else had assured me were evil). She told me to ignore all the advice about placing nose to nipple and to just

262

'As with so many things, when it comes to feeding their babies, women are damned if they do and damned if they don't.'

squidge my boob into the more manageable shape of a doughnut. I went on to breastfeed extremely happily for the next seventeen months.

But getting your baby to latch on is only the beginning. Those lucky enough to crack the technique then have to contend with judgement on the other side – waiters handing them a napkin to cover up feeds, shop staff 'politely suggesting' women feed their babies in a grotty customer loo (would you want to eat your lunch in a toilet? No, me neither), idiots tweeting that public breastfeeding is no different to Page 3 (yes, this really happened – I gasped when hundreds of people, a high-profile journalist among them, retweeted it). Men who would cheerfully gawp at sexy boobs in a paper or magazine, but suddenly feel 'uncomfortable' on seeing breasts do the job for which they were actually designed. As with so many things, when it comes to feeding their babies, women are damned if they do and damned if they don't.

I'm genuinely pleased that two out of a dozen or so girlfriends avoided these pitfalls and managed to hit the breastfeeding jackpot and enjoy a textbook experience feeding all of their children. I know from personal experience that when breastfeeding works, it is wonderful. But for everyone else, it can be unbearably hard. Many women will give up, not because they think breast isn't healthier, not because they're not aware of the benefits to themselves. But because they are exhausted, they are depressed, their baby is underweight, or they are desperate to stop spending every waking hour worrying about this one thing that absolutely does not define you as a mother. There are a million other ways to bond and to show your love. If attempted breastfeeding is consistently making you sad, then it is not serving your baby, and you should feel no shame in reaching for the formula. It's an act of kindness to the whole family. And don't let anyone, however well meaning, tell you any different.

Is it postnatal depression?

Almost sixteen years ago, I was standing in a warm London kitchen, preparing dinner, my freshly bathed, massaged and carefully pyjamaed five-month-old baby sleeping soundly in his cot downstairs. My very nice husband came home from work and found me chopping mushrooms in a steady, efficient rhythm, and kissed me on the head, entirely unaware that I'd spent the previous fifteen minutes wondering idly how long, if I were to seriously cut myself, would it take for me to bleed out, and

264

whether this would mean the baby would be left alone for a worryingly long spell. I was not actually suicidal, but the resigned, dispassionate nature of this internal monologue scared the life out of me, and I realised I couldn't safely take another day of pretending (a week previously, I'd calmly declared I was going to retrain as a barista for reasons even I didn't understand). I placed the knife down on the board, looked my husband square in the eye, and said firmly, 'I am going mad. I promise I am definitely going absolutely mad and I need help.'

I wasn't exaggerating. The one and only thing clear to me was that I genuinely felt insane. Since the birth of my much-wanted baby, and the death of my father just a few weeks later, my life had felt like an interminable movie I was watching from behind a thick sheet of tracing paper. I did all the stuff I was supposed to do – the stuff I had been looking forward to doing: the baby's nappies were changed regularly, the surplus breastmilk was pumped and frozen during his naps, the shopping was put away, the house remained relatively clean. But I myself was drowning, not in the workload, but in a disorientating tidal wave of grief, boredom and regret. First came the fear of meeting other mums, in case they could 'see' I was really bad at this (I now know almost all new mothers think this). I would keep the curtains closed all day, every day, scared that someone might spot me through the window and try to pop in for a cuppa. I never answered the doorbell without first checking the peephole for the postman. Weeks would go by without me and the baby going any further than our back garden, and yet at weekends, in the company of others, I was the life and soul.

I was horribly lonely and isolated (I was the first in my friendship group to have kids – it's amazing how instantly the invitations drop off), and yet I couldn't bring myself to pick up the ringing phone. During these days (so long ago that social media didn't exist as we know it), I stayed in my pyjamas, eating too much, flicking through magazines, consumed with jealousy and sadness for those still in an office producing them. I'd finally get dressed and made up just an hour before my husband came home in the evening, then lie about what I'd been doing. Gradually, my condition worsened and I developed extreme paranoia. I became convinced that if I left the house, I'd be mugged or attacked, or my house would be burgled. If I walked the dog, she would be stolen and I'd be unable to leave the pram to run after her abductors. I thought my husband was going to die if he popped out for so much as a paper on a Sunday morning. I cried constantly in private, and yet publicly I couldn't convince anyone that I was anything but fabulous.

Clearly, I had a very bad case of postnatal depression. But I hesitate to say that because I'm not sure the term is helpful, or even begins to do it justice. Certainly, the euphemistic colloquialism 'baby blues' should be put in a lead box and booted off Brighton Pier. Because PND is really just depression, and when I say 'just', I actually mean real, deep, scary, lonely, hopeless, debilitating and seemingly unending sorrow that can have a horrible effect on the entire family, but especially on the mother at its helm. For some, it is dangerous and life-threatening (mercifully, I never had an urge to hurt or abandon my child – though I quite understand those who have what must be terrifying thoughts of that nature), others may feel safe but are consumed by an unprecedented level of sadness, loneliness or anxiety that robs them of their quality of life and, temporarily, of their relationship with their baby.

What is unique about postnatal depression is that it's an affliction that strikes at the exact time when the world thinks women should be at their very happiest, their most in love with life and those around them, at a time when they're starting a new job – the one job in the world where no training is given, and that comes with a zero holiday or sickness leave contract. I felt bereft of the job I was good at, the people I worked with, the adult conversation and the confidence boost of a task well done. I felt useless, lacking and ashamed that I had woefully miscast myself in a role that was supposed to make me feel the most satisfied and enriched I'd ever been. I felt guilty that I was unable to enjoy my lovely, healthy and adored baby when he was relying on me, and when so many women struggled to conceive one of their own. I look back and feel guilty that I'm no longer sure who I was grieving for more acutely – my dead dad or the old me.

But I was fortunate. I was able to recognise my need for professional help. The one tiny upside to my bereaved state was that I had a small inheritance to at least begin to pay for emergency psychotherapy that, over the course of two and a half years, gradually led me into recovery. Many women are much less fortunate and get neither the help nor the understanding they need.

The pain and the mental isolation of postnatal depression can easily cause women to decide not to chance another baby in case the worst happens again. One woman I know has barely had sex since her last child was born five years ago, another decided with her husband to opt for a vasectomy – to them, surgery seemed like a walk in the park compared to the threat of another eighteen months of fear, panic, tears and grave marital instability. But however a mother copes, it's important to remember that while any depression – postnatal or otherwise – is real and terrifying, it always, always comes to an end. It gradually lifts. My relationship with my eldest son is as happy and adoring as that with my youngest, with whom I mercifully didn't suffer at all, and I truly love being their mother.

I wouldn't dare tell anyone how to 'cure' their own PND, because there is no silver bullet to fix the problem. But I will say, for me, recovery came via a combination of one huge decision to get therapy, and a million small ones: opening the curtains, going for a three-minute walk around the block, deleting my card details from dozens of websites where I constantly self-medicated with things I neither needed nor really wanted. And perhaps most importantly, the act of saying 'I am completely bloody mad and I can no longer cope'. It's hard and shaming to effectively shoot down the myth of magic motherhood and say, 'Actually, this is quite shit. I am quite shit,' or even, as I did, 'I am going absolutely mad.' But I know from experience that to say it is the very opposite of bad parenting. In putting your own happiness first, in ensuring that you don't endanger your life or your family's stability, you are loving and caring for your child in a way that is nothing short of heroic. Forget the veg-puréeing and the baby-signing. This is what good mothering really is.

267

Life &
Finances

'It's the extremely satisfying knowledge that you can change a plug, replace a fuse, make a roast and a lump-free gravy, and could probably survive on a desert island by utilising the well-planned contents of your handbag.'

If I'm really honest with myself, my proudest achievement in life – or at least, my most unexpected accomplishment – is my ability to be a functioning adult, having transitioned from childhood prematurely and with zero training for the job. My assumption, based on my upbringing and several adult episodes of financial mismanagement, was that I always would be useless at balancing the books. Like lots of people at the time, I grew up in a house with 50p coin meters fitted to the back of the television and at the fuse box. When the coins timed out, the electricity cut out until fed another. Later on, and with coin meters outmoded, our gas, electricity and phone were billed and consequently cut off quite often. I'd come in from school, flick the light switch and . . . nothing. I never asked why it wasn't working. I instinctively knew the bill hadn't been paid and we'd just have to wait until payday for light. Similarly, food. We'd have vast quantities of delicious things for a week, and then nothing at all for the next three. Lunch money would fail to materialise, and so from the ages of seven to eleven I bought two white baps each morning for 16p from the local bakery, to eat at school and make my pocket money go further, then gorged my grandparents out of house and home at weekends. This general sense of chaos, organisational apathy and dysfunctional feast or famine was all I knew and how I always expected life to be.

And it was for a while. I lived mainly off plain pasta and potatoes for at least three years in London and struggled to fix an abode. It can be hard for anyone to acquire adult life skills, but it strikes me that those who've never seen adults adulting particularly well are ironically in a similar boat as those who've been so well looked after as to have been denied the incentive to learn the basics – paying bills, avoiding debt, being properly insured, progressing at work, booking holidays, packing a suitcase or keeping on top of internet passwords and so on. Too little or too much parenting both cost the child in adulthood. It took me a long time to reset the dials and while the carbohydrate addiction remains, I've become relatively good at managing my life, work and finances.

I can't stress enough that when I talk about finances, I'm not talking about income. It's infinitely harder to manage money when there isn't enough of it to pay for the bare essentials, never mind for anything on top. But it's also true that many people who earn plenty of money find themselves penniless each month because they are unable to manage their expenditure and debt.

I'm as far from a financial expert as one could imagine (if you're looking for proper grown-up money and investment advice, my cupboard is bare. Instead, I recommend *Black Girl Finance: Let's Talk Money* by Selina Flavius and *Clever Girl Finance: Ditch debt, save money and build real wealth* by Bola Sokunbi), and I wouldn't know how to buy a single share if my life depended on it. What little I can claim is that I am organised and fiscally responsible out of fear of ruin. I pay my bills because I can't bear to ever be cut off again and I pay my taxes on time not only because it's the right thing to do, but also because I believe I will certainly go to jail if I don't. My house's loo paper supply is never allowed to deplete to fewer than thirty-six rolls and I do the work I'm paid for because I assume that otherwise I will end up out on the street – no man, bank balance or position will ever quell that instinctive sense of instability, and I'm not sure that's as bad a thing as it sounds. With no real training, I am pretty good at being a grown-up because all I ever wanted was to become one.

The novelty has yet to wear off. The practicalities of adulthood are occasionally tough (literally no one enjoys opening windowed brown envelopes), but where others see financial responsibility, I also see delicious fiscal autonomy. Learning how to do stuff for oneself is empowering. From filing your receipts and complaining about bad service to changing a tyre and checking on an elderly neighbour, we learn how the world does and doesn't work, how to treat people and expect to be treated in return. You make do and you learn fast. Paying off a debt alone can create a huge sense of accomplishment, and nothing feels as wonderful as the first car you buy yourself. Meanwhile, 'Oh, I get my dad to sort out my insurance!' might seem like a winsome affectation for a thirty-five-year-old, but the grim truth is that those parents or more worldly-wise friends to whom you cede responsibility for the grown-up stuff won't always be around – in some cases, by choice. And until you get to grips with adult tasks, you won't appreciate the simple satisfaction of having changed your gas supplier or successfully looked after a spider plant. You'll also look like a bit of a dick. Of course, it's not all about money. Adulthood is about deciding how you want to live your life, whether that means adopting a dog without needing permission, inviting whoever you like to stay, having full command of the remote or deciding to fry chips at 3 a.m. It's the extremely satisfying knowledge that you can change a plug, replace a fuse, make a roast and a lump-free gravy, and could probably survive on a desert island by utilising the well-planned contents of your handbag.

These are just some of the things I had to learn, very often the hard way, while growing up far too quickly. But crucially, I'm still learning. I've been scrappy and combative online, when the flip-closure of a laptop was a healthier response; I spent decades in the wrong mortgage. Life is an amorphous thing and its admin changes with it. Priorities, income, circumstances change with our needs and wants. And so some of these things won't be at all useful to you, others may come in handy in five years. Some things may seem so obvious to you as to be laughable, but may be handily gathered to shove under the nose of someone who has yet to grasp the nettly responsibilities of adulthood, and must learn that it's high time to do so.

What to take to a festival

A weather-appropriate tent
In warm, dry weather, a pop-up tent will generally do, but in unpredictable weather (in the UK, especially), you'll need a proper, pegs-in-the-ground tent with decent protection from the sun, wind and rain. Whichever tent you buy, BRING IT HOME AT THE END OF THE WEEKEND. Leaving your tent for someone else to deal with is environmentally irresponsible and rude. If you no longer want your tent, donate it to a homeless or refugee charity.

Sleeping bag
The tapered mummy-type ones are cosier than the rectangular variety, which let in draughts. You don't need an expensive one fit for an Arctic expedition if reclining briefly, half-pissed, in Reading.

Inflatable mattress or lily (plus foot pump to inflate)
A thin layer of air beneath your sleeping bag makes an enormous difference to comfort and sleep quality, and the mattress can be rolled up tightly when deflated. Again, take it home.

274

Spork
A double-ended spoon and fork. It saves you having to use environmentally unfriendly disposable cutlery and can be rinsed easily at the water fountains.

Groundsheet
Many tents come with integrated ones, but it's useful to have a small one to fold up and carry around, so you can sit on it and relax in the arenas without getting your bum wet. This also saves you from having to bring a folding camp chair, which is always a huge pain to carry through crowds.

Torch
The pitiful light of a phone isn't enough to find your way back to your tent. Maglites are the best – you get lots of light from a small unit.

Wellies or other waterproof boots
Lace-up hiking boots are easier to remove without dirtying your hands, and are less sweaty in hot weather. Wellies are easier to hose down, so take your pick.

Phone and portable charger
One with at least three charges' worth is ideal. If you're prone to losing your phone, consider spending a tenner on an entry-level pay-as-you-go handset for festivals only.

At least one roll of loo paper – preferably two
They won't live on a holder, so squish them flat.

Antibacterial cleaning wipes for Portaloos
Even if you plan to hover (do plan to hover).

Biodegradable wet wipes for hands and face
I like those by Simple, but baby wipes will do.

Hand sanitiser
Carry it everywhere.

A properly waterproof coat with hood
Ideally one from a company that specialises in rainwear, rather than a mainstream fashion company making nice anoraks.

A couple of old carrier bags
In case of wet and muddy clothes.

Sun-protecting hat
Essential. Naked sun and booze can make you feel sufficiently ill to miss a whole day of music.

Two pairs of socks for each day (in case of wet or muddy feet)
A fresh pair of evening socks when showering facilities are scant can be almost orgasmic.

A warm sweatshirt that can be wrapped around your waist when it gets hot
One with a hood gives you an in-built groundsheet for your face.

Tights or thermal leggings
Even at the hottest Glastonbury, I still end up needing to layer some opaques under my shorts in the evening.

Belt bag/bumbag
One needs to be secure and hands free.

Reusable aluminium water bottle

Glass probably won't be allowed through security and you can keep refilling from water fountains onsite.

A backpack

Never bring a wheelie suitcase. It won't wheel through mud and soft soil and you'll end up carrying it across site. I see very unhappy-looking people do this every year.

High-protection sunscreen

Try to pack a large one for morning dousing, and a mini to carry around.

Essential toiletries

Toothbrush, toothpaste, cleanser, deodorant, dry shampoo, insect repellent, tampons, minimal makeup if worn and so on.

A microfibre towel

These fold up much smaller than a regular terry towel, and absorb more water post-shower. I use Aquis.

Apple AirTags

Optional but incredibly useful. These allow you to always find your tent (and anything else with a tag in it), however dark it is, or however drunk or far away you are, just by looking at your phone.

Earplugs

For when you're ready for bed but others aren't.

Debit cards

Debit cards and some (but not a ruinous amount of if lost) cash.

Sunglasses

At least one pair and ideally not designer unless you can cope with them falling off at a crowded gig and being trampled upon.

Essential medication

Plus a few painkillers, cystitis treatment and some Imodium (just in case) placed in a waterproof sandwich bag.

Parking ticket

I once arrived at Glastonbury having entirely forgotten to book my parking ticket. It cost me two hours and all the good spaces before it was sorted. Get this done in advance.

Your ticket
Heaps of people forget this.

Don't bring

Playsuit
I will never understand why these are so popular at festivals. I guarantee its hemline will end up soaking up floor-wee.

Suitcases
See above. They will not wheel through mud.

Thick clothing layers
These take up acres of packing space and can't be adapted as the weather changes.

Glass bottles

Anything suede
A useless material at the best of times, but inevitably destroyed on a festival site, whatever the weather.

Native American headdresses, Indian subcontinental or Southeast Asian bindis
Unless you are Native American, or from Indian or Southeast Asian culture. People's cultural heritages are not a cute fancy dress opportunity for Instagram.

Super-precious jewellery and watches

iPad
Especially if you plan to drive everyone in your vicinity mad by holding it up to film an entire Chemical Brothers set, when there's a BBC camera crew already streaming it live to the nation. Yes, I am still bitter.

How to remember countless passwords

Passwords were once the bane of my life. Here's a method for composing them which is honestly a lot less complicated than it looks – and once you've got the hang of it, it'll allow you to have a different password for every website you visit without having to write down or commit to memory a single one.

You're going to start by coming up with a key. This bit will be the same in every password you use. I suggest you make it at least eight characters long and incorporate in it those pesky requirements: an upper case letter, a number and a special character. Some sites require them, some don't, so if they're present in your key, you can forget about coming up with them. The key could be based on anything personal. Avoid common security question answers; think a bit laterally. Let's say you pick your first address after you left home, I don't know – 83 Acorn Drive. Let's say your landlady there was called Marge. Condense that to 83ADMarge. Bung a special character in the middle – how about a left bracket? (Exclamation marks are a bit route one, aren't they?) So: 83AD(Marge becomes your key. That's going to appear in all your passwords and once you've set up a few it'll become second nature.

Next, we personalise the password to each website, based on the website name. You need a rule that will govern how you do this, and this is up to you. Let's say you take the first two letters in the site name, swap them and between them insert the number of letters in the website name plus two. I know, I know, but honestly, once you settle on a rule and do it a few times, it's easy. So, in this case, say you're devising a password for Amazon. Swap the first two letters – 'am' becomes 'ma' (make everything lower case for consistency, because you know you've already covered any upper case requirement in your key) and insert between them the number of letters in 'Amazon' plus two. So 'ma' becomes 'm8a'. eBay becomes 'b6e', Lovehoney becomes 'o11l'. Whatever floats your boat.

Now add your key to this bespoke prefix. So add the 83AD(Marge key to m8a and, hey presto, your Amazon password is: m8a83AD(Marge – which, let's be honest, is a bit more secure than 'Password', isn't it? Your eBay password is b6e83AD(Marge. For Pinterest it would be i11p83AD(Marge and so on.

The beauty of the system is that every website you visit will have a complex, unique password. As long as you remember your key (repetition will massively help) and your rule, you're golden. You may have to decide with a site like Theaa.com whether you take 'theaa' or 'aa' as the site name, but as long as you're consistent, it shouldn't be a problem.

How to queue at the supermarket

Choose the checkout with the massive, full trolley everyone is avoiding. The steady rhythm of scanning a large number of items is actually quicker than the stop-start of multiple customers with one basket each. Invariably, it's the chatting and muddling around for purses and loyalty cards that slows the checkout process. Multiply it by three or four and it'll take longer than one Mum BigShop.

How to split finances and money with your partner

A 2018 survey by solicitors Slater & Gordon identified money worries as the leading cause of marital breakdown. Differing financial priorities and approaches to spending and saving invariably strain a relationship, so once yours reaches the communal expenses stage, it's wise to have a fair and transparent system in place.

Add up all your bills and shared expenses and split them down the middle. Then agree on an adjustment for any imbalance in your income (if one of you earns vastly more than the other, a fifty-fifty split is palpably not fair). Allocate direct debits accordingly, or open a new bank account and arrange for your individual accounts to pay into it. Do not under any circumstances surrender your own bank account for a joint one. You must protect your credit rating and financial independence for the future. However idyllic your relationship – and long may it remain so – keeping a 'running away fund' is a sound policy, not just practically but psychologically.

279

How to stay sane on the internet

This may seem very much like a case of physician, heal thyself, since progress on this book halted no fewer than three times as I sought professional therapy and treatments for mental health issues caused by online defamation and abuse.

Online upset most commonly prompts nice, sympathetic people to shrug and say 'just ignore it', and although that appears insensitive and simplistic, in the end I'm afraid it's true that the only aspect of online animosity that a subject can control, to any degree, is the management of one's reaction to it.

Social media has been so transformative that most of us are still getting to grips with our relationships with it, but the learning curve has been huge already. Here's what I've learned:

What to do if someone on social media consistently makes you feel angry, uncomfortable, resentful or sad

I cannot stress this enough: go through your social media follow list now and unfollow or mute anyone who – for whatever reason – grinds your gears. 'Hate-following' – that is, following someone purely because you dislike what they have to say – is bad for everyone involved. Bad for you because you are knowingly and deliberately triggering a negative reaction – either internal or external – in yourself towards others; and bad for them because it's mean-spirited and, frankly, indicates a problem in the follower, not the followed, who is simply being themselves (or, as is much more likely, a tiny part of themselves) online. No one has to like anyone; no one can be liked by everyone; it is normal to be turned off by some personalities. It's also normal to express one's displeasure privately to friends. Where it gets weird is in the wholly voluntary decision to share virtual space with someone you can't stand, purely to snark at them or about them in a public space. And everyone – including me – has done it, to some degree (Donald Trump's Twitter follower count was proof enough). But no more. Life is finite. Hate-following is like forcing yourself to live in Alaska, then moaning relentlessly about the cold.

Mute

I do this often. Muting allows you to become oblivious to anything the muted account posts, either widely or specifically to you. It's effectively the act of inserting your AirPods as someone shouts or simply chatters in your face as you try to walk to work in peace. I sometimes mute people I like, usually temporarily and not necessarily for negative reasons, but because I'm not personally invested in a subject (Wordle, the Superbowl, diets, Mother's Day). I also mute people I don't especially like but have to be polite to because they are spouses, relatives or colleagues of friends I encounter in real life. Muting works just as well for the perpetually argumentative too. If you're not in the mood (and I rarely am nowadays), and they don't take the hint, let them shout into the abyss while you watch penguins playing on slides.

'Hate-following is like forcing yourself to live in Alaska, then moaning relentlessly about the cold.'

Don't respond

The hardest act of all, but the most worthwhile – and it took me years to realise. For most of my life online, I've had the pleasure of speaking with thousands of interesting, opinionated, funny and smart people from every walk of life. They have challenged my thinking and opened my eyes to other perspectives or causes. A number of them have moved from Twitter and become a big part of my real-world life (including my own husband). But I've also encountered a significant minority of nasty, threatening, scary and wilfully troublemaking people. Whether bored obsessives or ill-tempered opportunists, all internet users acting in bad faith have one objective: to get a reaction. And we have all done it, to some degree or other. Some people insult or publicly drag others for wider audience approval (retweeting a deliberately controversial Piers Morgan tweet, say, with a withering prefix), others make a direct attack on their quarry in the hope of receiving a reply from the wounded party. And when we feel wronged or attacked, it's almost unbearably tempting to compose a full and forensic rebuttal. I've done it a million times. But the only person it will ultimately satisfy is your aggressor, who not only knows they have your attention, but also that of a gathering crowd. Appearing not to have noticed them lets a fire burn out, and although that may feel frustrating at the time, believe me when I say you'll feel fantastic in the morning.

282

Value the good guys

A famous TV celebrity once told me that she'd one morning realised, while being roasted by someone on Twitter, that she spent about 90 per cent of her time online dealing with a tiny minority of miserable sods. She was so distracted by their snarky comments and insults that she was rewarding bad faith from trolls while ignoring interesting, positive people with manners. This is an extremely easy trap to fall into, which ultimately makes us complicit in the toxic business model of social media platforms: drama pays. Her observation rang true. After that, I made a point of responding positively to at least five nice people for every one acting in bad faith. Within a few months, I was almost always ignoring the latter. Most people are nice. Engaging more with the majority is life-enhancing, worthwhile and gives much-needed perspective to the online experience.

Ask yourself: is your anger indiscriminate?

Most internet trolls start from a position of hating someone, then they retrofit everything their hate figure says to fuel the villainous narrative.

Something X says passes without comment, while the same thing said by Y will be twisted and manipulated and served to reinforce every prejudice held against him. Again, it's important to realise we all have the capacity to treat others this unequally. People we like are given a pass; people we hate are closely scrutinised and dragged over the coals. True, some people may have already made their bed so badly that it's hard subsequently to take any seemingly right-thinking pronouncements at face value. Nevertheless, it is healthy to notice when we react less to what was said than to who said it.

Is your anger proportionate?

When someone says something on social media that makes me cross, I now think, 'Why am I following someone who makes me feel this way?' and either mute or unfollow, depending on how I answer the next question: 'Is my anger actually about me and how I'm feeling today, and not about some stranger's tweet?' Let's be real: there is hardly ever any need to become properly furious at a social media post. If we feel that way, it's overwhelmingly likely that we're really furious about something else.

Is your input necessary?

The belief that one's negative personal view of something must be known is a state of extreme arrogance and insensitivity. For years, I turned down, as a matter of course, any TV or radio show that invited me on to trash-talk some celebrity's makeup or frock. It struck me as hugely unhelpful and old-fashioned and, well, a bit grubby. And yet online and in relation to people on the telly, I'd act like it didn't matter and snark and bitch along with everyone else. Times have changed, but so too have people, I think. There is now an implicit belief that the online rules of engagement are different to those in real life.

Do you realise you're talking to a person?

A couple of years ago, a journalist I'd only met once found herself in the middle of a Twitter storm when a column she'd written about plus-sized women went viral, justifiably angering many. Thousands of negative retweets ensued. Having read the piece and broadly agreed that it was an unhelpful one, I unthinkingly retweeted someone else's negative analysis of it. I thought no more about it until a couple of months later, when the journalist wrote a follow-up column about how she had struggled with body image issues her whole life and understood, with the benefit of hindsight, that she'd written the column during a bout of mental unwellness and extreme self-criticism. She described how the resulting onslaught had felt, how it still affected her. Now, I'm certainly not saying that voicing one's dismay over a published tweet or column is trolling or deliberately unkind (it happens every week to every journalist, myself included. It goes with the job and is perfectly fine). People are free to openly dislike whatever they read, of course. But what I am saying is that in the rush to join the chorus of disapproval over some tweet, TV show, article or podcast, it's extremely easy to forget that behind the tagged account is a person with feelings, a family, and the same emotions and capacity for mental disquiet as anyone else. That event in particular, though nowhere near the first like it, changed forever how I view viral events online. I wrote to the columnist, apologised for my retweet (she hadn't noticed it because there were so many thousands of them) and decided there and then that I'd never have cause to send another. I took the view that it just wasn't necessary to voice my negative opinion when voices are already so numerous as to be overwhelming and mob-like – especially when it added to the sheer awfulness of another human's experience that day, week or month. These things frequently do.

It is fine to disagree

I'm both sorry and relieved to say that being on either end of an online argument is essentially pointless. There is neither the requisite inclination nor the character limit to engage in nuanced, helpful debate online. Tone of voice can't be heard, facial expression can't be seen, the sense of humanity is lost and so only anger and frustration at the inherent wrongness of an avatar remains. I may be incorrect, but fourteen or so years in, I believe quite strongly that people very, very rarely change their minds about issues that are important to them because someone online challenged them. I also believe that strangers don't need to agree or meet any consensus. I don't expect everyone to share my politics because I'm not fifteen years old. If someone is using intolerable hate speech then I'm extremely trigger-happy with the report button and it's satisfying to get multiple messages each week, informing me of the perpetrator's ban from a platform. But for everyday disagreements, it's fine to just say, 'Yes, I hear you. I don't agree and that's fine,' muting if necessary (often it's not). I do this a lot nowadays for the sake of my own mental health and it's game-changing. Reasonable people will take it at face value. Unreasonable people will feel furious at being stymied. Either way, your day is better for it.

Remember you curated your social media

Almost everything you see on social media is a result of the people and content you yourself chose to follow. If you hate what you see, then it's time for an audit and edit. Look for new people to follow who make you happier.

How to pack a suitcase

I was once a compulsive over-packer. Socially embarrassed and obsessive in my desire to fit in, I packed for every eventuality, dress code, weather and whim, and ended up looking ridiculous as I lugged a giant suitcase onto a coach or train for a simple weekend away. At least three-quarters of my clothing would go unworn and need to be unpacked and put away on my return, when I least felt like doing it. Many years recovered, I'm convinced that this sense of anxiety is what causes most people to overpack. Their unordered thoughts convince them they've forgotten something crucial (ever spot random items like a scarf or spare sunglasses on the way out of the door, then throw them into your already-packed travel bag, to be on the safe side? That was me, too). The secret is not to strive for a changed personality, but to take your time and be able to show yourself your methodical workings as proof that you really are packed. Here's how.

285

Make a list

Sounds obvious, but I don't mean some running shopping list of random stuff you might bring. Those almost always result in forgotten items. Instead, I always make a structured, timetabled, sectioned list that divides my trip – whether a mere business overnighter or long-haul holiday – into days, events and demands, and includes everything I'll need for each. It takes half an hour and saves hours of faffing and deliberating. For example, a day might include several hours on my feet (comfy shoes, a crossbody bag), a work dinner (a smarter top) and a steam room (swimsuit), so I subdivide that day's list into three. I include everything I will need for each, right down to the socks on my feet. Even when days are much of a muchness and the same items are duplicated often, I still list them separately wherever I plan to wear them, so that nothing gets forgotten. Finally, I make sections for non-clothing essentials, such as medication, charging cables, hair tools, period pants, a camera, laptop and so on.

Clear a workspace

Try to find a space you can commandeer in the days leading up to a trip. For a weekend away, a small tabletop is ideal. For a holiday, a sofa or bed – the point is to clear a space that isn't a suitcase, where all your items can be laid flat and remain visible. Gather all the items on your list and place them on the workspace, ticking them off the list as you go. Place them in category piles – tops, bottoms, underwear and so on. Having everything laid out separately like this heads off any anxieties about under-packing, and identifies areas in which you've visibly overdone it. Do this for as long as you can spare the space.

Be realistic

Following the list should keep you on the straight and narrow, but if you're someone who can't not throw in extras to be on the safe side, please consider the following: wherever you're going and however many pairs of shoes you pack, you will need (and probably wear) no more than two. If travelling somewhere warm, you will need no more than one thicker jumper or sweatshirt for your flights and chilly evenings. You absolutely will not change your nail colour mid-trip. You will not try a whole new eye makeup look for the first time. You will need two lipsticks, maximum – a nude and a red (if you wear it). If it's to be boiling hot, the last thing you'll want to do is blast your head with a hairdryer. Unless camping, you won't need to take towels. And remember that shops exist globally. If something is really that important in life, it will be available locally.

Some things you shouldn't forget

While sweating the superfluous, there are a number of essential or useful items that are often forgotten. It's easy to pack a great outfit for every eventuality and forget socks, a belt and hair ties altogether. Pyjamas, if worn, are similarly overlooked. Make sure you have a charger to match every electrical item (lots of gadgets, from portable speakers to cameras, share the same fitting so you may be able to double up). And pack a dirty laundry bag to keep any unworn clothes fresh.

Secure your toiletries

An exploded shampoo is the worst start or end to any holiday. Decant your liquids and lotions into smaller bottles and either sellotape or clingfilm the lids to contain possible leaks. Move any forbidden items, such as tweezers, razors and nail scissors, into your checked luggage pile to avoid confiscation at airport security. Any powder compacts such as bronzer can be protected from crumbling with the insertion of a cotton wool disc or two. If you're a flannel user (I never cleanse without one), pack a couple in a plastic sandwich bag so you can use one on the morning of departure without having to leave it behind (this is also useful for swimwear, since children always want to eke every last second's pleasure from the pool).

And roll...

When everything on your list is in your workspace, you're ready to pack. Starting with your clothing, lay each item flat, folding T-shirts and skirts inwards to form a narrow rectangle, and trousers or jeans down the middle, then roll the garment as tightly as possible into a sausage shape. Keep rolling the sausages, setting each aside on the bed. The only items that should not be rolled are shirts and collared dresses.

Pack smart

Pack your shoes in one side of your case (if you don't have shoe bags, place them in pairs, sole-down, in those free elasticated shower caps you get in hotel amenity kits – they're the best footwear protectors), along with your bulkier items like gadgets. Consider carrying your sweatshirt or jumper in hand luggage, since aeroplanes are invariably freezing. On the other side of the case, lay collared shirts across the case opening, the sleeves and tails hanging over the side of the case. Now take your sausage rolls and place them as tightly as you can on top of the shirts in the case. Arrange them, Tetris style, until everything is packed.

287

Fill all negative space

Suitcases aren't your only source of space. Sun hats maintain their shape and take up less room when stuffed with balled socks. Shoes can house deodorant, mosquito spray, playing cards, compact cameras, sun lotion (tape down the lid) or fans. Even underwired bra cups can store soft items like knickers or swimwear. Wherever there's a cavity, there's storage.

Wrap up

Bring the dangling arms of your shirts back into the case, draping over the pile of rolled clothing, as though giving them a hug. This is the best way to minimise creasing in transit.

> *Things to pack in a carry-on for flights:*
> - Passport, boarding pass and landing card
> - Antibacterial wipes and hand sanitiser
> - A jumper, sweatshirt or thin blanket
> - Wallet with payment cards and currency
> - Hair ties
> - A hydrating facial spritz or moisturiser
> - Water bottle (this will need filling after security)
> - Essential medication, even if you won't need it on the flight
> - A small cosmetics bag, if you wish to apply a little makeup before landing
> - Clean underwear, socks, T-shirt and travel toothbrush, in case your luggage doesn't land with you
> - Earbuds/headphones/AirPods
> - Book, e-book or magazine
> - Mints or gum to freshen up before landing
> - House keys
> - Anything very valuable that would be heartbreaking to lose, like jewellery
> - Laptop, tablet or anything else with a lithium-ion battery not allowed in checked luggage

288

A note on travelling with debit and credit cards

I did one trip to New York, where every purchase involved a declined transaction and an extremely expensive call (with waiting time) to the bank to get my card unblocked again, before the whole exhausting process began again. I spent at least 20 per cent of each day dealing pointlessly with a problem caused by nothing other than what my bank wrongly picked up as 'suspicious activity'. Since then, I haven't had a single issue, because as soon as I arrive at a UK airport to travel, I buy something small (gum, paracetamol, a magazine or similar) in an airport shop with each of the cards I plan to use abroad. This calms the paranoid bank algorithm and reassures it that it really is me – not my stolen details – on the move.

How to book a city break hotel

As useful as online hotel comparison and booking websites can be, if you are planning to stay in any major city for more than three nights, email the hotel direct. City hotel bookings are overwhelmingly for short breaks and business trips where full changeovers are frequent, and the rooms are priced accordingly. The reservations team will almost always knock off some money for a longer stay requiring less admin. I have never failed to get a significant discount in New York, and have usually paid less than even the comparison websites offered.

How to start a new job and feel useful

'Turn up, work hard, don't be a pain in the arse' – this could save whole terms of 'careers guidance' and is absolutely key to success in the early days of any career, regardless of job title, qualifications, experience and contacts. People give jobs to those who knuckle down and make life easier for everyone else. Do remember that no one accomplishes anything on the first day of a job. Instead of panicking that you don't look sufficiently industrious, spend the day emailing those with whom you'll be working closely and try to schedule a date where you might go to lunch together or grab a coffee to become better acquainted. Investing your time in unfamiliar people, rather than unfamiliar tasks, is almost always the most productive and ultimately constructive use of those first days. If you can financially afford to start a new job midweek, this can be very helpful. Five whole days in an alien environment is challenging, so if it can be broken up sooner with a weekend to gather your thoughts, that will set you up for a solid second week on the job.

289

How not to lose your temper

Plenty will make the argument (loudly, I expect) that losing one's temper is a healthy, positive act. But for whom? On the very rare occasions I've done it (I could count the instances on one hand), whatever release and righteous fury I've believed myself to be experiencing in the moment has quickly made way for regret, shame and remorse at how utterly pointless and needlessly upsetting the whole thing is for anyone present, myself included. If those you live with are equally as content with shouty confrontations, then great. Colour me repressed. But having grown up with an angry, shouty parent and lived, at times, with a couple of angry, shouty men, I can say from considerable experience that a mismatch of temperaments can be traumatic, anxiety-inducing and ultimately fatal to relationships – romantic, platonic and familial. Those living around a shouter can involuntarily enter a state of hypervigilance, where we tiptoe around issues in fear of triggering a tantrum. The commonly expressed belief that losing one's temper is a form of healthy honesty is wholly one-sided – the rest of us are inhibited from being our honest selves for fear of tampering with the internal wiring of a timebomb.

What is surely relatable for many of us is the occasional, deeply necessary, urge to let off steam. But there are ways of decompressing that don't involve other people at all. I'm a big believer in leaving the room (and preferably the house) and swearing blue murder in the car, a quiet spot in the park, a street where nobody knows me. But if and when trapped at home, make it clear that you are angry about a feeling, a mood, an event or a thing, not with a person. Stay on topic, being specific about offending behaviours rather than personal about someone's character. Explain your feelings, register your annoyance, make clear your desire for change and apology. But don't say something nasty. People all too often become frustrated with the rules of argument and just toss a grenade that cannot be un-thrown and, whatever the pre-existing goodwill on both sides, the relationship can't recover.

A final word on aggressively angry people. They get angrier. A new partner with a vicious temper is always a huge red flag. Don't ignore it, or assume that what is manageable today will always be so. Bad tempers have a habit of escalating, as the aggressor is emboldened and those on the receiving end try, frightened and intimidated, to become smaller and quieter to accommodate them. Boundaries stretch until no longer fit for purpose. Never stay with anyone who makes you believe that you are hard to love. If a partner's temper frightens or unnerves you once or twice, then try to imagine it appearing every week of your life. Then ask yourself if you could live with that, not the one-off your angry partner may in all sincerity believe it to be.

*'Never stay with anyone
who makes you believe
that you are hard to love.'*

How to ask for a pay rise

It's not easy asking for a pay rise; here are some useful pointers to bear in mind. Employers don't care that you have bills to pay, or a car to maintain, or extra mouths to feed. They need to hear why your specific work calls for more money, which duties you're effectively performing for free, how much money you're either saving, or bringing to, the business, what added value you're bringing to the role that would cost significantly more were another person in the job market to fill it. Be forensic, dispassionate and methodical and show clearly how you've come to your proposed salary increase figure. Then be prepared to negotiate.

How to arrive at a party

If you're attending the party of a close friend, arrive on time to lend a hand with last-minute arrangements, and to ameliorate any anxiety they'll usually have that no one will turn up. For all other parties, thirty to forty-five minutes after the start time is ideal, since there'll be no awkwardness and people won't yet be so drunk that you'll never be able to catch up. If the party venue is someone's home, bring a bottle and some ice. Ice is cheap and always the first thing to run out. Avoid bringing flowers as it forces your host to stop looking after the party and start trying to find (and worse still, clean) an appropriate vase.

How to be at a party

I'm a dreadful mingler and so I find this rule of three helps remove any guesswork and allay any guilt: introduce yourself to three new people or three small huddles of people, depending on your courage levels. Ask three (well-spaced, not machine gun-fired) questions and be interested in the answers. Stay for about three minutes per person before feeling perfectly polite in moving on. You may very well have relaxed and decided to stay longer, which is marvellous, but three minutes is respectable if you don't.

How to leave a party

When do you think, after an event, 'Thank god I stayed an extra hour'? I'm saying never. FOMO is almost always unwarranted. In leaving anything well before the end you actually miss nothing but the certain brutality of a hangover. Much more enjoyable to channel Anna Wintour and leave the party in full swing and in full command of your faculties. Long gone are the needy days of doing a full lap to say goodbye to everyone (note to anyone still in the zone: with the loveliest will in the world, people really, really don't care). Now I waste no time and make a 'French exit', just slipping away silently, because the thought of another drink and the 1 a.m. train home is never as appealing as a proper face cleanse and the opportunity to knock an episode of *Grand Designs* off the Sky planner. It propels me forwards and into a taxi, where, frankly, I can usually see what I'm missing on Instagram.

How to treat a friend to a meal

If you're treating someone special to lunch or dinner, open the menu and make a point of saying how delicious the most expensive thing on the menu sounds. Your companion will immediately relax in the knowledge that they can eat whatever they like (it's almost never the most expensive thing on the menu anyway).

How to be off sick

I love an occasional day spent indulgently under a blanket, fresh box of tissues resting on my boobs, a steady stream of hot tea and the unusually guiltless pleasure of a copy of *Closer* magazine to ease the suffering. It's when the more mindless the television, the more restorative its effects, and when three chapters of an easy book represents quite enough graft for one day. It's a time to feel self-compassion (and yes, some self-pity), to languish behind the firewall of an out of office, a rare opportunity to enjoy looking like total crap, wearing old pyjamas and a grubby ponytail, with a moustache of lip balm under a reddened nose.

Many people, of course, don't have the option of calling in sick and are forced to prioritise their professional commitments over their health. Employees with lousy contracts and few rights (often the poorest workers in society), as well as the self-employed – whether working as taxi drivers, journalists, designers, musicians or plumbers – will invariably lose income or at least significantly increase their workload should they take a necessary day off. I haven't been paid for a sick day in years, but at the same time, my greater flexibility means I could always dash to school more easily to collect a pukey child than many employees, who frequently have to face the sighs, tuts and pass-agg comments from unsympathetic bosses.

It's a reminder that calling in sick is a privilege that shouldn't be abused. Pretending to be ill when you're perfectly fine is often as stressful as facing an unwanted day at the office, and a sort of purgatory, where neither activity nor inactivity can be fully enjoyed. It's hard to relax while worrying about what your colleagues are thinking, how ill you need to appear tomorrow morning, whether you should wheeze through an essential Zoom call. Unless you plan to make like Ferris Bueller and tick through a bucket list, then there's no fun in it. The perfect sickie is one where you are almost, but not quite well enough to go in. Where you can get to the bath without crying, where your Heinz tomato soup stays down, where a hot water bottle soothes the not entirely unpleasant ache in your tummy, and where walking to the bus stop is impossible, but shuffling to the kettle is not. Under these circumstances, it should be enjoyed as the best kind of gift – one that you didn't ask for.

If the sickie is too frequent, or fails to hit the spot, then the problem is perhaps not your body, but your job. Instead of hiding from the problem in front of *Antiques Road Trip* and *The Karen Carpenter Story*, time may be better spent on unfiltered, uninterrupted, slightly feverish thoughts on what we really want. A girlfriend of mine realised, when lying on the sofa in a germ-infested dressing gown, that she was thoroughly miserable with her (now ex-) husband and instead of only alleviating the symptoms of her anxiety, stress and exhaustion, she also needed to address the root cause.

Even when all is well, sick days have a shelf life. The difference between cosy, blissful boredom and flat-out cabin fever can be a matter of hours. There's a moment you realise you haven't spoken to anyone in three days, that the house is a mess, that you've watched Australian customs officials confiscate one too many carrier bags of overripe fruit, and can no longer live with the smell of your own hair. In a flash, you're reminded that feeling un-useful, inactive and out of the loop is tiring in itself, and ultimately pretty depressing, and that the easier path is back to work.

How to speak publicly

I speak publicly for a living. The majority of my income comes from hosting live events and broadcasting on the radio, social media, podcasts and, very occasionally, the television. But it still sometimes makes me nervous. A few years ago, I was invited to address the Oxford Union. I accepted because I was flattered to be asked to do something so prestigious and because I

'I take the broad view
that if something
is scary, I should
probably do it.'

was immediately intimidated by an institution that had previously hosted world leaders, politicians, prominent activists and Hollywood icons, and I take the broad view that if something is scary, I should probably do it. Fast forward to the day itself and to me, sitting in my car, telling my husband that he must tell the Union secretary that I am wholly incapacitated by the failure of my perfectly functioning kidneys, or by an extreme attack of the asthma I don't have. It was very unlike me and I am forever grateful to Dan for telling me to piss off so I was forced to go ahead. So go ahead I did, only by leaving the dinner table while everyone else was eating pudding, and sitting on a lidded lavatory to completely rewrite my speech on the back of a fortuitously lengthy Muji receipt (thank god for three-for-two on socks). The moment the debate began, and a man began to say something about beauty that was absolutely reductive, patronising and untrue, my husband said he saw my eyes flicker in fury and instantly knew I'd be okay. There were other measures that got me through this, the most nervous I've been in my life, and it was good to be shaken from my relative complacency and reminded of their importance. These are, for me at least, the best ways to push through the fear and deliver a good presentation – whether a bridesmaid's speech, PowerPoint presentation, product demonstration or eulogy for the deceased.

Don't drink

Many occasions include a pre-event drinks reception. However nervous you feel, and however robust a drinker you believe yourself to be, do not accept a glass of anything alcoholic before you've done the hard bit. I accepted occasionally in the early days and although I probably got away with it, I would love to go back and say no, if only so I didn't mentally replay the tapes now and wonder if I sounded a tit. Even if you feel perfectly normal, alcohol always causes some disinhibition. Nobody wants to tell an unplanned anecdote to a roomful of people and have someone (inevitably) preserve it on voice memo for a later tweet. Booze also blunts the sharp corners of one's thinking. It causes most of us to end a sentence later than we should have, to drop the stitch of a thought we otherwise never would. I once interviewed someone who was definitely on the tipsy side and it changed my own habits forever. The only time I will now ever drink onstage is when the main interview is over and we've moved on to questions, purely because I think it makes the audience feel more relaxed and welcome in asking them.

Know your stuff

This really is three-quarters of the picture. Everything is so, so much easier, and people infinitely more confident, when the preparation has been done. Having been on several book tours, I can say that there is nothing more excruciating to watch than an interviewer attempting to bluff their way around the very apparent fact that they didn't read your book in advance. It is infinitely harder than just skim-reading the damn thing. Conversely, if I'm doing, say, a department store tour, where I colour-match hundreds of women to their perfect foundation, the fact that I know every Bobbi Brown shade like I know the nooks in my own house means that I feel almost invincible and the whole thing is enormous fun. Whatever the occasion, making it your business to know exactly what you're talking about will always, always make for a great speech and a much happier you.

Look good, but comfy

This is where serious business types will roll their eyes. I believe strongly that looking your best is an important part of presenting your best. I would no sooner go onstage with crap shoes as I would with a length of damp toilet paper attached to their sole – though nor would I wear pretty ones in which I couldn't confidently stride out from the wings. Clean, smoothed clothes, neat makeup (if you wear it) and styled, dry hair (I'm horrified by how commonly men and women go to work with wet locks) are all vital. But I also believe there's huge value in wearing something that just makes you feel great – a dress with a particularly flattering neckline, a belt that looks a bit special, a pair of earrings bought for a personally significant occasion. Whatever it is that gives you that edge, use it. I wore pearls and stilettos to the Oxford Union – I figured that at least if my speech died on its arse, the photos would not bring further shame on the family.

297

Rehearse

I'd be lying if I said I rehearse the events I work on, but I do think that if a presentation is super-important, or takes you out of your comfort zone, it is helpful to have a run-through. Get your kids, partner or dog to listen to you, or make a video on your phone and watch it back. Then do it once again, but no more unless you've made major changes, because over-rehearsal can make you inflexible and unnatural, to the point where just one unplanned word or sentence later can needlessly throw you off. Leave yourself space to improvise, to read the room on the day. A modest amount of rehearsal will give you a structure in which to comfortably enjoy yourself.

Don't have your phone onstage

I don't care if you're just reading from a document. Holding your phone and glancing at it even once onstage looks absolutely bloody awful. If you need notes (absolutely fine), make the effort to print them out on paper. I usually then cut my notes into discussion points and stick each onto a separate plain postcard, which I hold in a neat stack.

Laptops are also bad. I once attended an event hosted by a male celebrity who sat with his stickered computer open on his lap. It felt to me like an anxiety dream. No woman would ever have the confidence to look so sloppy and unprepared to a crowd of people – and quite rightly. The only exception to the no-tech-onstage rule is an iPad, since it looks roughly the same as a piece of paper, and a clicker for a PowerPoint presentation where appropriate. If you need more gadgetry than that, have it laid out on a separate table and approach it only when needed.

Be yourself

In my twenty-five-odd years' experience of interviewing celebrities, it's almost always been the case that the very best in the business (Claudia Winkleman or Andi Oliver, for instance) are the most authentically themselves. It's easier to say 'be yourself' than to hear it, I do understand. One doesn't want to start noticing every instinctive gesture, linguistic tic and habit. But what it does mean is avoiding adopting new ones that aren't you. Don't start using business speak that doesn't suit you, or expressions more common to other age groups, if they jar. Don't feel like you need to change your voice and accent unless you are a natural 'subconscious mimic' (a completely normal type of person whose gestures, voice modulations and accent automatically adapt to reflect those around them) – in which case, let it happen. The less you're thinking about doing things in a new way, the more you can focus on doing things well.

Know you deserve it

When I look back at the hideous, quite literally emetic, pre-show nerves of the Oxford Union, I think that at the root of my anxiety was some gut feeling that this wasn't 'for the likes of me'. It wasn't a conscious belief, but I think deep down, the fact that I left school at fourteen, didn't come from money and had never mixed with these sorts of people made me feel instinctively out of my depth. But here's the thing about imposter syndrome: all the evidence points at your being entirely qualified and entitled to do whatever it is other people invite you to do. I actually had more experience in the subject under discussion (the beauty industry) than anyone else in the chamber. The society knew this and just accepted it, so why shouldn't I? If you're asked to toast the bride, it's because she knows you know her the best and will not let her down. If you're asked to present the findings of your project, it's because you ran it. If you're asked to share your expertise, it's because you have it. So accept the invitation for the sincere compliment it is.

How to write a will and why you should

True story: I one night became absolutely furious about the woman who will marry my husband after I die and one day leave all of my extremely hard-earned money to her own children, not to the two sons for whom I've worked like a dog all these years. The fact that I'm not ill, my husband is several years my senior and the woman and her children don't exist is neither here nor there. Scenarios like this happen every day, often to grieving families who would never in a million years have expected such outrageous behaviour from an ostensibly decent person. Inheritance brings out the very worst in people. Everyone believes they are right, which is why we must remove from the process any ambiguity, speculation and third-party opinion.

299

If you read this heading and thought I was about to show you a nifty and cheap way to protect your children's or partner's inheritance, by downloading some DIY document from the internet, or spending a tenner on some ready-written 'will pack' at WHSmith, I'm going to disappoint you, but please bear with me. Yes, these things are available. Yes, they have doubtless served a purpose to many, and no, you won't be short of satisfied customer testimonials. But speaking as one of five siblings locked in a seemingly perpetual cycle of unravelling the knots of sheer fuckwittery of multiple, albeit beloved, dead relatives, I beg you to pay a small amount of money to a solicitor and get a proper will drawn up. The pain of an unclear will, an out-of-date will, an incomplete will, an unsigned will, or – worst of all – a non-existent will, is a tedious, extremely expensive, depressing, stressful and frustrating administrative task for those left behind to complete, often unsatisfactorily. It is a really terrible burden delivered at an already horrible time. The need for a will has nothing to do with being poor or rich – I have never been in a position where I stood to inherit even a tiny fortune. In reality, a will can make the difference between a pair of spectacles going to a loved one to whom they mean the world, or being thrown into a bin bag on the street. A will is about saving the bereaved from the infinite logistical complications and practicalities surrounding the estate of a person who has – like all people do at some point – died. The last thing your grieving friends, family or partner needs is a huge, complicated job that exists only because you didn't get around to doing a very simple one. If you don't take the precautions now, then whatever you'd like to happen when you're gone probably won't. Set aside £150–250 and make an appointment at your earliest convenience. Then make tweaks as life changes.

How to say 'No'

Kids are great at saying no, but instead of nurturing the impulse where appropriate, we scold and punish them out of it until they end up as adults, fearful of giving this perfectly reasonable and often highly necessary response. It's hard to undo, but we desperately need to find the confidence. No, I don't want you to touch me; no, I won't cover for you; no, I won't be giving you my number; no, I don't want to do you that favour; no, you can't come for Christmas; no, I can't take on any extra work; no, it's actually not okay; no, I'm not coming to the party; no, I can't/won't lend you the money; no, I didn't orgasm; NO NO NO NO N-O. A firm, clear, polite but negative response is among the greatest of all life skills and yet, still, most of us take decades to acquire it, because it makes us sound disagreeable and we're too scared that we won't be liked. It is an unavoidable truth that no one but, say, Julie Walters and David Attenborough, is liked by everyone, and not being liked is not a sign of an unpleasant person. Your 'No' requires no justification or even explanation. You need not grapple for reasons to explain why you said it. You can be polite and gracious and, if it makes you feel better, throw in a sorry, as in: 'I'm sorry, but no, I can't.' But there's no need to elaborate – the conversation is effectively over in one syllable, and that is plenty good enough.

How to tip

If you can afford to, it should be 10–15 per cent for servers, 10 per cent for taxi drivers. Three to five quid for your hair washer (depending where the salon is), 10–15 per cent for your hairdresser, beauty therapist or manicurist, unless they're the salon owner, in which case, none is expected unless they're a one-woman band.

How to get a cab to stop for you

If the pavement is crowded with cab seekers, walk further so the busiest traffic will reach you first. If you're in a large group, split in two (few drivers will want to pull over while you organise yourselves into batches according to who has keys, who lives near whom, who needs to stop at a shop and so on). Make sure you're not holding any food, drink or a cigarette – it will put off heaps of drivers who won't want any residual smell or spillage in their cabs. Walk in the direction of traffic towards your final location and outstretch your arm confidently, stepping forward to the edge of the pavement. Only ever climb into a licensed taxi with a proper light and number on the plate, door or partition. Or call a reputable company to avoid all the above. It is perfectly fine to say you'd rather not talk (I often say I need to listen to something for work – not that I'm obliged to explain myself), but if the conversation ever makes you feel at all uncomfortable, take a quick photo or make a note of the licence plate, which you'll find on the back seat, and WhatsApp it to a friend.

How to take a compliment

When someone pays you a compliment, do not say:
    'Oh I feel so scruffy/fat/tired-looking at the moment.'
    'Have you seen THIS though?' and point at a spot, graze or cold sore.
    'Ugh, I didn't know what to wear. I feel like I've worn this loads.'
    'I don't/I'm not, but bless you!'
    'Oh, it was dirt cheap in the sale!'
    'Really? I think I look terrible!'

However, do:
Take a moment to actually hear the words being spoken, smile and say:
    'Thank you very much!'

Try it. It is polite and makes the compliment-giver feel good about their decision to be nice. And with practice, it works on you, too. Try also to pay it forward – receiving a compliment reminds me that I should pay two myself that day.

301

How to not hold a grudge

I find it very hard to hold a grudge, though that makes it sound as though it's something I'm trying to work on. I'm not. As someone wise once said about lingering resentment and the decision not to forgive: it's like drinking poison and waiting for your enemy to become ill. I just don't see what practical benefits grudges offer the holder. You spend stacks of your time thinking about how cross you are with someone, while they skip through their life feeling happy and free. This doesn't seem remotely fair to the aggrieved party and so I mostly reject it out of hand.

I'm certainly not suggesting that you or I develop amnesia over any ill-treatment we receive. I log things mentally, always. As Maya Angelou so wisely said, when someone shows you who they are, believe them, and having had my fingers burnt, I rarely seek to resume closeness – especially when no apology appears. But I don't brood on it. Life is too short: while I need not tolerate these people in my own life, I am content to leave them to theirs and wish them well.

How to finish a book you're not enjoying

Don't. At this point in history, there is an inexhaustible supply of wonderful books. Just the classic novels still on my list will safely see me off to natural causes, before I even start on contemporary fiction, memoir and philosophy. I give fiction three chapters. If I'm not experiencing a state of flow by then, I now invariably take the view that dogged perseverance is eating up the time I could spend on loving another book. It's frustrating when everyone you know is so sure you'll love something and it leaves you cold (Barbara Pym, in my case – I can never keep up with who's who), but much more disheartening to struggle on. Pass it on and pick another.

How to put down your phone

Phone dependency may not be life-threatening, but I do worry that the digital revolution has caused us to become so used to getting everything we want, whenever we want it, we have forgotten that time is finite. That for every hour spent reading fake news, watching Vimeos or gazing at other people's avo smash on toast, all of which we will immediately forget, we are robbing ourselves of an hour's worth of real, meaningful memories. It needn't be thus. If you want to have a healthier relationship with your phone, there are a few simple steps you can take.

Recognise the problem

When you wake up in the morning, what do you do first – go for a pee, or check your smartphone? Is your last interaction before sleep with your partner, or a touchscreen? Ever zoned out of a conversation with someone who's made the effort to visit, while you side-eye messages and updates from someone you barely know? Ignored the pilot's airplane mode request until the second before take-off? Or later? And have you ever wondered how long a post-coital cuddle should acceptably last before you can pick up your phone again? These are classic signs of compulsive behaviour and dependency and shouldn't be shrugged off as part and parcel of twenty-first-century living.

Change your habits

- Apps are painstakingly designed to keep us on them for as long as possible, in order to gather our data and expose us to targeted advertising. Delete your most-used social apps so whenever you're tempted to use them, you have to decide if you can be bothered to log in on the websites. This acted as an extremely effective deterrent when I decided Twitter was negatively affecting my life.
- Disable notifications on WhatsApp and Messenger, and move these apps away from your home screen so the myriad colourful icons aren't constantly staring at you, pleading for attention.
- Download an app that tracks your phone use and sets offline targets (most people, I've realised, don't have the foggiest idea how heavy their phone use is. It's sobering data). Decide on realistic targets (in my case, two hours a day) – going cold turkey is impossible in this day and age.
- Plug in your phone away from the bed. Apart from rendering it harder to pointlessly scroll first thing after waking and last thing before sleep, it makes for a more effective morning alarm – one you actually have to get out of bed to switch off. I've read lots of experts suggesting you leave your phone downstairs, but knowing I couldn't call the police if I heard burglars, or pick up an urgent phone call in the middle of the night, means I'd never sleep, personally.
- Read newspapers only on your laptop, or in print form.
- Leave your phone in another room while watching TV.
- Never look at your phone while eating, especially if children are present. It's the worst manners and sets a really bad example.

303

Lead by example, not lectures

If you manage to make significant inroads into your phone usage, you should notice improved productivity and concentration, quite possibly better sleep and a brighter mood. But you'll also notice something else – just how much time everyone else is spending on their phones. When I first tackled my addiction, I quickly appreciated the extent of the problem around me. I once went for lunch and noticed that at one point, I was the only person around a table of six not on their phone. I became frustrated with my husband, who I'd constantly catch checking Twitter or football results when I thought we were watching TV. As I'd attempt to engage verbally with phone users, I was acutely aware of how distant I too must frequently have seemed – and how unkindly I would probably have taken to a telling-off. Understand that every adult in your orbit has to make the decision to put down the phone themselves. But by all means have a stern word when a friend or partner's phone becomes the third wheel in a joint activity, and don't make a secret of any progress you recognise in yourself. Letting them see how your experience has improved is perhaps the best persuasion you can offer.

304

Give yourself room

Like crash diets, total digital abstinence is neither healthy nor achievable. I wanted a lasting, meaningful change in habits. I made the decision to never scroll back through timelines if I could help it – to only look at what was in front of me when I had the time – and found that, actually, I was entirely FOMO-free. I didn't reinstall the apps, either, and my social media activity very happily plummeted back to what I'd describe as healthy levels of engagement. You don't have to throw your phone in a river. Just set reasonable limits, stick to them and control your use long enough to recognise the sharply diminishing returns of endless scrolling. It's embarrassing to admit phone addiction. But it's an admission that most of us, at some point, should make and many of us are identifying the need for change. Something to think about when, the second you finish this sentence, you pick up your phone to see if, during the last four minutes, Baby Animal Pics have updated their Twitter feed.

Where camera phones make life better

It's tempting to blame smartphones for the relentless intrusions of modern life – and I frequently do – but there are ways to use your omnipresent phone camera and photo albums for good. Always take pictures of the following:

- Your parked car in vast multi-storeys, including the marked floor and row numbers.
- Skin moles, in order to track any changes.
- Any paper receipts for expenses claims.
- Your location at a gig so your friends (or you) can find your spot. If at a large festival, this won't be enough (saying you're waiting at the veggie burger van is of no use when there are thirty of them). Better still, download the what3words app, which gives your friends your exact location, anywhere in the world.
- Cloakroom or dry-cleaning tickets.
- Post office receipts with vital tracking information.
- Complicated wiring behind the back of TVs or computers. When you unplug everything to redecorate or move house, you'll have a visual record of where each cable goes.
- E-tickets and Covid passports. Logging back into an app is time-consuming, and even impossible in a shaky wi-fi zone. Screengrabs require no connection and scan just as well.
- The licence number of taxis. I snap the interior licence plate of any late-night taxi and WhatsApp it to my husband or friends.
- Colours that appeal. If you see a vegetable, scarf or flower that would look great on your bathroom wall, snap it and save it for paint-shop-matching at a later date.
- Chargers. As soon as you open the box on a new electrical device, whether a camera, hair straightener or power pack, take a photo of the gadget, box and charger together, so you can identify the right lead later on.
- Baby scan photos. Sonographic photographs of unborn babies are printed on thermal paper and fade over time. Take a digital image of the print-out so it's never lost.
- A rented flat or car. Don't allow a landlord or car hire place to withhold any of your deposit by claiming you caused already present damage. Take plenty of timestamped pictures before moving in any of your stuff.
- Valuables. Insurance claims are faster, easier and fairer if you have a photographic record of your valuables in situ. Snap everything and send the files to a relative or friend offsite.

What to do with large credit card debt

I have one credit card with zero balance and I've currently no idea where it is. Fear prevents me from ever borrowing money again. It wasn't always thus. Miserable and chaotic while paying for my stressful and expensive divorce, and to raise two kids alone, I managed twelve years ago to rack up a fortune in credit card debt. I still shudder to remember the card company ringing me repeatedly at 4 a.m., demanding that my minimum monthly repayment (of interest only) be settled, having bounced again. Alone with two kids, I was charging petrol, solicitors, food, clothes – you name it – to a credit card I had at that time no hope of clearing. I will never do that again. There is nothing one can buy, nowhere one can go, that feels as good as being debt free. Mortgages aside, debt is suffocating, frightening and anxiety-inducing. It can make you feel guilty, hopeless and out of control. If your borrowing is making you feel this way, can I suggest you do the following:

1. If your credit rating still allows, apply for a 0-per-cent interest credit card. This interest rate will probably be fixed to a term of six, twelve or eighteen months and apply only to balance transfers rather than purchases. Choose the longest term you can get.

2. As soon as your new card is active, transfer all debt from older, interest-accruing cards, stopping any interest dead.

3. Keep the physical card somewhere safe, away from your computer and purse. If you have someone you can really trust (perhaps a parent), you could give it to them for safekeeping.

4. Do not ever, ever use the credit card in an ATM machine. Withdrawing cash with a credit card is among the most expensive ways to borrow money, triggering a hugely inflated interest rate. Use direct debit for bills such as rent and utilities, and debit cards or cash for essentials like groceries and bus fare.

5. When all your balance is transferred to the new card, you will have one predictable repayment to make each month. You absolutely must pay it to protect your 0-per-cent interest rate, and your credit rating, so set up your direct debit for payday. These repayments will be deducted in their entirety from your balance amount, so instead of constantly fighting the fire of interest, you'll see a monthly reduction in money owed.

6. You will likely need to speed up this process with as much over-payment as you can manage. Do not buy anything on credit. Return any unused items for refund and redirect the cash to your new card. Cancel any holidays – you won't enjoy them properly while in debt. Take your lunch to work, carry coffee in a flask, don't eat out or engage in expensive socialising. Sell non-essentials on eBay if worth some cash, then transfer your PayPal balance directly to your credit card.

7. If you've yet to hit zero when your 0-per-cent term expires, repeat steps one to six until it has. Remember that this process will only be possible if you've maintained your payments and are still eligible for credit, so protect that monthly repayment with your life.

If you can't obtain a 0-per-cent or low-interest credit card

If you are in good standing with your bank, you may be able to take out a loan. This will likely be cheaper than a credit card and will at least allow you to pay more than just interest each month. If the bank won't help, and you have no family members or loved ones able to step in with a loan, you will need to consider a debt management service. Before you become sucked in by Google ads offering debt resolution (these companies usually charge a fee you could be spending on debt repayments), do consult one of the many charities and services set up to help those living in debt. StepChange.org is one, but your local Citizens Advice Bureau will have more suggestions. The bureau staff deal with all sorts of people with debt every day and are experts who've seen it all. There is no need to be embarrassed.

Can you manifest wealth?

You will find hundreds of YouTube videos and too many self-help books suggesting that one can simply 'manifest' wealth and success by sticking up a mood board, chanting daily affirmations and wanting it enough. I find this stupid to the point of offensive, and am troubled by how many people are buying into what now appears to be a major online movement. People are not poor because they are not thinking positively enough. They are often born into poverty, unemployment or mental or physical ill health, or fell into it when a family member died, or needed full-time care, or they had to take an extended period off work. Positive thinking and a pretty collage of cruise liners and Cartier watches will not summon from the sky a large pot of cash and wild career success for people on any level of a wonky playing field, much less those at the lowest. Life is complicated and routinely unfair. Wealth is either inherited or acquired through different combinations of good luck and hard work. If 'manifestation' is merely a euphemism for the focus, positivity and drive required to exploit any luck and work towards your goals from wherever you start off, then fabulous. I believe it is helpful. But we must be honest about it to others and stop acting as though it's some faux-spiritual magic trick they've yet to master.

Some advice on overspending

If you're not overburdened by debt but still looking to shop more responsibly, these tips might help get you started.

Use debit cards
I believe that the true impact of spending can only really be felt by many of us when the spent funds are removed from our current accounts immediately, so I don't spend money on credit cards, ever. I say 'ever' when, in fact, I mean 'now'. The aforementioned credit card debt was enough to put me off them for life.

Do have a credit card somewhere

The only credit card I do have is somewhere in my house and never in my handbag unless I'm travelling and there might be an emergency – even then, I lock it in a hotel safe rather than taking it to the shops. If you're able to keep a credit card, it's useful for true emergencies and for maintaining and improving a credit score. Credit card companies will often cover your purchases against non-delivery, counterfeiting and the like, so are worth using when in doubt.

Pay in local currency
It's tempting to choose the 'pay in pounds' option while shopping abroad, but it is almost always more expensive than paying in local currency. Your bank will do the maths for you and the sterling amount will appear quickly on your banking app.

Don't apply for store cards
These are invariably very high-interest credit cards that somehow fool us into thinking they're something more fun that doesn't really count. I've no idea how they manage it, but resist at the cashwrap.

Know your danger zones

Almost everyone is more likely to spend at one time of day than they are at another. One of my friends has such a stressful job that she does the vast majority of her unnecessary spending during her lunch hour, as she attempts to self-soothe and wind down. I'm a night owl and so I was unsurprised, while going through my online shopping orders recently, to find that almost all of mine is done unthinkingly late at night. Knowing when your spending happens allows you to keep it under control. Now, if I'm scrolling past 10 p.m. and see something I like, my policy is to sleep on it and revisit in the morning, whereupon my desire has usually passed.

Engage in passive consumerism

Equestrian wear, mobility aids, toddler furniture, the kind of massive, ghastly pashmina wraps not seen outside of Fulham wine bars since 2001 – you name the catalogue, I'll pore over it, cuppa in one hand, Sharpie in the other. Catalogues from which I have no intention of shopping, but which arrive daily for my attention, soothe my soul. I can enjoy the at-home browsing without the expense. Might I actually have use for a banana isolator and grape scissors? How does that model feel about posing on a commode? These are the things I ask myself when I've spent days searching in vain for meaningful answers to infinitely more complex questions. Likewise, shopping-but-not-shopping online – the act of sating your impulses by filling your basket but never checking out (I've lost count of how many pairs of personalised Nike trainers I've designed, and I've barely run a yard in my life) is like window shopping without having to get on a bus.

Make your own coffee

It has now emerged that paper coffee cups are not, as we'd all assumed, recyclable (just one in a thousand is recycled because the plastic laminate on the cardboard is too hard to remove). And so all along, while I'd been turning my nose up at plastic bottled water, I'd been happily slurping a daily takeaway coffee and contributing to the problem. So I treated myself to a thermal cup from Bodum and now take a homemade cup of tea or coffee everywhere – to school, on the train, on dog walks or long car journeys. It's nice to feel I'm not contributing to landfill and gratifying to find my coffee is still hot, 100 miles later.

309

Takeaway savings account

I'm a renowned glutton, so the arrival of Deliveroo, Uber Eats and Just Eat – services that turned all my favourite restaurants into takeaway joints – seemed to answer my prayers. But as I crept, fatter and poorer, towards one particular New Year, I realised the honeymoon period between me and the overworked, overpedalled and underpaid delivery man was over. And so I decided that every time I craved a takeaway on a weeknight (my Friday-night curry is precious and has been ring-fenced), I open my bank account app instead of Deliveroo, immediately transfer £20 into my savings account, then decide what to cook.

How to buy a car

I love driving and always have. Cars, however, bore me to tears. Unlike all the men in my family, I have zero aptitude for mechanics, nor do I possess the most basic knowledge of motor cars. I just want one that works, has a decent stereo, is comfortable and doesn't cost too much to fill with petrol – and this sort of pains me, since I pride myself on being able to shop well for anything. For years, I'd just ask a big brother or a husband and do as I was told, but now I buy my cars with no input from anyone. For this, I have my friend, the consumer journalist Lesley Jones, to thank. She knows a frightening amount about cars and has taught me everything I know about shopping sensibly for new wheels, whether new or second-hand. And now I pass on her wisdom to you:

1. Go online and play on configurators, which will help you create your perfect version of the models you like and get a feel for your deal-breaker specifications. Do you need heaps of luggage space, child space, air conditioning, auto-transmission, a sunroof, an upgraded stereo? The possibilities are nearly endless and, as with a new house, something will have to give. What's a need-to-have and a nice-to-have? What's truly going to make your life easier and your drives more enjoyable?

2. If you're buying new, carwow.co.uk is a genius site that will log all your wants on a model, then link you with dealerships all over Britain that will fight for your business, sending direct messages detailing their best price. I bought my last car like this, on Lesley's advice, and would now never buy a new car any other way. I saved over £2,000. There's no need to go into a showroom and haggle if you don't want to. They'll even deliver the car to your door if you want them to.

3. If it's a second-hand car you're after, view all the YouTube videos and reviews you can of that model. These will give you a good idea of the must-have options, or identify the best model of your chosen car for your specific needs. Search on Autotrader.com, using their filter to add words to your search – 'sunroof', 'automatic', etc.

4. Private vendor listings on eBay, Gumtree and the like will typically be cheaper than the same car bought from a used-car dealership, but the latter may have guarantees and warranties for peace of mind that may be worth the extra to you.

5. If you see a bargain car advertised as Category A, B, N, S, C or D, it's been classified as damaged in some way, from a minor bump to a near write-off, and then repaired. Be wary of this and always get a second opinion from a mechanic, to ensure the work has been carried out properly and the car is neither unsafe nor a potential money pit in future.

6. Always ask around first before you start trawling sites. Sometimes a friend of a friend will come up trumps with a hardly driven gem their great-uncle is keen to let go. This has happened to me previously and if you're not dead set on a certain make or model, you can land a brilliant car that would ordinarily be snapped up in minutes.

7. Remember to factor in your insurance premium. You may be surprised to see what you can afford, but the four-figure insurance premium could suck all the joy from the drive.

8. Similarly, the bigger the engine, the bigger the yearly road tax and the insurance premium. Anything modified (for example, if a previous owner had the suspension lowered) is going to cost you, too.

9. Put all feminist principles aside when buying a car. If you can honestly say you have no idea about mechanics, engines and how to tell if it's in decent condition, just take someone along who genuinely does, even if it is a tyre-kicking mansplainer.

10. At the same time, don't imagine that the car world is still a man's one. Most dealerships have women on the sales team, all of whom will know their stuff. I bought my last car from a woman and can truly say that it made a positive difference to the whole process.

11. Think carefully about colour choice, especially when intending to resell somewhere down the line. Classic colours like red, charcoal, silver, navy and black will appeal to more buyers at resale than pink, yellow, orange or lime green. Also, do you really want to look at a vivid colour every single day? There's a good chance you'll tire of it.

How to avoid school reunions

I'd sooner die, but if you're wobbling guiltily on the brink of attending, remind yourself of the following:

If you liked them enough then, you'd know them now

I can think of little worse than travelling 200 miles for the privilege of hanging with people who at best don't remember me or at worst played a direct role in my desire to leg it out of school at the earliest possible opportunity. As an adult, I deliberately avoid women who remind me of schooldays, so why would I volunteer for a refresher course in the real thing? I now choose friends on the basis of shared worldview, values and sense of humour, not because we were once trapped together in a building that smelled strongly of feet.

It can be done virtually

I understand the universal desire to hark back to simpler times, to shared experiences and horror stories. But it needn't happen face to face. My husband is part of a growing WhatsApp group that now includes some twenty of his year-mates and lets him dip in and out of conversations at leisure, rather than sitting awkwardly at a formal dinner trying to identify the man engaging him in conversation by picturing him without a beard. I too get the occasional impulse to discuss memories of our pathetic riot and consequent imprisonment of a supply teacher in the geography cupboard, or the teacher who walked his cat on a lead. But I can do all this with my oldest friend, or one of the measly five school pals I've accepted on Facebook. I like them all but see no reason to sit with them in a pub, each of us mentally calculating who looks older and more out of shape than whom.

It no longer matters

Reunions can act as an exorcism of demons, I'm told. And perhaps there's an argument for taking away the power of bad memories by revisiting the scene of the crimes. I understand the temptation to go back, flicking the Vs. The guilty hope that the raving beauty who laughed repeatedly at your big ears has no remaining teeth, that the person who mockingly called you 'ginge' went on to have five redheaded kids who hate him, and that the teacher who said you'd never amount to anything is now hosing offal from a warehouse floor. But the rewards are fleeting. God knows what setbacks have since befallen them, and to engage in extreme levels of schadenfreude arguably makes you as much of a sneering arsehole as

312

those you left school to escape. For a formerly unhappy schoolgirl, the only outcome greater than success is the realisation that you simply no longer give a shit.

How to split bills

Add your chosen tip percentage (let's say 15 per cent for argument's sake) to the total and split equally between everyone. Anyone who starts snarking about someone else having eaten a side-dish or pudding they themselves didn't should not be invited next time. The only time one should make exceptions to this rule is when someone (e.g. a pregnant woman or recovering alcoholic) doesn't touch a drop of booze and the bar bill extends beyond an averagely priced bottle of wine – in which case, ask for a food bill and a booze bill and divide the latter only between the drinkers. Parents bringing children to an otherwise childless group should always make a gesture to acknowledge their increased spend, by throwing in an extra amount to roughly cover their additional cost (for god's sake, don't open the calculator app). All that said, if there is a significant mismatch in earnings within a friendship group, a choice of restaurant that is affordable for everyone is polite and correct. If a more affluent member of the group is particularly keen or insistent on a high-ticket eatery, then they should always treat the friends for whom it would otherwise be prohibitive, with the minimum of fuss and embarrassment.

313

How to avoid spoilers

I'm always curious as to how spoilers are so ruinous to TV viewers not engaged enough in a programme to catch up in a timely manner. Sure, some people work evenings and nights (been there), some have important social occasions or gig tickets they've been waiting months to use. We've all found ourselves in the unavoidable position of missing something we love and having to avoid all reports of it until we're safely in front of the box. But why is it everyone else's job to wait until you deign to settle in for Bread Week? Neither your schedule nor your social priorities are the rest of the country's business.

Nor, I'm afraid, is your social media compulsion. Even if you set up hashtag filters for unwanted updates on your favourite shows, the reality is that modern television is made for online discourse. This is not some matinee theatre performance of Agatha Christie's *The Mousetrap*. Big shows want, and need, to be shouted about. They have their own Twitter accounts, place hashtags in the bottom corner of the screen. Scenes are planned, plotted and written for the sole purpose of getting viewers to pick up their smartphones.

And when, as far as the spoiler police are concerned, would be an acceptable time for chat about something that has already aired? It's hard to know. A friend of mine was once roundly scolded for discussing the end of *The Sopranos*, which had been broadcast over a decade earlier. What next? Fury over the revelation that Den and Angie divorce, Scarlett O'Hara gets dumped and the sailors survive aboard the Battleship *Potemkin*? My husband and I once discovered a crucial upcoming *Breaking Bad* plot point, just by glancing into the window of a printed T-shirt shop. I was gutted but accept that the risk of revelation is the price paid when something looms large enough in the public consciousness to become a shared cultural event.

So if you really want to avoid spoilers, take a road-safety approach. Assume everyone else is a bad driver and that, as careful as you are, the only way to stay entirely protected is not to leave the house. Switch social media off until you can catch up – if that's not practical, then accept the risk. People simply don't have some sixth sense for when you're ready to watch the bloody telly. And speaking of *Sixth Sense*, Bruce Willis is a ghost. Don't tweet me.

How to have a relaxing Christmas

Almost half of us wish we could skip Christmas, reportedly. And not necessarily because of the expense, which I could understand, but because of the stress of celebrating, hosting or attending the festivities. As a Christmas obsessive, though, I can honestly say that the end of the year is my most relaxing period by far. Here's how I keep my blood pressure steady.

Skip the 'Christmas drink'
As a nation we have an unfathomable obsession with trying to see each of our friends before Christmas, to the point where our diaries are nose-to-tail engagements with people we can see at literally any other time of the year. Why? There's no more reason to stockpile drinks with friends than there is to buy enough groceries to feed the nation – everything will still

'Going out for a brief walk, even if only to the offie to score more Baileys, wakes up my brain.'

be there when it's all over. Instead, give your friends the gift of a night off this Christmas when, instead of constantly rushing off for a glass of wine in a bar full of braying corporate pissheads, they can go home and wrap presents bra-less in front of *Selling Sunset*. Save your get-togethers for January, when everyone is bored, skint and desperate for good cheer.

Christmas style: just say no

Each to her own, but Christmas is the one time of year when I absolutely cannot be bothered with fashion and beauty. The act of making an effort seems to be the very antithesis of the festive period's appeal. Besides, glitter is playing havoc with the sea (every time you wash it off, it goes down the plughole and, ultimately, into the ocean to harm aquatic life) and there's something a bit bleak about all those sparkly party dresses hanging sadly in the wardrobe post-NYE. Instead, I get out my cosiest jumpers, most festive red lipstick and team them with sheepskin slippers and a cheerful pinny. That said, I do treat myself to a pair of amazing pyjamas every Christmas, and justify the splurge on the basis that I'll be wearing them for at least twenty hours out of twenty-four. The point is that they feel quite posh, as though I've dressed up when I've actually done no such thing.

Move around

The best thing about Christmas, for me, is the lying under blankets in front of a terrible made-for-TV movie on Channel 5, motionless but for one arm moving in and out of the Ferrero Rocher caddy. But there are limits. I've learned that if I don't do at least some moving around every day, then without even realising it at first, I get sad and sluggish. Going out for a brief walk, even if only to the offie to score more Baileys, wakes up my brain, puts colour back in my cheeks and, most importantly, punctuates the day so the holiday doesn't blur into one continuous, over-too-soon veg-out session. Just the act of wrapping up warm and going to the pub or beach means I can come back in again with even greater appreciation for my sofa and slippers.

It's just a roast

If you can cook a roast, you can cook Christmas lunch, or dinner as it is in my case, because I never finish on time and don't feel in the least bit sorry about it. My graft, my pace. Likewise, I take the view that if I don't want to eat it, I don't have to make it. This means bread sauce (yes, that is wet bread and milk. For sociopaths) is bought from the supermarket, microwaved, decanted from plastic to china, covered in freshly ground black pepper and ground nutmeg, and plonked on the table. Also, cranberry sauce (yes, that is actual jam for meat) comes from the Colman's factory and you'll like it or lump it. Last Christmas I didn't bother with anything much traditional and made a porcini mushroom lasagne instead. Cooking the lunch is underrated. What seems like a chaotic sweatbox is actually a safe haven from moaning in-laws and racist uncles. Put on some music and leave them all to it.

Parties are optional

I'm here to tell you that, obligatory work dos aside, you absolutely do not have to attend Christmas parties if you don't want to. If you're really tired after a busy year, don't go. If you feel uncomfortable around any of the guests, don't go. If you're stressing about how much a cab will cost, don't go. I love a good party but if they're not fun for you, they have failed in their objective, and no one ever regrets a bubble bath and an early night with an audiobook (try Meryl Streep reading *Heartburn* for maximum pleasure).

Presents

Shopping for gifts is my favourite thing, but if it makes you panicky and anxious, rethink your whole strategy. Oxfam Unwrapped gifts (pig manure, anyone?) are fun, extremely quick to purchase online and so worthy that no one could ever complain. Vouchers are only boring if grabbed thoughtlessly at the Esso checkout. Vouchers from my favourite shop, Presentandcorrect.com, are as quick and easy to buy as Amazon's, and allow the recipient to spend the Christmas holidays porning over obscure stationery. Even Secret Santa is easy – go to a cheap tat shop and snap up the worst items a fiver can buy (one year my friend Nic bought me a Michael Gove mug). It's much funnier than attempting to be tasteful.

How to deal with a tight friend

We all have one. She or he is the one who gets in the first, memorable round and never goes near the bar again. The one who goes to the shop for a pint of milk and asks you to cough up the quid, who forgets every pound you've spent on them, but remembers every penny of their own outlay. They're the slowest to find their wallet, but the fastest to spring from a taxi. The only way to deal with them is swiftly. If someone is brilliant and fun and otherwise kind, but tighter than a pop sock on a marrow, then for the sake of the friendship, you must notice their tightness out loud, and with good humour, making it clear that you won't tolerate it. A smiley but incredulous, 'You want to split £1.50 for the parking? Surely you're joking?!' is the vibe we're after. A more direct, but still good-natured 'It's definitely your round, Rob' is also perfectly acceptable and fair. The straighter down the line you are, the better it will be in establishing healthy boundaries and laying down a code of conduct for the friendship. All of this is very different, of course, if someone is just broke. If you have a friend with very little money, you need to be either creative in finding very affordable things to do together (walks in the park followed by a cup of tea, for instance), or cheerfully generous in paying for pricier pastimes for you both. That's what friendship is.

How to turn forty

University – travel – career – cohabit – mortgage – marriage – babies (or whichever pick-and-mix version of this you happen to buy into) is not just a conventional pattern, it's a handrail through life that suddenly ends in middle age. At that point we are all on our own without a map, left to our own devices to seek continued happiness. The important thing is to keep developing, not just living. Here are some things to consider as your fifth decade looms:

Remember, this is their problem, not yours

Other people are a bit mad about the idea of turning forty, but don't let them project that onto you. Before my birthday, I went for a pre-party blow-dry. When I told the young female hairdresser I was about to turn forty, she gasped as though I'd just confessed to a case of the clap. Later, a taxi driver said, 'God – and you're celebrating?!' I'd heard countless similar comments in the preceding year (I'd been rather proudly saying I was 'almost forty' for a good eighteen months), to the point where I suppose I should have stopped owning up. But I refused to pretend, just because other people were weirded out by something that is an inevitability for everyone lucky enough to have survived their youth. Forty is an arbitrary figure that proves nothing other than you've been alive at least one day longer than when you were thirty-nine. You are about halfway through life and that is always cause to reflect. But to engage with the daft mystique of one number is to perpetuate it.

Let it go, let it go

This is an opportunity for a life audit. Things that are no longer important in your life: the charts, staying an extra hour at the party, substandard friends (there's not enough time to see the great ones as it is), pretty but uncomfortable clothes, having everyone you know agree on political issues, wooing people who don't like you, confronting friends who've upset you, amassing belongings for their own sake, whether or not people approve of who you fundamentally are. These can be replaced with things which become hugely important for the first time: having a proper pension, exercising, framing photographs you love, social occasions centred around sitting down, mates who'd help you dispose of a body if you needed to, holiday accommodation that's at least as nice as your own house, living in the moment, reliable thermostats, maintaining harmony in good relationships, good pillows.

Own it

You are now closer to old age than you are to childhood, so you can no longer blame your poor decisions, judgements and misfortunes on the relative crapness of your formative years. Your mistakes are now yours, not your parent's or teacher's. That's a tough pill to swallow, especially if you're not prepared. Therefore, if you've yet to start processing your childhood and past relationships, then it is now imperative that you do so. I know professional therapy can be woefully inaccessible to many (though if there's anything non-essential you currently spend your money on that could pay for it, I'd strongly recommend the switch – it will be your most worthwhile investment), but there are lots of online support groups and forums for specific issues, as well as dedicated charities. Whether you grew up around domestic violence, or suffered the loss of a sibling, or lived without a father, or are now considering living without your family at all, there is a community out there that understands and empathises with many of your feelings. Seek them out. Google credible psychology books and read voraciously on your issue. Get to know yourself properly, both as an adult approaching middle age, and as a child who may still be hurting. Being kind to the latter is essential in finding happiness as the former.

319

Enjoy not being fancied as much

Those who joke that no one will fancy you after forty are a little bit right, but missing the point. It turns out that many people see forty as some sort of attractiveness cut-off point, meaning they were never going to

'You may realise that being fancied has gradually become much less important and it will feel quite brilliant.'

be someone you could grow old with anyway. Your age acts as a handy filtration system for dickheads. They pretty much all stop noticing you. But what will emerge is a large number of good, divorced men and women embarking on round two, who know how to have relationships, how to iron their own shirts, how to have good sex with people old enough to remember Frankie Says Relax. You may realise that being fancied has gradually become much less important and it will feel quite brilliant.

Pay respect to your body

There's no way to sugarcoat it – your forty-year-old body is probably not what it was. You will no longer be able to lose half a stone between now and Saturday night by eating fewer crisps and more apples. Neither will you bounce back from hangovers – getting drunk on a weekend effectively means kicking Monday and Tuesday in the arse. You may get more headaches than before, enlarge the text on your Kindle for an easier life, and find eyeliner more challenging to put on slackening lids (embrace sexy and smudgy, rather than sharp and bold lines). You will occasionally look at old ladies with shopping bags on wheels and quietly wish Whistles would make them cool. You will consider joining a gym, realise everyone in them is about nine, and take up yoga on the living room floor. On the bright side, if your partner is male and over forty, he will have apparently zero ability to tell the difference between a size 8 and a size 14. You will feel utterly stupid about how disparaging and downright mean you were about your young body.

321

Bear in mind, the nines and ones are worse

A preoccupation with actually turning forty, as you may come to see in retrospect, is like entering an endurance event and obsessing over the starting gun. According to a major academic study in 2013, people of ages ending in nine are more likely to have an extra-marital affair or attempt suicide than those of other ages, including those ending in zero. It seems that the dread and perceived crisis of hitting the next round number is far worse than the reality. So any anticipatory fretting you're going through at thirty-nine may prove much worse than whatever actually happens once forty ticks around. Many of my friends found thirty-one, forty-one and fifty-one worse still. The year of celebrations ended, and they were metaphorically left in a messy party venue, wearing a wonky paper crown. Forty-one is unexceptional and marks the beginning of the journey towards fifty, and I do understand the feelings of deflation. But at that age, I found it essential to live in the moment – not in anticipation of the future one may or may not be lucky enough to see.

How to change your mind and allow others to change theirs

Appreciate the power of 'I don't know'

Many real-life conversations begin with 'I'm not sure' and yet on adversarial news shows and online the implication is that if one is sitting on the fence, then one must be ignorant and uninformed. In fact, the more you know, the less sure you feel about anything. It's usually nonsensical for anyone to come down hard on either side of almost any worthwhile debate. Conviction is admirable, but time and again we see that iron-clad certainty isn't really working.

Allow others to change their minds

In the 2020 documentary *Beastie Boys Story*, surviving members Adam Horovitz and Mike Diamond discuss the band's evolution from hard-partying frat-rats to thoughtful, socially conscious artists who make a point of calling out misogyny and inequality. Diamond recalls an incident when Horovitz was accused of being a hypocrite. His response was perfect: 'I'd rather be a hypocrite than the same person forever.' If someone who previously espoused a view with which we disagree then changes their mind, resist the temptation to catch them out, to embarrass them with the paper trail of their altered thinking. Welcome their ability to reflect and change rather than screaming 'hypocrite', and hope not only that you can display the same open-mindedness, but that others won't punish you with your erstwhile opinions when you do.

322

Saving properly

There are hundreds of proper, expert-led financial resources available online and in-person. You don't need advice on the big stuff from me, someone who unironically prefers fifty pence pieces to pound coins because they're more interesting-looking. But when it comes to saving, I will offer this advice: pay yourself first. Your earnings are split into two columns. Column A is for the non-negotiable essentials: housing, heating, water, food and travel to work. These need to be paid for in order for you to live your life. Column B is up for grabs, so who in that non-essential list should get paid first – the shop owner, the pub landlord, the taxi app developer, the pizza

'You will feel utterly
stupid about how
disparaging and
downright mean
you were about your
young body.'

place proprietor, the fashion company shareholder? None of them. You should. It's your money and you need to be paid before anyone else claims a bean. So pay what you can afford before any incidentals directly into a savings account, so that older, perhaps more well-off, perhaps less well-off, Future You can still pay for Column A. 'Trying to save' can feel too foggy a term to be motivating and effective. 'Pay yourself first' is clear, unequivocal and obvious when you think about it. So do it.

How to fail, and make the best of it

We live in a culture where failure is seen as something to be avoided at all costs. But just as children should get chickenpox and be allowed to play in mud so a bit of bacteria won't harm them later on, young women must experience small failures to ready themselves for the big stuff that can, and definitely will, go wrong. Frankly, it's a kindness to fail now. I've seen so many people who've only ever known a charmed, secure, smoothly run life go into full meltdown the moment even the tiniest thing has gone awry. Failure is not only inevitable, it's essential.

The only true failure is not to learn from it

Failure is the most powerful way to learn lessons, evaluate what it is you really do and don't want, and feel the incomparable sense of self-confidence in knowing you can pick yourself up off the floor, out of tear-sodden pyjamas and back into the world, harder and stronger than before. There's no use telling yourself never to fail, so see failure as an inevitable opportunity to make things right. It's a crucial life skill. Some are broken by failure and others make the best of it. A quick inventory of my closest girlfriends demonstrates that I can only truly be close to the latter type. All have messed up (rehab, bad relationships, work disasters, seen dissertations get pissed up a student bar wall), made the wrong decisions to dire consequences (unprotected sex on day eleven, choosing not to get contents insurance, an extra-marital affair) or just had really bad luck. But none of us has let it define us; we've all picked ourselves back up and vowed to do differently next time failure comes around – because we know it always will.

Fear of failure is far more debilitating than failure itself

Trying to avoid failing stops us from succeeding, because no worthwhile success comes without risk. It's invariably a case of the bigger the reward, the scarier the task. In denying ourselves the opportunity to fail, we're actually stopping ourselves from experiencing the pure, undiluted joy of

'Trying to avoid failing stops us from succeeding, because no worthwhile success comes without risk. It's invariably a case of the bigger the reward, the scarier the task.'

'I love a well-timed cancellation. The joy of hearing from a friend with what is clearly a matching disinclination to leave the house is pure and infinite.'

true success. Not to take the plunge is the biggest failure of all because we only regret the things we didn't do, not those we did.

Full-time failures are really tedious company

There is no one duller than a person who wangs on about life having dealt them a cruel hand. Seriously, these people are impossibly draining and so comfortable at their own pity party that repeat failure is not only a foregone conclusion, but also a lazy way of never aiming for success. Don't be that girl. In one year, my closest friend was made redundant, diagnosed with cancer, and bereaved when her partner was killed in a terrorist attack. And yet she still put herself directly in the line of failure to launch her own small business, because otherwise she wouldn't be living. Some failure is inevitable, but it's never the beginning and end of your story unless you allow it to be.

How to be bored

I revel in boredom and value its often unexpected productivity. The true state of boredom allows us to enter the recesses of the imagination, as if unearthing neglected toys at the back of the cupboard under the stairs. It's a mental colonic, clearing the way for new thoughts and ideas. I know that if I'm finding it difficult to concentrate, and painful to work, then I've probably not been allowing myself to be sufficiently bored in the preceding days. My brain isn't used to being left unattended; my synapses cluck for stimuli and prevent me from focusing, when I just need to turn down the noise for a bit, empty my mind, and re-alphabetise my spice cupboard. Conversely, avoiding boredom prevents us from ever truly being present in the moment and, if you'll forgive a rare display of hippy thinking, mindfulness is essential to happiness. If you're constantly distracted and stimulated, then how can you possibly enjoy the unadulterated here and now of your life? In obsessively seeking an exciting existence, we're neglecting the one we already have.

To me, boring is beautiful, a sublime state of grace. A day off without plan, expectation or forced stimulus is as good for the soul as fresh air, multivitamins or excursions to the Science Museum, and yet, it's the one childhood condition we parents are expected to feel guilty about inflicting on our young. When did it become law that children's weekends and holidays had to involve doing so much? Sporting activities, street dance, guitar lessons, expensive trips to theme parks, high-octane sessions at softplay, and barely veiled pressure to maintain academic momentum. In showering them with frenetic activity, we're depriving them of the imaginative self-reliance born from crashing boredom. It's as important a skill to master as the three Rs.

My mum and dad worked hard in an era – the 1980s – where, let's be honest, attentive parenting meant running the odd bath and plonking three edible meals on the table. Weeks of the holidays went by with nothing happening at all, bookended by the pouring of Coco Pops and the beginning of *Crossroads*. This almost continual boredom compelled me to cut up old Sunday supplements and catalogues and glue them into my own magazine. I got out my pens and drew, I read, I wrote stories, I opened pretend shops, made horrible things to eat, invented imaginary friends, made up dances and entire worlds with my big brothers (I once stayed all day in my bedroom, frozen in terror, because they told me a member of the IRA was in the living room, but still). My boredom sparked a career choice, a love of books and a lifelong obsession with film.

A love of boredom also has distinct social benefits. Having acquired this essential life skill, your kids will never be the restless person on an otherwise chilled holiday, fidgeting and moaning while everyone else dozes contentedly beneath a Jilly Cooper novel (there's no one more boring than someone who is constantly bored). They'll never see bad weather as some worst-case scenario in which nothing worthwhile is possible (handy in British summertime). They will know the unmitigated joy of a rained-off Saturday on the sofa, an empty library, the peaceful contemplation of long car journeys with only pylons to stare at, and the comforting, mindless construction of a thousand-piece jigsaw of Victorian Dorset. They'll know that life still glides smoothly along when the stabilisers of constant stimulation are removed, and that happiness comes from within yourself, not from those outside. They'll learn that there's always something nice to do. You just need to be thoroughly bored to work it out.

328

How to cancel

I love a well-timed cancellation. The joy of hearing from a friend with what is clearly a matching disinclination to leave the house is pure and infinite. To cancel something you know would be perfectly enjoyable can still feel like playing hooky, giving a gift to oneself, being afforded an unexpected moment of infinite possibility. But don't push it. Cancellations are not an excuse to abandon good manners. There are rules:

- Don't accept invitations you've no intention of honouring. Cancellations only work if you once truly planned to go. Stringing someone along is something else entirely. Wherever possible, if you know you're not going to go, say you can't go from the off.
- Don't delay. As soon as you know you won't make an engagement, cancel – or, at least plant the idea by alerting your companion that future cancellation is likely. People should always be given the chance to make more stable plans.
- Don't assume you won't be missed. This is a very common display of low self-esteem that, in practice, reads as arrogance. Never fail to show on the assumption no one will notice you're not there. They absolutely will. Contact your host in advance, or, if you really couldn't anticipate your cancellation, contact them immediately afterwards with an apology and explanation.
- However, do not text to cancel in the couple of hours before a party. It's an extremely stressful time for the host when they will receive what feels like everyone's cancellations, leaving them convinced that their party will be disastrous. Don't make it unnecessarily worse when it's too late to do anything about it.
- Don't cancel on someone who is newly separated and never, ever, ever those newly bereaved. A widowed friend of mine once told me that cancellations were the most devastating part of day-to-day life in the aftermath of his wife's premature death, that just a scheduled cup of tea with a friend, or a trip to the cinema, was very often the only thing getting him through the month. What is an insignificant engagement to one person is a lifeline for another. I've never forgotten it.
- Don't tell mad lies. You will either get busted or feel guilty. Faking cystitis, diarrhoea or something similarly low-level but temporarily debilitating is, I think, the furthest one can respectably go. Anything that sounds alarming, serious or involves older people or children is a no-go and ultimately bad karma, I think.
- Don't underestimate honesty. With the right friend, there is much to recommend saying, simply, 'I am so tired. I cannot be arsed,' or 'I'm so grumpy this week. I am really lousy company.' It saves time and is a feeling very often shared by the cancellee. It also affords you both the opportunity to change tack – I've seen many a night out become a very satisfying home visit and takeaway. Sometimes we don't want to cancel at all – we just want a rethink.

329

'There's no way to sugar-coat or intellectualise the simple fact that I can no longer be arsed. I like my house better.'

- Never cancel weddings unless unexpectedly taken ill. The fact that people don't turn up to weddings is astoundingly selfish. Space is almost always at a premium and any no-show has invariably been invited at the expense of another who could have come after all. It can cost upwards of £100 to accommodate a wedding guest, and so apart from leaving gaps in the table plan, failing to show results in significant financial losses to the couple.
- Make the delivery commensurate with the occasion. A text or WhatsApp cancellation is fine for a casual rendezvous with multiple people; a one-on-one date is more respectfully cancelled with a lengthier email or, better, a telephone call.
- Pay for your cancellation. If any costs are incurred (unused cinema tickets, for example), you must cover them.
- Don't take the piss. Repeat cancellers are a total pain and demonstrate a lack of care and respect for a friendship. Three consecutive cancellations would be enough for me to have stern words with someone.
- Put on your makeup. You will then probably want to go after all.

How to stay in

Something happened around my thirty-fifth year: I stopped wanting to go out. In crept a sort of mild social agoraphobia, where invitations to lovely events landed in my inbox and my heart immediately sank. Gradually, it's got worse. Very often I'll decline previously tempting offers and not waste everyone's time (I used to attend several gigs a month. Now I see two a year, at best). Sometimes I RSVP yes out of a sense of duty, then long for a cancellation; often I'll go because I genuinely know it'll be a great night with people I love. But increasingly, my instinct is to just stay in and make a nest on the sofa ... There's no fear, anxiety, or any other legitimate reason for my avoidance of social engagements. There's no way to sugar-coat or intellectualise the simple fact that I can no longer be arsed. I like my house better.

Give the gift of staying in
You may feel that as much of an obligation as it is to attend a friend's party, hosting your own is even more unavoidable. What would your besties think if you stayed in on your own birthday with your feet up? You know, I wouldn't worry. A few years back a friend decided that she was going to

celebrate her birthday by not throwing a party. I raised a glass from my bed and felt nothing but love for her kindness. By not attending someone else's bash, you give yourself a little gift. By not hosting your own, you spread that joy to every member of your exclusive list of non-attendees.

Especially on New Year's Eve

I am in no way a New Year's Eve pooh-pooher. I love to mark the calendar change with bubbles, snacks, the hugs and kisses of loved ones and, critically, the option to be in bed within an hour of the new year commencing. Frankly, once you've enjoyed the sensation of not being sandwiched into an overpriced venue or virtually inaccessible public space, of watching the fireworks on TV instead of wandering the city, stilettos in hand, desperately seeking a taxi, there's no going back.

A gentle concession to sociability is to offer a few local friends the option to see in the new year at your home – but make it a loose and open invitation, which crucially requires no RSVPing or excuse-making by anyone who is no more minded to traipse out pre-midnight than you are.

Don't underestimate the virtual meet-up

A legacy of the pandemic that I think will retain some value is the Zoom get-together. For me, the regular small-scale screen chat with friends is proving an enduring and rather lovely means of social engagement. The key here, I think, is numbers. Two to four faces on your screen makes for a relaxed evening during which everyone can share their news without fighting for attention. Bigger, though, is not better. The more friends squeezed into a single Zoom, the more chaotic and stressful the whole thing, and the more the dominant parties will leave the less vocal feeling marginalised. Remember that in a physical meeting, a big group will naturally devolve into smaller conversations – something a typical online meet-up will not allow.

... But also: go out

Clearly, the hermit's life is one I can't wholly indulge. I adore my friends and need to see them regularly to maintain my sanity. It resets the dials. And after all, if you never go out, you can't enjoy coming home again. Almost without fail, the most gratifying moment of my evening is the sense of achievement in having caught the 23:37 train home to Brighton (nicknamed 'The Nana Express' in my house). Coming a close second is texting my husband from the cab, the message often consisting of nothing but the teacup emoji, so I know a full one will be waiting as soon as my shoes have been kicked off in the hallway.

How to deal with unwanted gifts

I love buying presents more than I enjoy receiving them. My self-consciousness is such that for a long time I'd feel anxious about what to do with my face in response to any gift, even if I loved it. When I didn't, I'd put it away, retrieving it only when its giver visited. I very, very rarely do this now. Because money is precious; it's awful for someone to part with their hard-earned cash, only for their present to end up inside a plastic storage tub in the loft. The whole point of their financial sacrifice was to give you something nice that will be enjoyed. So now (as well as providing gift receipts with anything I give others), I say, 'Thank you so much. It's so generous of you to give me this. However, it's very similar to something I already own/it's too big/it's too small/I've seen it in another colour that would match my kitchen perfectly, and so could I possibly swap it for something I'll get heaps of use out of?' Post-swap, I then thank them specifically and genuinely for the replacement. It's the right and respectful thing to do, with one caveat: when a gift has cost little, but has been given with great thought and emotion, then smile, hug and keep it. Whether or not you like the item is neither here nor there. The real present is the love and thoughtfulness with which it was gifted. Enjoy it.

333

What to do if you receive a scary tax bill

It's a common occurrence in the fast-growing freelance community: an unexpected tax bill for an amount you're sure you don't owe, and you're even surer you can't pay. Please listen to the truest advice I can give: you must speak to the tax office at once. Ignore them and three things will certainly happen:

1. They will become annoyed and ever more insistent, and will be less reasonable when they finally catch up with you (and they will).
2. They will be wholly unable to help you find a more manageable way to pay what you actually owe.
3. Crucially, they will assume that their (often wildly inflated) calculations are correct, when they were only ever a jumping-off point, and proceed to base any future calculations on the wrong numbers, thus causing you a lifetime of identical headaches.

You absolutely must bite the bullet and call HMRC as soon as you possibly can. The bottom line is that tax officers are reasonable human beings who need to collect their money. They would sooner have it than not, and will generally work with you to find a realistic way forward, even if that means breaking down the amount into small instalments over a longish period. They can only do this if you let them in.

If you are self-employed and in the extremely fortunate position of turning over £85,000 per year, you must also register for VAT, add 20 per cent to any invoices, then hand that money over to the VAT office every quarter. I mention VAT here because, unlike income tax, there is none of the wiggle room described above. VAT is not your money and never was. You didn't earn it, only collected it on behalf of the government, and you must therefore pass it on, on time, no excuses. Any understanding and compassion extended by the self-assessment crew will never materialise from the VAT gang. I know from having lived briefly as flatmate to a man being hounded round the clock by HMRC that, truly, not paying your VAT is to open the gates of hell. You will rue the day you stole from them. Pay them.

How to buy a home, and get a mortgage

I've been lucky enough to buy my home after many years of renting, and although I don't believe home ownership is the be-all and end-all (Europeans don't understand the UK's obsession with it), it has, for me personally, been of immeasurable importance to my sense of stability and emotional security. After the people I love, there is nothing more important to me than my house. If home ownership is your goal, there are some things to consider.

- Rent will almost always be more expensive than a mortgage, but there are many more forgotten expenses that can tip the balance in the other direction. On top of the house price, you may have to pay for stamp duty, will certainly fork out for conveyancing fees, surveying, mortgage fees and more, which can reliably comprise up to 7 per cent of the house price. Plus estate agent fees if you're selling, too. New owners tend to spend around £5,000 on new goods – and that's before you factor in bills you may not currently pay as a renter, such as council tax and water rates. So make sure you see beyond the seductive rent-versus-mortgage figure.

- There are several types of mortgage. Trackers follow the Bank of England's interest rate; discounted mortgages offer a predictable, reduced repayment amount while you're setting up home. Some mortgages allow you to overpay if you're feeling flush, others don't but do let you switch to another offer within an agreed timeframe. The brilliant Moneysavingexpert.com, an independent financial adviser or decent building society will help you find one that works for your lifestyle, but even if you ignore all other else my strong advice is this: Do. Not. Get. An. Interest. Only. Mortgage – unless you have absolutely no other choice. However more manageable the lower monthly repayment sounds, however appealing your financial adviser makes it seem, however confident you are about coming into money later on, or in making serious equity on your property, just don't bite. Get a repayment mortgage that sees your balance dwindle, albeit by a very small amount, each month until you own your house in full. Interest-only mortgages require only that you pay the interest off your loan for the mortgage period (usually twenty-five years) then settle the true cost of the house at the end of the term, either using a repayment vehicle such as an endowment policy, or via some unknown means (ever found yourself with an unexpected six-figure sum? Me neither).

335

- What can you really afford? I would always try to stretch one's budget as much as is safe. What I mean by that is that if you can sacrifice some non-essential expenses to obtain a better flat or house with a slightly bigger mortgage, then this decision is likely to pay off. This absolutely does not mean living beyond your means and putting yourself at risk of failing to make mortgage repayments – nothing is worth that. It means that prioritising your home above socialising, holidays and shopping – at least in the beginning – is absolutely worth it, for the health of both your finances and your soul. After the people you love, nothing will have a greater impact on your emotional wellbeing than your home environment, so it's worth tightening your belt in other areas to get the right one. The more valuable your home, the more money you're likely to make in a rising market, and for most people income increases over time, so a property that feels a little out of reach will likely begin to feel more comfortable later on.

- What's your deposit? The single biggest obstacle to home ownership is the ability to secure a cash deposit. It's true and depressing that many young people are simply waiting for someone to die to make home ownership a possibility. Most mortgage companies will need buyers to contribute 10 per cent of the purchase price as a statement of intent and to protect lenders from future losses. Some lenders will agree to less, buyers wanting to rent out their future property will probably have to find more, so it's important to know exactly how much you'll need from the get-go. Remember that it's not possible to borrow money for a mortgage deposit from a bank or building society, so unless you have access to pots of ready cash, you'll need to tighten your belt and save for it. While you do that, take good care of your credit rating. Just one forgotten parking ticket can jeopardise your future home ownership, so be diligent in managing your bills.

- If you have a traditional and secure job, then congratulations. An increasing number of freelance workers make mortgages a little less straightforward. If you work for yourself, it is extremely important that you invoice your employers regularly (ideally monthly, like someone earning a salary) and keep all the paperwork to demonstrate the regularity of your payments. Have all your tax returns at the ready. A mortgage lender will want to see stability and reliability.

- Mortgages are chicken and egg. You can't get one till you've found a property, but you should get a 'mortgage in principle' offer from your lender. This lets you know what you can afford and puts you in a position to make an offer if the right property comes up. The offer in principle will be subject to surveys by a lender-approved surveyor. A basic valuation report is to reassure the lender that they'll be able to sell the property if it's ever repossessed. A fuller report will check the property more thoroughly, and is worth every penny if you're very keen to proceed. Whichever you choose, you will have to pay for these, whether or not the purchase goes ahead.

- Be nosy. Try to get under the skin of a property you're viewing. Try the taps and shower, because there are few things more miserable than trickly water pressure. Inspect any suspiciously fresh decoration – is it literally papering over the cracks of a shoddy building? Check behind furniture, under rugs, in gutters. Get the low-down on the boiler and find out when it was fitted. Ask about neighbours (sellers are legally obliged to tell you if they've lodged any complaints about them) and revisit the property at the busiest and noisiest time (such as when a local school finishes for the day, or when people are leaving for work in the morning) to see it at its least idyllic.

- What's it worth? Scotland has a different offer and bidding system to England and Wales, and buying a home at auction anywhere is different again, but however you reach your purchase price, always base it on how much similar homes in the area have sold for, not what they're asking for. This information is available easily online.
- Hire a conveyancing solicitor. They will check on all the things you can't readily access or understand, such as any proposed planning issues, or boundary rights. They'll also handle the transferring of funds between lender, you and your vendor, ensuring that everyone gets their money at the same time. Expect to spend at least £1,500, probably more, on your conveyancer and their various costs.
- Consider a removal company. Most people can move themselves into their first home, since they're likely to have accumulated fewer belongings. But if you have lots of stuff (I do), or items that are valuable, consider paying a removal company, who'll know exactly how to pack securely and will be insured properly against breakages or loss. They also move the right boxes into the right rooms, so all you need do is unpack at your own pace. I have only once moved with removal experts and I swore then that I would never again attempt it without them. They are worth every last penny.
- Know your exchange from your completion. In England and Wales, exchanging contracts means everyone is now legally bound by their agreement to complete the sale or purchase. This is the big moment. Until then, anyone can pull out of the buying chain, however unfair and costly their decision to others. Completion is the last and most exciting bit, when everyone gets their money and hands over the keys, and it usually happens on moving day.
- Get your utilities sorted in advance. Most traditional utility companies can now switch you on remotely on the day of arrival, though some will need to send an engineer to meet you at the property. Ironically, the exception to this rule is internet connection, which seems to take forever to become active, so make sure you've plenty of credit and hotspot facilities on your mobile phone.
- Clean everywhere. It's much easier before unpacking. Then choose one room to live and eat in. Spend the first day making that room cosy, assemble a usable bed and forget the rest for now. This allows you to unpack and arrange at your own pace, while offering sanctuary from chaos and preventing existential crises and absolute despair.

337

'There's nothing like noticing the same sequence of tracks you heard a couple of hours earlier cycling round again to abruptly remind you of your own mortality.'

How to compile a playlist

I love playlists and loved mixtapes before them, and frequently compile them as gifts. Knowing how to put together a playlist is a valuable life skill – I've DJ'd at friends' weddings, anniversaries and landmark birthdays and it's lovely to feel part of a celebration. In analogue days, there was but one rule of compilations: don't repeat an artist. Now, freed from the restrictions of a ninety-minute cassette, you have all the time you want. But that means more rules. Here are mine.

Keep it short

If it's an introduction to an artist or genre for a friend, keep it to an album's length. Forty-five minutes or so is ideal. If they're going to buy whatever you're selling, that's enough to get them interested. You might love those three alternate takes of an obscure early B-side and that seventeen-minute club mix, but the uninitiated just need the bangers. Or at least, the twelve to fifteen tracks you'd genuinely put on a 'best of'.

. . . Or make it long

On the other hand, if you're making a playlist for a party, make it long enough to be playing before the first guest arrives and still going by the time the sun's coming up over your empties-and-reveller-strewn patio. There's nothing like noticing the same sequence of tracks you heard a couple of hours earlier cycling round again to abruptly remind you of your own mortality. It's like the playlist is tapping its watch and reminding you about that 9.30 a.m. you've got with that woman from HR. Within such a long playlist, that old rule about no artist repeats goes out of the window – but try to avoid the same artist coming back within the hour.

Be vibe-appropriate

If your party playlist is soundtracking a kitchen disco, think in club-night terms. Start upbeat but modest – you don't want everyone danced out by 9 p.m. – and build to bangers. If you're planning more of a chatty, sit-down do, keep it backgroundy and not distracting, with ambient tunes. Resist the temptation to drop in a 'Hung Up' or 'Dancing On My Own' unless you want a row of restless legs on your sofa.

Mix up decades

Seventies New Wave into The Strokes, Amy Winehouse into Sixties soul – unless you're hosting a theme party, you can hurtle through time without your playlist jarring if you juxtapose things well, putting newer tracks alongside their influences, subtly phasing in and out of genres.

Indulge yourself in-car

Your car, your rules. Try to avoid those adrenaline-pumpers that will make you inadvertently press the pedal to the metal. But anything that encourages a tuneless singalong is to be encouraged – though you might want to wait till you're on the motorway before you press play on that one.

Add and subtract

Not every playlist needs to be furnished in one go like a show home – another advantage that digital has over old-school tape is that you can edit an ongoing list as the mood takes you. Keep open a playlist of, for instance, cheer-uppers for when you're feeling low (or, conversely, tearjerkers for when you want to wallow in a gloomy mood) and when you overhear something in a shop that's a perfect fit, Shazam it and bung it on that list.

How not to cry

I am a terrible combination of teary and emotionally repressed, which, in practice, means I cry easily, then want to flee the country in shame. I hate it so much that I still think about a couple of particularly mortifying cries, one of which was while sitting in an executive boardroom, having just been shown an upcoming TV commercial. Weirdly, I tend not to cry at sad things – more when I feel emotionally overwhelmed, but in any situation, the following works if a blub threatens at an inappropriate moment.

In the first instance, push your tongue firmly against the roof of your mouth, maintaining pressure until the tears abate. If that doesn't work, reach up with your hand and also discreetly apply pressure to your earlobe. If neither works, nip to the loo. Naturally, if I'm in the comfort of my own home and pyjamas, when such catalysts as a military tattoo, lame dog or male voice choir appear on screen, then I let the tears run free.

How to live with regret

'I have no regrets' is a phrase one hears often in everyday life, and I am generally mistrustful of anyone who lives theirs without ever admitting they wish they'd made another call. Who has lived such a flawless life that they don't wish they'd done something differently? It's the sort of throwaway cliché, much like 'everything happens for a reason' (no it doesn't, shush), spoken by people looking to live with as little personal responsibility and insight as possible. My own regrets are infinite – from choosing to hang out way longer than I should have with a group of unkind friends, to smoking my first cigarette in a hot boy's battered-up Citroën at a festival, because I thought it made for a cool scene straight from a French New Wave film. I made bad choices because I was an idiot, ignorant, young or unthinking. But my self-judgement over each of them has been essential to my principles and self-awareness thereafter.

Regrets are important in changing future behaviour and I'm not convinced anything does so as powerfully. They prompt you to do better next time, however insignificant they are in the broader scheme. I deeply regret not packing sunblock for a trip to the Gower Peninsula to celebrate my friend Rachel's sixteenth birthday over thirty years ago. Drunk on cider and giddy on company, I got horribly sunburnt and permanently damaged my skin. A tiny and wholly personal punishment, but the point is, I have been way more diligent about sun protection than the average adult since.

My idiocy in not speaking much to my grandad on what was to be his last Christmas Day cannot be repaired. My selfish teenage brain getting my father's big retirement party date wrong hurt his feelings and there will never be an opportunity to make it right. But these experiences have meant that when a friend has a significant birthday, or someone I know only casually gets married, I think of its importance less through my own eyes, more through theirs. I keep in touch with friends when we're both busy because there'll come a day when one of us won't be around.

341

Remember also that every act has a consequence, and even without actively correcting our future behaviours, one mistake can ultimately lead us somewhere better. One friend's marriage to the wrong man ultimately delivered her to the right one, and three brilliant children. My (quite rightly) getting the boot from a tabloid newspaper well over twenty years ago led me down a path to the career I always wanted.

Instead of refusing to look backwards and harping on about living with 'zero regrets', we should give our regrets room for processing, without allowing them to overcome us. Because ultimately, regrets should have a shelf life. Left to fester, they damage soul and body, taking away more than they bestow. There comes a point, after learning from our mistakes, when we must draw a line in the sand, forgive ourselves, pledge to do better and refuse to let life be governed by the past.

Friends, Relationships & Family

'If I were to draw a roadmap of my life, friendship would be the A-road, branched by twisty, often perilous lanes onto which I sometimes detoured and got lost.'

There's a scene in Madonna's behind-the-scenes documentary *Truth or Dare*, when a dancer asks her who is the love of her life. She waits a couple of beats, pretending defensively to need time to think about it, before croaking, sadly, but resolutely, 'Sean . . . Sean', referring to ex-husband Sean Penn. I was sixteen and in a dreadful relationship with a much older man when I saw it at the cinema, and as with practically everything Madonna does, it caused me to think and reflect. Who (aside from Madge, of course) was the love of my life? Who would one day make me feel complete, lost, found, as though I might expire without him by my side? Who, in my life, would be The One?

I was still asking myself the very same question twenty-five years later, as I sat, laptop to laptop, across a bar table from my partner, a peerlessly lovely and clever man who makes me laugh aloud every day, is incapable of letting down my two children and me, and whose joy when anything good happens to any of us is so pure that I've been forced to reconsider everything I'd learned about romantic love in the preceding three decades. And yet, I realise I've still not engaged in the fantasy. I've been too many times around the track to think the concept of The One anything more than the kind of fatalistic balls spouted by numpties who claim that everything happens for a reason. 'I don't think I have a love of my life,' I said to him, knowing I could with impunity. He looked up with the international expression for 'DUH' and said, with typical grace, 'Your friends, obviously.'

We both knew I didn't need to disagree, that he wasn't seeking any disingenuous assurances to make him feel better. If I were to draw a roadmap of my life, friendship would be the A-road, branched by twisty, often perilous lanes onto which I sometimes detoured and got lost. My friends are my family, my confidantes, my support system, the people who make my world seem the right way up. And I don't mean the nice friends with whom I simply enjoy a thoroughly pleasant evening and a few too many drinks. Those people are splendid and vital, but I mean the core friends who immediately notice when my general mood has shifted .5 of a millimetre to the right and make it their business to find out why. I mean those who've held back my hair as I've redecorated a bathroom floor (cheers, Jase), or travelled 300 miles with a Valium and DVD of *Showgirls*

345

to avert my personal crises (thank you, Sarah); girls who've forgiven my cock-ups and mortifying faux pas, my moments of wild irresponsibility, occasional selfishness and poor life choices – and to whom I offer all of this in return, as our lives and challenges shift and vary.

They've told me when I'm making a mistake and still feathered the nest for when I return, war-wounded, having belatedly discovered they were right. There's zero jealousy, no tolerance for serious fallouts (we'd simply bang on one another's doors until it was sorted), only honesty, acceptance and concern. As a collective, we've lived through every conceivable heartbreak, mental or physical health crisis, family drama and some really terrible haircuts, affording all of them due gravity while never forgetting to make rude jokes at one another's expense. They are the myriad girls and smaller number of boys who, when I've been going through some messy trauma, have pulled me closer, not pushed me away in discomfort and disgust, for whom I never have to download catch-up notes, even when several months have passed between meetings. They feed my very existence and without them I would starve, wither and die.

By contrast, it's an unequivocal truth that I would not expire without my wonderful husband. I could definitely live without him. I would hate to, I have no intention of doing so and if we, for some as yet unimaginable reason, didn't make it, I would be sadder than I can bear to think about. But the kind of romantic love I need manifests itself not in co-dependency, or in the surrender of self, but in a mutually uncomplicated, free-willed decision to be together because it's much, much nicer than being apart. I could go on without him if I had to. What I can't and couldn't do is live without my friends. They're not a substitute for love, they allow me to feel it. They don't get in the way of my romantic life, they augment it, as we share and compare our relationships in a safe space. My ability to be vulnerable, flawed, wrong or smitten in their company equips me for a better time at home. And my other half knows it. He doesn't care that I still don't believe in The One, that after a lifetime of knocks, the only thing I truly believe in is The Eleven. Whoever shares my romantic life has to know and like himself enough to understand and respect the fact that he'll always come a very close second. And at least in that sense, I know I'm living the dream.

In the beginning, he'd often tell me I was 'lucky' to have such amazing friends. I know I am extremely fortunate to have met them, but the ability to retain and maintain any great relationship, platonic or romantic, long term, is much more about judgement than luck. I'm not lucky to see my friends – I prioritise it, like I prioritise important work meetings or family events. I'm not lucky that they confide in me – I've worked hard to create a safe place for them to turn. It isn't by chance that my friends can trust me, and I them. It's entirely by design. My point is that friendships and relationships are work. They require constant effort and maintenance to grow and mature. And I really think I'm only good at them because I've been so appalling at being a family member. For as long as I can remember, I have understood that my chosen family are my one chance to have the support network so many others enjoy from birth.

And so what follows is some of what I've learnt along the way, via serious illness, family conflict, the partner abuse of people I love, heartbreaking bereavement, will disputes, estrangement, cancers all over the place (curable and not), relationships with bad men, a divorce from a very good one, a second marriage with the right one, a miscarriage, two kids, depression, a friendship group for whom I would do anything, friends who weren't friends at all, friends I truly loved but lost avoidably and unavoidably, poverty, affluence, many screw-ups, countless 'sorrys' and a whole lot of sex – very much not in that order. I've heaps still to learn, but when the subject is your all-consuming passion, every lesson is a joy.

347

How big an age gap is too big in a relationship?

Age gaps feel smaller the older both parties are, of course. I cannot bear to imagine either of my teenage kids in relationships with someone twelve years their senior, as I was at fourteen. It's repellent and dangerous. But when it comes to mature adults, only those involved can decide where their ick factor kicks in. If unsure, it's good to consider how important the following are to you:

Life stage

Age is just a number, but life stage is of critical importance in relationships. Someone who is, for example, twenty years older than you but fortuitously in sync with your desire to buy a house, have children, go clubbing, or travel across Europe in a camper van is a great find and there's no problem. But more often, a much younger or older partner will be at a different life stage and you'll need to think carefully about how this will work. I know of one couple who staggered on for years as one party went clubbing and slept in late, while the other retired and rose early to raise the unplanned child she'd wanted so desperately. No one had been dishonest about their lifestyle preferences, but the mismatch was ultimately untenable and they split amicably.

348

Cultural references

These may not matter to you, but for many of us, shared references from music, television, film, fashion and politics are the underpinning of daily discourse. A mismatch of life histories and context can make both parties feel less understood and age differences feel too pronounced. For example, I was already wavering on my decision to accept a dinner invitation from a man much younger than me, but when the sound of Pet Shop Boys' 'West End Girls' on the Gap instore sound system prompted him to ask me who was 'covering East 17', I knew immediately that there'd be too many conversations we'd never be able to share, and cancelled. Couples born into the same generation may have a greater mutual understanding and more shared experiences. It's also undeniably true that people from two different generations can have more in common personally than with someone their own age, but it's worth asking yourself how important a commonality of context is to you. There's no need to feel bad or talk yourself out of your position.

Physical health

An active younger person and an inactive senior is a broadly unfounded stereotype (my older husband loves orienteering on the downs in blustery winds, whereas I'd sooner nap), but it is true that if one of you is active and the other is unable or unwilling to be, then you may have a problem. Sex is an important consideration – one partner may feel they've had plenty, and their appetite has dipped in later life (similarly, a mismatch of libidos can happen at any age and in any direction). That's unlikely to change drastically, so consider whether this is a price of admission that you're willing to pay. If you're athletic generally, you may take the view that you can do your hiking, cycling, dancing and swimming either alone or with friends, but the emotional connection you share with your more sedentary partner is irreplaceable. But think it through first to avoid conflict and heart-wrenching dilemmas later on.

How to support a friend going through IVF

Difficulties around fertility are varied and complex in their emotional effect. What are more consistent are the mistakes made – albeit usually with the best will in the world – by those around them. If you know someone wanting and struggling to become a parent, here are some important things to consider:

They know more than you

Bearing witness to someone's difficulties is usually more helpful than offering advice. People going through IVF or any other fertility-related treatment know far more about their own bodies than anyone. They will have researched the subject into the ground, discussed it at length with qualified experts in the field and considered it all far more than they'd have liked. Don't be tempted to add to the avalanche of information with recommendations of treatments you've read about or seen on TV. Instead, be a safe haven from the exhausting tirade of unsolicited and unhelpful advice.

Don't mention the pregnant friend who 'just needed to chill out'

Having spent many an evening in the company of a friend with fertility issues, I know how often this nameless bloody woman is cited by strangers as the cautionary tale for all involuntarily childless people everywhere. Yes, it is absolutely true that some couples become pregnant naturally when they withdraw from fertility treatment. Yes, it is widely thought

'Bearing witness
to someone's
difficulties is
usually more
helpful than
offering advice.'

that stress can negatively impact one's reproductive health. What is also true is that there is absolutely no way of predicting or controlling if or when this will happen, and so telling someone that all they need to do is relax for a baby to be made quite naturally is singularly unhelpful and, ironically, extremely stressful to hear.

They know adoption exists

Suggesting adoption to someone in treatment carries the inference that IVF or medication isn't going to work, at the very time when a couple may be struggling to remain positive. It hurts. In any case, people undergoing extended fertility treatments have already thought about adoption, fostering and any other option potentially available to them, and almost certainly have a greater understanding than biological parents of the potential difficulties and stresses of the adoption process. If they decide to embark on it, it will not be because someone else suggested it. Don't go there.

IVF is extremely expensive

After any free treatment has been exhausted (depending on your location), fertility healthcare becomes very expensive. It is common for couples to be priced out of treatment altogether, while those able to keep going will feel the strain on their finances. Be cognisant of this when making plans with a friend in treatment, considering the affordability of restaurants, trips and holidays before booking. There's no need to make a big deal of it, but letting your friend know you see the pressures is kind. If you happen to be able to treat them, here and there, then that's one way to approach it.

351

Your moaning is hard

It is completely reasonable and healthy for parents to moan about the kids they adore, just as it's fine to complain about a spouse you love, or a job you enthusiastically applied for. No one feels positive about everything all of the time and we all need to let off steam when inevitably annoyed by the things we'd hate to be without. But ask yourself, truly, whether the person who should hear your parental gripes is the person struggling to start a much-wanted family? It is extremely hard for people who desperately want children to hear other people criticise their own. However much we understand intellectually that a moaning parent isn't really ungrateful for their child, when times are tough and sensitivities are high, that is inevitably how it will come across, and it can smack of injustice. When your kids drive you mad, vent at other mothers. And please, please never try to make someone feel better by joking, in relation to their infertility, that they're welcome to take your kids off your hands. If light is to be made of someone's fertility woes (and I'm all for gallows humour), then it must come from the person in treatment, not from someone with kids.

Watch the question count

When someone is undergoing protracted fertility treatment and people care about them a great deal, the sheer admin involved in answering their well-meaning requests for an update can feel like a part-time job. Giving everyone a download of information on your progress, feelings and next steps can be absolutely exhausting, and so any friend who gives you the day off from reading the news will be a godsend. Let it be known that you will always clear space to listen, but back off until they choose a time that suits them. In the meantime, they will definitely tell you if there's been meaningful progress, so there's no need to ask.

What to do if you hate how your partner dresses

For the most part, you'll need to lump it. All you can do instead is be honest but tactful, making sure you compliment your partner lavishly whenever they wear something you actually like, perhaps explaining what you like about it and making styling suggestions ('You look great in a proper shirt/I much prefer how those looser trousers look/that suit would look nice with trainers' and so on). Go shopping together and be positive about things you like, encouraging your partner to try new things. You can buy them gifts of clothing at your own expense, but these must come with no implied sense of obligation for them to like and wear them. But beyond that, if your partner isn't asking for help with their wardrobe, you'll have to respect their decision and pray that wearing socks comes back into fashion (seriously, British men, what the hell?).

How not to break up with someone

A couple of years ago, a girlfriend of mine met an ostensibly normal, funny man on Tinder. They met for a drink, then a week later, dinner with a dessert of heavy snogging. They decided to arrange another date soon and in the interim – and at his instigation – embarked on a WhatsApp rally that continued through practically every daily waking hour and several beyond. He hadn't felt like this in years, he said; 'you're so special', he gushed. He sent photos of his family and cat, sweet pictures of a lone plate of breakfast eggs with a 'wish you were here' and sad face emoji, nightly bedtime kisses and links to concerts he wanted them to see. Meanwhile she, very much enjoying their chats but feeling somewhat bemused by the strength of his affections, simply looked forward to their next meeting and the possibility of a shag. Then, forty-eight hours before it, he vanished. No responses to her texts, no explanation as to why he'd cut her off, no assurances that he hadn't been killed in a road accident. That was it, they were done, and she never heard from him again.

It's called 'ghosting', and according to YouGov, there's a one in ten chance you've experienced it, along with dozens of my friends. It's when someone abruptly withdraws all contact from a romantic partner, avoiding them thereafter, as though the relationship had never actually occurred. According to a 2012 study published in the *Journal of Research in Personality*, ghosting is the 'least ideal' way to break up a relationship (well, duh), presumably because it leaves its victims in great confusion, anxiety and with a profound sense of incompletion. All-important closure has been denied and, for want of a more scholarly term, it is absolutely bloody mentalising.

It may have a newish name, but ghosting has been around forever. I recall it happening to me over twenty years ago with a colleague whose foot seemed worryingly fixed on the accelerator pedal. He pursued me doggedly and within three mediocre dates was saying, 'Meet my mother, come for Christmas, one of us should apply to move offices,' and various other insane and untimely suggestions. Then suddenly, he stopped speaking to me and studied the floor whenever I walked past him in the corridor. No explanation, no apology, just an impersonation of someone who didn't know me from a standard lamp.

The remarkable and infuriating thing then, as it is now, when I hear identical or worse tales of ghosting, is the arrogance in the assumption that you simply cannot handle the notion that someone with whom you've twice shared pizza might not want to spend the rest of their life with you. It presumes that any woman, so desperate to be wed and impregnated with the babies of a man she barely knows, will, in all likelihood, throw herself in the sea if a simple dinner date has no legs.

This seems such a spectacularly arrogant and patronising misapprehension that it must be tempting for my girlfriends to wear badges saying 'not looking for a husband and baby right now, thanks'. Because really and truly, we are not – least of all with someone we're not sure about.

'If too much digital courtship occurs between dates, a real-life person can rarely live up to expectations, which can trigger an emergency gear shift.'

Time and time again, I find my ghosted friends, while warm and relatively keen on their date, had no plans beyond 'let's see what happens'. Even if they've hoped for kids one day in the future (and so what?), they've been a million miles from the single woman stereotype, scrapbooking bridal mags and vandalising condoms. And even if long-term commitment is an irrational fear for some men, then why repeatedly and needlessly drop love bombs as though they've finally found The One? Perhaps charitably, I wonder if there's an element of hoping to fake it until they make it.

And should someone feel the need to cry sexism or misandry and deploy the hashtag #NotAllMen, I can pre-emptively assure them that every man I know is similarly baffled by ghosting and wouldn't think to engage in it. And I daresay, yes, that there are women who behave similarly badly. I just don't know any, while I do know over a dozen girls and gay men who've been ghosted. Far from it revealing some genetic anomaly in men, it's the recent normalisation of the behaviour that's wrong.

Digital communication certainly provides daters of any gender with all the tools for this dysfunctional relationship pattern. The degree of separation afforded by WhatsApp, texting, emailing and Messenger can unnaturally accelerate a relationship, and the selective and frequent sharing can easily make us believe we're on a fortieth date, despite having met only twice. If too much digital courtship occurs between dates, a real-life person can rarely live up to expectations, which can trigger an emergency gear shift.

355

If dating blogs are anything to go by, ghosting has become increasingly commonplace since the advent of dating apps, and is now so prevalent as to be the default. People who fall foul are left to imagine all manner of terrible things about themselves, replaying conversations, reinterpreting messages, wondering if they went temporarily insane, when the truth is much clearer. There is simply no way he liked you enough, or, as Carrie in *Sex and the City* would say, 'He's just not that into you.' And that is perfectly fine. No one is for everyone and there's great freedom and self-acceptance to be found in the realisation that there was nothing you could have done differently. You were just not for him, and, by default, he was definitely not for you. Of course, there are acceptable ways of expressing that, either bluntly or gently, which brings me to the next truth: he lacks manners and empathy. He thinks this is an admissible way to behave towards another human being, and so again, he merely jumped before he was pushed.

- After one to three dates: dumping electronically is fine.
- After four to six dates: the same is true, as long as you're content to be thought of as a bad person.
- After more than six dates: do it face to face.

Seven failsafe ways to occupy kids on a rainy day

1. Painting nails
   Spread newspaper over the kitchen table and bring out as many shades of inexpensive nail polish as you have handy. Allow the child to pick their shades and, depending on their age, either paint their nails for them or allow them to paint their own and yours (accept your fate and just remove it later). Allow them to pick four songs to sing along to on Spotify while you wait for the paint to dry fully, before it's safe to leave the table. Or move on to toes. You can extend the task by making a price list or signage for your nail parlour. It never fails.

2. Customise catalogues and magazines
   Grab as many old catalogues and non-precious magazines as you have, get the pens out and make your way through them, designing tattoos on the bare skin of models and celebrities, placing people in unpopulated interiors, drawing worms, maggots and spiders into artfully styled plates of food, and popping hats and jewellery on animals. Cut out the best ones and mount them on blank paper or card to send to family.

3. Make a horror film
   My son seems to come home from every babysitting gig with a very unscary horror film that whiled away at least two hours of time with his charge. All you need is a smartphone and, if you like, a very simple editing app such as Splice. Ask the child what would scare any absent adult (rather than them) the most, then encourage them to find props – sheets, slime, Halloween masks and so on – to make a five-minute film to 'terrify' a beloved adult, then send it on WhatsApp.

4. Make Rice Krispie cakes
   The easiest cakes in the world, with no baking and not much waiting required. Truly, some of my happiest childhood memories are of making and eating these. Melt a pack of butter and a bag of

356

marshmallows in a large saucepan. Pour in enough Rice Krispies to coat them in mallow gunk and bind them together in a sticky but malleable lump. Divide with clean hands into small paper cupcake cases, each filled with a clump the size of a golf ball. Leave to set while you melt chocolate on a low heat in the microwave or in a bowl over a pan of hot (but not boiling) water. Spoon a dollop of melted chocolate onto each cake and leave to set (about an hour). A small child can do everything except the saucepan work with minimal supervision. There's an easier and quicker version of the recipe, where you just pour the cereal straight into lots of melted chocolate and leave it to set, but it's less delicious than the above (my mother's recipe) and I always feel the simpler version doesn't kill enough time to be worth making all the mess.

5. Write a ransom note
Pretend you've kidnapped your pet or a favourite toy and write a ransom note, using mismatched individual letters from the headlines in magazines, papers, food packaging and comics. The gorier and more menacing, the better. All the cutting and sticking takes much longer to do than you imagine.

357

6. Make gift tags
Take out all last year's Christmas cards (I always keep mine for this purpose) and cut around the robins, holly sprigs, reindeer and so on to make round or square gift tags for next year's presents. Punch holes in the tops and feed string or ribbon through each. It's surprisingly time-consuming, a satisfying way to reduce waste and very easy for any child old enough to hold craft scissors.

7. Produce a chat show
Sit together and write up twenty questions to ask your guests ('What will the story of your life be called?' 'What is the best present you've ever been given?' 'Which dinner should be banned?' 'What are the best and worst smells ever?' and so on), then take it in turns to be host and megastar, interviewing one another. Throw together costumes for extra busywork, then film the whole thing on a phone and WhatsApp it to friends and family.

How to throw a party with different groups of friends

As someone who seriously reconsidered my acceptance of a proposal of marriage I'd welcomed, purely on the grounds that the agreed nuptials guaranteed the cross-contamination of families and disparate friendship groups, believe me when I say that whatever your own concerns in this area, I see you and feel your pain acutely. Despite my abundant sympathy and understanding, I am here to tell you that the problem is probably you (and in my case, me). You are worrying too much because you are probably someone who, owing to early life experiences, is hypervigilant when it comes to group dynamics. You are probably someone, also like me, who will always panic at the thought of people not getting on, or the exposing nature of having everyone you care about in the same room, with their attention on you. It is a nightmare scenario for some of us. However, it is not normal. Unless there are real and insurmountable differences between two groups (if their deeply held religious views are in unfriendly opposition, for example), then you should feel calmer in the knowledge that most people just want to get on but don't much care if it doesn't happen. They'll go home and say to their partner, 'X's husband was a bit weird. He said something odd, I can't remember now . . . it'll come to me . . . I'm making a cuppa – want one?' And then they will forget. Alternatively, if you are the sort of person who (quite normally and healthily) presents myriad versions of yourself across diverse audiences – work colleagues, family, old friends, newer acquaintances – then you might understandably be perturbed at the prospect of presenting a single, unified persona when all of those diverse groups are gathered together.

358

If you really can't get past the fear, then rethink your event. I split my hen into two weekends, not because there was much chance of my friends not getting on (they're all wonderful and polite), but because I knew that unless I made things more manageable for me and my neuroses, I wouldn't be able to enjoy what should be a fun time. So half my friends came to Brighton Pride and out dancing, while the others came on a separate, chatty weekend in the countryside. Weddings aside, most things – birthdays, engagement celebrations, weekends away – can be carved up safely into sub-events without offending anyone. Good friends will understand completely and want you to feel comfortable. And there's a lot to be said for having a small-enough gathering to be able to give loved ones some real attention. A restaurant table for sixteen-odd people, for example, is a complete waste of everyone's time and money. Food takes forever to arrive and no one speaks to anyone but their immediate neighbours. And anyway, although organising a series of events might seem like a bigger headache than simply planning one big do, knowing that you don't have all your celebratory eggs in one basket and, instead, have a diary packed with smaller, more intimate fun times to look forward to can actually prove significantly less stressful. I milked my fortieth over a whole year in precisely this fashion.

How to choose godparents

For someone so godless, I am curiously devout in my belief in godparents. Mainly because I think it's extremely valuable and helpful for young people to have a long and loving friendship with someone of an older generation who is not their parent. Tradition dictates that a boy gets two godfathers and one godmother, a girl, two godmothers and a godfather, but I've been greedy and gone for two of each with both children. Obviously the most important criteria for any godparent is that you love them and believe you'll always know them, even if circumstances later interfere with the plan. Not being judgemental is an important quality in a godparent, if your child is to feel able to confide in them through childhood, teenage years and beyond. It may be a good idea to ask a mix of some very reliable and sensible friends (the sorts who could help the child in a crisis if you weren't around), as well as some fun, less-predictable types (the kind of godparent who can teach you how to throw a great party). Godparents from different backgrounds and cultures can also be hugely beneficial to a child's perspective. The important thing is that you ask those you believe will make good godparents – those who'll be supportive friends and counsels to your child – not those who simply believe it's their due, so don't ask someone simply because you believe you 'should' to avoid offending them.

359

Many people choose godparents on the basis that, should anything happen to them, the godparent would make a suitable carer and guardian in loco parentis. I did this, but if this is also your plan, it is vital that before agreeing anything else, you discuss this fully and carefully with the prospective godparent and any other blood relatives. When all is agreed, you must make detailed provision in your will to cover any financial and domestic arrangements, and to protect against any disputes. For everyone else, it is a matter of choosing someone you'd like in your child's life forever. Trust in them is vital, but the natural course of life means that it's perfectly possible to lose touch with one or two of your choices over time – especially if you had children early and people move away. This is a shame, but I take the view that if you've chosen well to begin with, those people will always leave their hearts open to their godchildren, should they ever turn up on the doorstep in need of a bed.

How to talk about cancer

Brave battlers, defiant warriors. We've all heard the combative metaphors. Except that despite how we choose to portray them, cancer patients are not embroiled in some mental wrestling match, where sheer strength of mind determines the speediness of their recovery or contributes in any meaningful way to the outcome of their treatment. Because they are ill. Positivity alone no more shrinks a tumour than snake oil, crystals and avo smash. What will make cancer even tougher, though, is the societal expectation of relentless optimism and a gung-ho, can-do mentality, even when it is at odds with someone's true personality, and flies in the face of medical fact.

While we patronise the one in two who will be diagnosed with cancer in our lifetimes, treating them like brave little soldiers for whom everything will come good if they simply refuse to accept otherwise, patients themselves are losing out on important discussions and vital planning. According to Macmillan, nearly two-thirds of sufferers never talk to anyone about their fears of dying because the pressure to see themselves as a 'fighter' proves prohibitive. Almost a third of cancer patients even report feelings of guilt if they can't stay positive about their disease. Thinking realistically about death seems to others like a concession of defeat when, in reality, it demonstrates an astounding strength of character.

This phenomenon of feeling guilty about accepting death, says Macmillan, may well account for just a third of terminal patients dying at home, when more than twice that figure would prefer to. In other words, instead of spending precious weeks or months making plans for their own deaths, and getting their affairs in order, a large number of patients are continuing treatment and entering hospital in an attempt to show those around them that they haven't 'given up' on conquering the unconquerable. Instead of encouraging people to engage in the important and worthwhile process of planning their final days, we are, undoubtedly with the best intentions, depriving them of the death – and remaining life – they want.

Even aside from the very real practical obstacle the whole 'fighting' analogy places before patients with terminal diagnoses, it's pretty offensive to cancer patients everywhere, who, in managing their treatment and recovery, can do little more than as they're told to. We don't decide which cancers hurt us, which kill us, which are sent packing by the drugs that doctors choose to prescribe us. We can only follow the suggestions of people who know better – turn up for the hospital appointments, take medication on time, eat and drink what's good for us, have the operations, scans and chemo. Nothing else is within our control. When cancer strikes, we have little choice but to put our faith in modern medicine and wish for the good luck needed to join the 50 per cent who make it past ten years of recovery.

I agree it's admirable to feel determined and defiant, and no doubt many find it helpful to see their cancer as a project to complete, a debate to win, a hostile territory to conquer. There is surely no right or wrong way to approach your own disease. Which is precisely why the party line used by so much of the media and charity sectors is so limiting. While it perhaps makes us feel less afraid, imposing a narrative on all patients prevents them from writing their own, deeply personal, often very different one. I know from painful experience that for every one sufferer bolstered by the idea that they're battling their disease, there's another for whom the effort of maintaining a brave face is exhausting and unhelpful. With restricted time left, there's a strong argument for living life as normally as possible, to feel like yourself despite inhabiting an increasingly unfamiliar body. If you're not a natural optimist, then how on earth is it helpful to anyone – yourself or your loved ones – to suddenly become one?

What is most disagreeable is that all this combat rhetoric by definition implies that people who die of cancer just didn't fight hard enough. Worse still, it unwittingly suggests a lack of bravery in 'giving up the fight' when very often, the toughest and most courageous decision of all is to cease treatment and face the inevitable. I've seen relatives and friends do this and, while I continue to grieve years later, I still feel awestruck by their dignity and immense bravery. Dying, though no one's

361

desired outcome, is not a battle 'lost' when the alternative is feeling undead – in pain, unmanageable suffering and unyielding exhaustion, with both patient and loved ones in acute distress. We are not giving up on those we love in respecting their readiness to leave, we are supporting them. Dying of cancer is not quitting. It is accepting.

How to support a friend when they're getting a divorce

I am divorced, and although I wouldn't wish it on my worst enemy, I accept that it was an enlightening and ultimately valuable time in terms of my friendships. I lost several, not because anyone took sides (there were no sides, just sadness), but because either I or they realised that our bond wasn't strong enough to weather the storm of such a major life event. And as much as that hurt at the time, now I realise it's okay. Some people are great friends but always destined to be transient. Others are for life, and sometimes the only differentiation between the two groups is in how they react to divorce, birth or death – ironically, the very times when we think we need all our friends more than ever. I've tried to remember what, during the worst of times, made the cream of my friendship group rise to the top and I've settled quickly and firmly for these:

362

Patience

Divorce takes ages. The umming, the ahing, the despair, the hopelessness, the fear for the children and for the immediate and distant future, the questions that can't be answered and the rehashing of conversations and events that led to this grim place. After the anger (which can be energising for a friend, who may feel purposeful and empowering during this phase), the rest of the process is incredibly slow and boring. This, in my experience, is where peripheral pals become frustrated or intolerant and drop off. And that's entirely their prerogative. There's little a divorcee-in-waiting can do about that, since the process can't be hastened by anyone. So if you want to show your friend that you support them, just stick around. Turn up. Be there. Stay.

Honesty

You are absolutely within your rights to say, 'I think we need to change the subject for a bit' – it is entirely fair and correct to remind someone who has been quacking on constantly about their divorce that you have challenges in your own life that also require some attention. It's okay to say, 'We've been over this a thousand times,' because you will have been. It's probably necessary to say, 'But what you said (or did) to him wasn't great either.' I will always accept honesty from people who love me, who have consistently shown up and gone out to bat for me. Being a friend in a trauma involves administering the medicine of reality. Being lied to, or simply told what you want to hear, arrests the progress of recovery. So be kind and compassionate, but direct.

Positivity

In the eye of the storm, many divorcees feel hopeless. They may be self-pitying, self-critical, pessimistic about their ability to find happiness again. They may feel they've caused their children lasting trauma, maybe even ruined their lives. Again, this may get tedious and can seem unhelpful and unrealistic, but it's all part of what is a deeply distressing process, and it will pass gradually. A good friend understands why their mate feels this way, but reminds them that it will definitely end, like everything else. Things will be better – perhaps better than ever before. There will be new opportunities and freedoms, perhaps an even closer bond with the children. Divorce is not the end, it's a new beginning. Talk about the future. Plan a trip or some nice experiences together. The important thing is that you don't get sucked into the vortex.

363

Pragmatism

If you know of a good family law solicitor, get the number. If you're a tech whizz who can set up a new laptop because a spouse has run off with the old one, swoop in and do it. If you have a close bond with the children, spend some quality time reassuring them. If you can cook, chuck a shepherd's pie in the freezer so that a newly single parent can have at least one less fraught night helming the house. Friends who help with practical tasks are every bit as valuable as those who listen and comfort.

Tolerance

It is extremely difficult to support someone who you feel is making choices you'd never make for yourself. They may be drinking more than seems healthy, repeatedly reconciling with an abusive spouse, making friends you don't like, dragging their heels over divorce paperwork, spending too much money or being overly critical of their ex. Whatever it is, there is little you can do except be your honest self – and even then, be prepared not to speed up the process a jot. Accept that you really don't know what you'd do in the same position, because you're not in it. Understand that this isn't your divorce to manage, even when you think the solutions are simple. When someone is letting go of their former dream, their once-certain future, nothing is anything of the sort. It all takes time.

Boundaries

Know that you are allowed to be annoyed and irritated by all the things you would previously have been annoyed and irritated by. During my divorce and while my children were visiting their father, I was once some six hours late home, where my friend Sarah was staying with me, because I'd got hugely drunk in a nearby beer garden with another friend. I was momentarily – and falsely – happy, and I selfishly made a choice to run with it, without a care for Sarah. She was rightly absolutely furious, and we had our first falling out in many years. We quickly made up, but I still think about it now. Someone in the midst of trauma still has a responsibility to their friendships, and you are being a good friend by pointing out where they are falling short. Don't ignore poor or inconsiderate behaviour, don't indulge delusion and unhealthy escapism. Point it out, but apply understanding and leniency. Your friend is in crisis and while her behaviour may be grounds for a talking-to, it probably shouldn't be a sackable offence.

And if you're the one getting the divorce ...

The most important thing to remember is this: don't be critical or mean about your spouse in front of your children. If your ex shagged his colleague while you were married, or doesn't pay his child support, or says unkind things about you, or routinely lets everyone – including your kids – down, then slate him to your friends, stick pins in an effigy or idly fantasise about driving an ice pick through his head. But make every effort to keep schtum about it to your kids. Your children are made of 50 per cent Mum and 50 per cent Dad – criticise him and you criticise them. I know it seems like the hardest thing in the world, but it is literally the most important thing in your entire divorce. To use your child as a sounding board for your frustrations – now or at any other time – is unintentionally abusive, and when things are calmer, you will rue the day you did it. To keep them away from the anger and bitterness is a huge act of love, you'll be proud of yourself for having done it, and I absolutely guarantee that your children will one day feel extremely grateful.

'Share your name when the baby is out and it's a fait accompli ... you'll be so busy and delighted that you can deny any motions for "Gary".'

How to choose a baby name

If you care about originality (and there's no qualitative reason you should – I still think Jack, William, Isabella and Grace are very lovely names, however popular they get), consult the top hundred baby names list online, so you know what to avoid. For inspiration, I'm a big fan of a baby name book, since it was just about the only book I could follow sleepily when pregnant. There's something very comforting and unchallenging about sitting in a massive nightie, saying only 'no, no, no, maybe, no, yes' for two hours at a time. But you could look at internet resources, your family tree, personal heroes and cultural icons – whatever works. My only hard-and-fast rule is this: do not tell anyone. Everyone in the world, however nice, will treat any baby name ideas as an invitation to debate and negotiate. They will say, 'Oh no! I was bullied at school by a Chloe! Chloes are bad news!' Or they'll tell you about the Luke they once dated who smelled like ham. They'll tell you there are fifteen Oscars in their daughter's class at school, or one Ava who's an insufferable brat. They'll claim your baby name is actually theirs, and secretly has been since they chose it when they were four years old. None of this matters. All that does is that you and your partner love the name and sincerely believe that your child will too. So share your name when the baby is out and it's a fait accompli. That way, you'll be so busy and delighted with your new family that you can shrug off any pleas to take the name of a dead relative, cheerfully refuse to 'sleep on it' and deny any motions for 'Gary' – three requests I genuinely had to field.

366

How to apologise

The willingness and ability to apologise sincerely marks the difference between a functioning, flawed human being and an inherent rotter. 'I'm sorry. It was wrong. I was a dick. I have either deliberately or thoughtlessly caused you or others pain/difficulty/mistrust and I really, really wish I hadn't. I know it wasn't okay, and am taking steps to ensure I never do it again. I hope you will forgive me,' is the way to do it. No ifs, buts, blame or disclaimers. Just say it, mean it and – apology willing – everyone can move on.

How to deliver bad news

Quickly. Do not say, 'I have something bad to tell you,' unless you're exaggerating about, for example, the unavailability of pepperoni as a pizza topping. If it's genuinely something bad, then taking a run-up at it while someone is feeling nothing but fear and dread makes a terrible time even worse. It's difficult, but do try not to dither. No one involved wants to be there, waiting to feel embarrassed, sad or disappointed, so the faster you get to the point, the better. Say something like, 'I'm very sorry to tell you that I am no longer happy and would like to separate/need to cancel the holiday/have seen your husband kissing another woman in the street.' You can express your unhappiness at being the bearer of bad news after you've delivered it when the other person has the opportunity to leave and regroup in private, or stay and seek comfort. Be there to offer it, but be careful not to give so much that you go back on your decision.

How to introduce a new partner to your children

Slowly. However hard you've tried to be clear and honest, it's likely your children will still be harbouring some small hope that you and their other parent will at some point reconcile. A new partner will definitely put paid to that, so it's important to handle any introductions tactfully and sensitively, introducing them first outside the home (a walk outside is much less pressuring than a face-to-face meeting in, say, a restaurant), then, perhaps a few meetings later, inviting the same partner round for tea and a film, with no sleepover. Perhaps it goes without saying, but it's unwise to have anyone to stay over until you feel as sure as possible that you can trust your new partner, and that your new relationship is serious enough to last. Seeing a parent with someone new is a huge deal to children of all ages – it's unfair to put them through the same emotional process repeatedly if you can help it. Look out for red flags: any new partner who is openly impatient about this necessarily delicate process is simply not the right person to join a readymade family and will likely never be able to accept the fact that your children come first.

How to respond when someone becomes very ill or dies

It's a sad truth that no one really knows what to say until they themselves need to hear it. So, as someone who has lost both parents, several friends and an unborn baby, allow me to suggest that what you should say is: 'This is absolutely awful and I am so bloody sorry you're having to go through it.'

Do not attempt to identify a silver lining – there isn't one.

Do not utter even a word about fate, or things happening for a reason, or presume any one detail of the death is of any relief or comfort.

Do not draw comparisons with your dead pet – no one cares.

Do assume the bereaved person has needs, even if they aren't expressing them. By all means, offer to help, but either be specific ('I would be very happy to make all the sandwiches for the wake/babysit your children for the next few days') or take matters into your own hands and leave a macaroni on the doorstep.

Don't cancel. When someone loses a partner, you may feel that calling off social engagements with them is a kindness, that the last thing they'll want to do is meet, eat and chat. But for many bereaved people, having plans is what gets them through. A cancellation may simply commit them to another unwanted night in their own head.

Do not, on any account, when someone you know has received a grave diagnosis such as terminal cancer, tell them you know a person with some herbal remedies, diet plans or cosmic ordering exercises that will reverse it. I know from bitter experience that this happens an astonishing amount and is breathtakingly inappropriate and distasteful. Similarly, never respond to someone's critical illness diagnosis by telling them which members of your family almost or actually died from the same condition. Lots of well-meaning people did this when my son was very ill and I have mentally struck them from my Christmas card list.

On identifying a controlling relationship

I've had three loved ones (two women, one man) escape coercive relationships or marriages and the victim's journey to identifying and changing their situation is a long, fraught and heartbreaking one. Their loved ones, with the liberty and clarity of distance, will likely see it much sooner. It starts with tiny, almost insignificant anxieties. There's fretting over photos of a lunch out being posted on social media, in case her partner sees her enjoying herself and accuses her of something. There's a request that friends don't 'say much' in texts, because he reads them all, when there's nothing remotely incriminating to say. There are the sudden cancellations because your friend 'needs to spend time with' her husband, the abrupt and inappropriate exits following hushed phone calls, the relentless questions from home ('what are the kids supposed to eat while you're out?'), all sent to cause guilt. The rare nights out as a couple, for which outfits and makeup have been vetted, and during which he invariably storms out early as a test to see if she'll do the right thing and follow him. There are financial commitments made on behalf of the victim ('you've got a better credit rating than me, you'll get a better deal on the loan/a better phone on your contract'). There are vital everyday functions ring-fenced by the abuser, from the hugely inconvenient – only he knows the Wi-Fi password or can switch on the heating – to the debilitating – only he's insured to drive the car or can access the bank account.

Then, in time, comes a more insidious dynamic, where the abuser perhaps senses detection by loved ones, and begins to describe them one by one as disingenuous, dishonest, lacking in morality and true concern. A victim can only truly rely on their partner; only he knows what's best for them; it's 'just you and me against the world, babe'. Work, too, doesn't deserve the victim's time and commitment and may need the push. His salary is fine for the both of you. There are the double standards, where a partner engages with impunity in exactly the behaviours he suspects, despises and punishes in his wife.

Then at some point, unless the tumour is excised in time, comes the gaslighting, where all of the above is dismissed as mere fiction, when the victim is accused of being 'exhausted/menopausal/hormonal/mentally ill' and of having imagined things. The victim's head is now a mess of paranoia, fear and guilt, where all trust is lost and all their statements and actions seem so risky that it's easier to shrink to fit, to say nothing, to do little except stay at home and attempt to balance precariously on the right side of the abuser.

There may also be violence. There may be alcoholism, drug abuse, sexual abuse, threats of suicide, custody battles or grave harm to loved ones. But we need also to understand that there may be no tangible, visible influence or threat. That coercive control takes hold gradually, almost imperceptibly, until it feels as much a part of the victim as the birthmark on her cheek. The challenge of starting again, with shame, less money

369

and shattered self-esteem, seems insurmountable. To deny children access to a parent they may adore, even an abusive one, seems cruel and selfish, even impossible. Assurances from friends that the children are learning dysfunctional abuse patterns that will negatively influence the rest of their lives are dismissed – they're fine, too young to notice, they'll only blame the parent with the audacity to break up their family.

Then one day, if the victim is lucky, something, perhaps another row, another put-down, another let-down, occurs. A tiny crack forms and a shard of reality shines through. The friends and family who refused to give up trepidatiously chip away at it, trying to shatter the whole facade, worried that they too are manipulating and bullying the victim, but spurred on by the fact that this has become the only language their loved one now responds to. They remind the victim of the abnormality of what life has become, of how quickly they themselves would identify the abuse of other people, 'more important' people, human beings that matter. Friends and family form a human crash mat and stand metaphorically under the window for what seems like an eternity, guiltily hoping for the situation to escalate to a point of no return, waiting for their loved one to jump from it, preparing to dress the resulting injuries, hoping they will heal. And truly, this is all they can do – love, continue to say 'this is not normal' and wait for as long as they can stand.

Gradually, the freed victim's brain fog clears. They can't believe what took place, are continually astonished to see men and women being nice to one another, affording one another everyday freedoms and respect. They wonder aloud, over and over, how it happened to them, an intelligent, discerning person, and why it took so long to leave. They ask 'why me?' and battle with the default feeling of guilt instilled in them over years of abuse. They are often mistrustful of new dates and relationships, while also struggling to understand how someone could have done this to another human, to the person who loved them. Was their bullying partner insecure? Were they abuse victims themselves, hurting inside, scared of being alone? Almost certainly. But mainly, the abusive partner did it because they liked it. Coercive control over another worked for them, gave them what they wanted, allowed them to experience the complex, messy, unfair world entirely on their own terms. They liked it until it was taken away, until their victim reclaimed control over their own life. One wishes they'd ponder the devastation, isolation and fear they caused, while experiencing it themselves in a prison cell. But, in reality, they will likely dismiss the victim as another 'psycho ex', move on and wreak the same havoc in their next partner's life.

When to tell someone you love them in a relationship

I can offer no cast-iron formula for the timing of something quite so personal as your first L-word drop. But my primary steer would be: tell someone you love them when you think you'll hear it back but not when you need to. By telling someone you love them, you're giving them permission to reply in kind. But you must also be prepared for them not to be on the same page without it causing irreparable hurt. It's fine to hold it in if you think you've got there first.

Never tell someone you love them for the first time during sex, because your partner will likely doubt the veracity of your claim. Don't say it out of desperation, or simply to placate someone who's expecting to hear it from you. If you do so and like does eventually turn to love for you too, the moment will be one of relief rather than joy.

Essentially, telling someone shouldn't actually be that tense a moment – it should come naturally as a relationship matures. So if you're overly nervous about telling someone you love them, it might be a sign that it's not yet the right time.

371

How to cope with working mum guilt

I once wheeled a suitcase straight out of a primary school concert into the parents' car park, where a taxi was waiting to take me to the airport for a five-night work trip. As other mothers were no doubt still mopping up their proud tears, I was boarding a flight, my facial muscles still aching from being contorted into full, ugly sobs over the sight of my youngest as 'Dancing Chimp Three', and wondering if I could bang out a 3,000-word interview between take-off and landing. There were no doubt other mothers absent altogether – women whose jobs deny them my freedom or flexibility, whose bosses neither get nor care how one's attendance at a crap nativity can feel like a matter of life and death; women whose incomes mean a day off guarantees an empty fridge or petrol tank. But I've missed special assemblies, countless football matches, a couple of sports days and a parents' evening, and I've never chaperoned a school trip. I was, and usually am, working and was very often feeling way more guilty than I should.

'Frankly, I'd do it
all again just for
the satisfaction of
delivering two good,
respectful, enlightened
men to the dating pool.'

During my years as a hard-working mother (some of them single and skint, more of them not), I've been given every encouragement to judge myself harshly – and so have my friends. The teacher who makes a point of saying, 'We don't see YOU here normally?!' crushing any residual pride you felt in managing to race from work in time for the last school bell. The classmate's mum who tilts her head to the side in sympathy at you being unable to attend another mothers' social event because you either have to be at work, or are so rarely free that story time with your kids, sex with your partner, sorting paperwork or putting on a whites wash is much more important to the family's health.

The mum who talks about your husband as though he's the Second Coming purely because he does exactly what she does – school run, lunches, extracurricular clubs – every day of her unlauded life. The men who tell you their own partner stays home because she 'really loves the kids' as though you're barely on speaking terms with yours. And I daresay that for every one of the tactless, seemingly mean-spirited guilt-mongers, there's an equally defensive working mum making patronising comments about cupcake baking and Pilates classes to a woman who stays at home in circumstances to which she can't herself begin to relate. When everyone is under attack, many will inevitably act out. But we don't want to hear it, any of it, any of us. We 'work' or 'don't work' because we feel we have to, need to, want to. All of us in paid work would do a little less if we could. But until we reach this nirvana, we are doing our best, raising our kids, attempting to keep our employers sufficiently happy that they don't move on to someone childless, young, perpetually available.

373

And despite knowing all this, your harshest judge and critic will be yourself. You will think about the time your child woke up crying from a nightmare and instead of being able to snuggle them up in your bed, you were in a shitty travel tavern fashioning supper from Diet Coke and Lotus biscuits. You'll remember hearing that your child had a bug and feel bad that your first thought was not for them, but for your boss and how she'd react to hearing you were downing tools for cartoons and cuddles. You will obsess over words you missed being spoken for the first time, over swimming strokes you didn't teach, wobbly steps you didn't get to clap, cuts and grazes that were already cleaned and plastered before you were even home to kiss them better. You'll recall the night you hit the twenty-four-hour Asda because it was 2 a.m., you'd just finished writing a report/chapter/evaluation and were way too broken to make flapjacks for the fete.

Speaking from the other side, the baby and toddler years behind me, I can say I would do it all again. Because gradually every working woman I know will stop worrying about their shortcomings and begin to feel proud of their strength and determination to keep food on tables and a roof over heads. I do, and I am glad that despite whatever else my sons missed out on (and part of the parenting experience is realising that all children feel sad about something you did or didn't do), they got to learn that women have a life of their own, that they are not defined by their children, that they work hard for their clan and make things happen, that they don't always need even an ounce of help from a man. They step up for their families whether at home or at work, and make sacrifices for the greater good. They make rent, pay bills, instil a work ethic, foster ambition, discourage entitlement, lead by example and set a high bar for what little girls, and the future female partners of little boys, can achieve on an uneven playing field. They show kids of all genders that the team is everything, and everyone must muck in while Mum earns a cheque or makes a home. Frankly, I'd do it all again just for the satisfaction of delivering two good, respectful, enlightened men to the dating pool. And in any case, everyone knows that whether it's a first step, tooth or word, it simply doesn't count until Mum has seen it.

374

How to talk to kids about porn

My children had a great sex education programme at school, covering all manner of social (as well as biological) matters. But however progressive and comprehensive such a programme may appear to be, there are gaps left by porn culture that aren't filled by school, and however distasteful it may be, it's down to parents to address them head on. Because when there's only three clicks of separation between a K-pop promo and graphic scenes of double penetration, I strongly believe that the health of their future relationships depends on it. You must separate fantasy from reality and unpick the myriad falsehoods of porn education.

I wanted my sons to know that if they one day have girlfriends (and it's perfectly fine if they have boyfriends), they are statistically unlikely to date women who expect anal penetration as standard and ejaculation always to occur in their faces. Their female partners won't moan constantly to maintain a soundtrack, won't keep their heels on while otherwise starkers, and are overwhelmingly likely to have pubic hair and boobs that

'Most girls don't have a hairless robo-body or a vulva as neat and dainty as a Parisian patisserie window display.'

flatten and wobble during sex. For their own sakes as well as womankind's, I wanted them to understand that she will not come in two minutes flat – a great deal more effort will almost certainly be required. They needed to know that everyone is not having threesomes, that most women who have sex with other women do it for their own benefit, not so nearby men can vicariously get their rocks off. Their sexual partners, however casual, shouldn't be expected to send nude pictures of themselves as though posing for a porn mag, and even if their partner is sexually experienced, or even promiscuous, they still need her permission for everything. Nor will she be locked, loaded and ready for action whenever a man is aroused. She, like all women, will have many aspects of her life that, at any given time, could be infinitely more deserving of her attention.

But what was equally important was that my sons didn't place similarly unrealistic expectations on themselves. Porn culture means that now, more than ever, boys need to know that the vast majority of men don't have penises the size of a standard rolling pin (or a wine cork, for that matter) – in fact, a good 80 per cent of them are in roughly the same average area. Most girls don't have a hairless robo-body or a vulva as neat and dainty as a Parisian patisserie window display. When they do have sex, even with a long-term partner, the chances of film-like choreography, where penetration magically and seamlessly occurs without any manual guidance, is relatively low. It's neither normal nor expected that a man magically recovers within four minutes of ejaculation, because real life doesn't pause for an extended camera break complete with dedicated fluffer and vacuum contraption.

They need to know that what is normal and to be expected is condoms as standard, bodily noises from both parties, a bit of a mess around period time, women being into it without screaming the house down, soggy tissues, embarrassing interruptions, laughter when something doesn't work or someone does a pratfall off the bed, the occasional need for lubricant and deciding you can't really be arsed because there's a brew cooling and *24 Hours in Police Custody* is about to start.

Young people need to know that real sex, with its imperfections and embarrassments, is one of life's greatest joys, and that porn sex is a foreign language that few people speak. But what I wouldn't tell them is not to watch it. Having myself known the illicit teenage thrill of watching *Fanny Hill* at a house party, I know that simply telling them not to go there is a hiding to nothing. I can't help thinking that when it comes to my own

376

kids, it would be less useful to tell them not to go near a vast expanse of water than it would to teach them how to swim.

Porn is everywhere, to some degree or another. Our sneaky VHS tape is now a limitless and free internet resource where every conceivable sexual proclivity is catalogued in graphic detail. Our overweight men shagging giggling women wearing a full bush and knee socks are now hard-bodied, nipped, tucked and modified *Westworld* characters performing untypical acts to which our kids are inevitably becoming acclimatised. YouTube has racier pop promos than the porn we grew up with. Silently accepting that our kids might have a crumpled mag under their mattresses won't cut it anymore. The genie is long out of the bottle and getting bummed senseless. We have to discuss porn with our kids in the same way we so readily tell them to call home and not to go with strangers. We need to tell them that this isn't reality, that it is not a sexual roadmap, and to fulfil our obligation to prepare them for adulthood. Because that is infinitely more hardcore.

Thoughts on estrangement from a family member

For some thirteen years until just before her very sad death, I was estranged from my mother. Previously, there were extended periods of one to five years when we didn't speak, before reconciling for a relatively short time until something happened and we mutually withdrew again. Because of my own estrangement, and my public support for Meghan, Duchess of Sussex, Jennifer Aniston, Drew Barrymore and various other high-profile people who've at some point become estranged from a close family member, I eventually opened a Facebook group called Necessary Family Estrangement, where anyone considering or implementing the same decision could meet others in the same boat. What I've learnt from the group is that although circumstances around family estrangement differ wildly, the reactions from people who've never themselves been in them are consistently unhelpful and would benefit from some perspective. Should you have made the difficult choice to distance yourself from a toxic family relationship, whatever the causes, you will be familiar with the stock responses. People – even the kind ones – are so horrified by an adult child's decision to sever ties with their parent(s), or to simply take an extended break, that they immediately tell you what they think you don't already, very painfully, know. They say, 'It's so sad!' (yes, it is); 'Is anything so bad that it can't be fixed?' (yes, it would appear it is); 'You'll be heartbroken when he's dead' (of course); 'Oh, I love my parents' (me too, but not at my own life's expense); and so on. I've heard them all. As people struggle to imagine something so at odds with nature and common experience, they invariably settle for judgement and decide you must be stubborn, petty, unforgiving or simply not very nice.

What doesn't seem to occur to the great concerned, however well meaning they may be, is that you may be happier, healthier and calmer without the family member(s) concerned in your life. Family estrangement, in my considerable personal experience, very rarely reflects a grudge. It's not about punishing someone, or teaching them a lesson, or refusing to back down. And it's certainly not about needing to win. Far from it – it is a loss so huge to everyone concerned that it feels much like a death. It's neither flippant nor entered into lightly. More often than not, estrangement is the last resort, a considered, painful decision to remove from your daily life behaviours and people (and it's easy to forget they really are just people, albeit with shared blood) that consistently make you feel unhappy, chaotic and upset.

Naturally, one always hopes that any broken family will one day be mended. Estrangement can last months or a lifetime, and even I've learnt never to say never. And it's no doubt true that the birth of a baby can spark forgiveness and reconciliation in some estranged families. But it can also very often galvanise an expectant or new parent into stopping the cycle of family dysfunction, for the sake of the next generation. Pregnancy and new motherhood can be a time when the victim of an abusive parent finally has someone they care about more, and takes action to protect their child in a way they felt unable to do for themselves. That isn't selfishness, it's responsible parenting. An approaching death, too, can expedite a reconciliation of sorts, but there are as many cases where staying apart remains the better plan. The estranger is wise to consider where an emotional upheaval would leave them, and whether they'd want, or be able, to cope if left alone in the fallout. For many, the estrangement marks the end of a protracted grieving period, and there is simply no more loss to feel. The variables are infinite and more nuanced than happy families can imagine.

If the thought of family estrangement horrifies or baffles you, then instead of judging, feel grateful that your family got that part right. Be happy that your situation isn't alien to others, that you'll be able to join in normal social conversation, that you won't feel embarrassed when you meet your partner's family, that you'll never have to lie about your plans for the holidays, that you won't feel like a freak for not having a relationship with those who raised you, from whom you are expected to tolerate anything. Be thankful and positively delighted that in your case, that's not much. And respect the heartbreaking decisions of others, trusting that they gave it a lifetime of thought.

On making sound memories

By the time our kids reach the latter stages of teenagerhood, most of us have a fairly comprehensive record of their development in the form of drawings, paintings, cards, school projects and of course photographs. But what even the keenest progeny archivists generally don't think to capture is a record of their children's voices. The incremental changes that occur in the way our kids speak, both in terms of pitch and vocabulary, can be so gradual as to escape notice and consequently never trigger the thought that moments in this particular developmental journey should be captured for posterity. It may only be when you call your pubescent son down for dinner and someone you momentarily take to be a strange man answers that you truly stop to think about the changes in your child's voice, by which time it's much too late to revisit the squeaky enthusiasm and sweet linguistic mistakes – ones you felt duty bound to correct, then mourned their loss – of their younger years. The habit of filming our kids invariably tapers off fairly dramatically post-infancy and the chances are that if you're relying on video clips for an incidental record of your child's voice, you might at best end up with an annually updated document of the sound of them blowing out ever-greater numbers of candles. So, once in a while, when they're chattering about their day or noisily immersed in a messy project, covertly press record on your phone and capture a few minutes of a voice or voices, which, melancholy as it is to consider, will a few months later have subtly evolved into something slightly more mature and impossible to otherwise revisit. While the clandestine approach will give you an unaffected snapshot of your little one, I also heartily recommend the more formal child interview. A record of your child describing, for instance, their day, what they can see around them, who their best friends are and how they picture their future has the potential to provoke tears and laughter in equal measure in years to come, when the pitch has long since deepened and the little voice

379

you sometimes thought would never stop quacking on has long since morphed into teenage monosyllables.

How to do Christmas post-divorce

Sitting in a solicitor's office one November day around a decade ago, my lawyer told me that proceedings were likely to be delayed because, at this time of year, family courts are rammed with separated parents arguing over festive arrangements for their children. It seemed extraordinary to me that while I was agonising over whether we'd even still have a house, and the eye-wateringly high monetary and emotional cost of resolving that in court, grown adults were putting both on the line to squabble over where Santa would leave his haul, and who'd get to pull the first cracker. Christmas, as we know, is a uniquely stressful time. Emotions run high around an event that has massive importance and meaning to many children. It's entirely understandable that adults already facing huge changes want to ring-fence festive traditions and enjoy their kids as much as possible. But as someone who's been there, both as the child of divorced parents and as a single mother myself, who has made a million mistakes but is now out of the eye of the storm, I know that there are practical, healthy and happy solutions for the family that don't involve people in black cloaks and white wigs. Here's what I've learned.

A date is just a number

We take it in turns to have our boys for Christmas Day, and the parent who misses out gets New Year's Eve. But Christmas Day is an arbitrary date – Jesus wasn't even born then, so don't give it too much undue meaning, which will only serve to make you feel worse. Young children don't care if it's the 21st, 25th or 30th, so whichever parent is sadly sans kids on the day should hold another Christmas during their custody time. Let Santa know it's all happening in advance, cook a turkey, play crap board games and pop *Elf* on the telly while you pour yourself a cooking sherry. If your Christmas falls in the days following the real one, you can get most of your presents and supplies for a lot less cash, too. Truly, two Christmases can be the best of both worlds and your children will adapt to it very happily.

Embrace technology

Zoom and FaceTime are a divorced parent's best weapon in the prevention of tears. It's completely reasonable for an ex and their new partner not to want you sitting in the corner all day, invading their privacy from a laptop screen, but pre-arranging one to three private calls (say, first thing and before bed) is the right thing to do for everyone. Children love showing the other parent their pressies, as well as checking in that the mum or dad is okay without them.

Restrain yourself

Don't cause your kids to fret. They should know that the absent parent would prefer to be with them on Christmas Day, of course. But if they think either of you will be sitting alone, weeping and heartbroken while they pull another cracker, then that will compromise or even ruin their time. Say you'll be okay, that you have nice plans and you'll be free to text throughout, but that you can't wait to have them home for round two. By the same token, don't ever ask your kids to choose which parent they'd like to be with. It's a horrible question laden with emotion, responsibility and pressure. Decide between yourselves, especially if your kids are little, then reassure them that it'll be lovely.

381

Know your limitations

If you can manage to spend any of the festivities happily together – even if it's just a school carol service or Christmas-morning cuppa – then that's a wonderful thing for your children. My divorced parents always had Christmas lunch together with us (and their respective partners) and it was very comforting, but I'm a very long way off being able to do the same for my own kids. Don't beat yourself up about it. If you can't be together and still provide a calm, safe, fun, love-filled environment for your kids (or if getting together is too geographically challenging), don't force it. Spending the day trying to avoid confrontation, or even travelling up and down a motorway, can be stressful and depressing for everyone. Divvy up the time fairly and do your own thing.

Make the most of adulthood

If it's not your turn, consider embracing the adult-only possibilities now open to you. On my no-child Christmas Eves, my husband and I do something fancy we never normally could, swapping hot chocolate and a panto for cocktails and a posh restaurant *à deux*. Similarly, you could hang out with friends who might not normally want to celebrate with kids, or even go away somewhere for a dirty weekend. I personally found this easier than trying to soldier on with the usual traditions, constantly aware of the two child-shaped holes in the proceedings.

Be a team

As someone who once discovered at 4 p.m. on Christmas Eve that my former in-laws had bought exactly the same presents as Father Christmas was planning to deliver the following morning (cue: one hour of insanity in Toys R Us while the security guard tapped his watch), I can say with some authority that it's really important to work as a team. Tell your ex-partner what you plan to buy for your child and avoid a game of one-upmanship. It's a dick move for one parent to give spendy smartphones, tablets and iPods, thus becoming the hero of Christmas, when they know full well the other can only afford socks and slippers. Don't be that person. My ex and I now always consult on presents to minimise duplicates, ensure we are spending roughly the same and, if necessary, even go halves on a special present together.

Don't go to court. Just don't

By all means, go to mediation if it helps devise a long- or short-term strategy for the festive period, but court is next-level dreadful. There are two justifiable reasons for thrashing it out there. The first is if the children will be unsafe in your ex's care – for example, if he or she is violent or abusive. The second is if your children will be truly emotionally distressed if away from you on Christmas Day. You feeling gutted or like you've been treated unfairly is not a sufficient reason to spend fortunes putting the whole family through this. It's horrible to be without your kids on Christmas Day. I've been there; I've cried and wailed. But everything – the Christmases and the break-up – definitely gets so much easier and you will think much more clearly with the benefit of hindsight. And I guarantee you'll then look back on a decision to bring in lawyers, and realise that you'd temporarily lost your mind.

It's not about you

Christmas means more to them than us. Be grateful your kids have two parents on the scene when many people have no choice but to go it alone. However frustrating, infuriating, unjust and downright heartbreaking it all feels, your kids just need to feel happy. The rest is just tinsel.

How to have sex when pregnant

As everyone rightly asserts, every pregnancy is different. But when it comes to sex, a lengthy crowdsourcing session with my friends reveals that pregnancy and childbirth have been causing the same common system glitches for generations. It's naive to imagine that being confronted with the functionality of reproduction will not somehow affect its recreational purposes, and our avoidance of discussing prenatal and postpartum sex does nothing to manage our expectations. Bravo if anyone manages to breed and bone in blissful tandem, but they are the chosen few. The rest of us biological mothers will almost certainly experience at least one of the following before, during or after a baby:

Sex drive goes bananas – in either direction

In the second and third trimesters of my two pregnancies, after the sheer exhaustion and perpetual queasiness had lifted, I was, to put it mildly, as horny as a toad. Suddenly, everything caused sexual thoughts – soft-rock power ballads, friendly shopkeepers, adverts for cat food. However incongruous and improbable the trigger for my rampant libido, I was reliably up for acting on it. Many of my friends were the same, others the opposite or unchanged, of course, but an extreme sex drive seems to occur often enough in pregnancy for it to be a very definite Thing. It can be brilliantly fun, or only mildly inconvenient, unless you're unlucky enough to have a partner suffering from another common pregnancy syndrome . . .

383

Some men lose their desire

Mismatched sex drives aren't ideal in any relationship, but during pregnancy, the chasm between them can be frustrating in the extreme. I know of several male friends who felt freaked out at the thought of penetrative sex during their partners' pregnancies, for all sorts of irrational or unfounded reasons, from worrying they'd harm the baby to feeling anxious not to appear disrespectful of motherhood. Some tell me they also felt under new pressure – to provide enough cash for everyone, to be a good, reliable and stable parent, to be seen as flawlessly supportive of the entire pregnancy – and, understandably, none had done wonders for their libido. One can use foreplay to keep the campfire burning for you without going the whole nine yards for him. And if all else fails, a pregnant woman can at least live vicariously through . . .

Dirty dreams

Oh man, the expectant-mother sex dreams. Filthy, graphic, vivid fantasies that would somehow still make for porn so woefully un-arousing that blue-balled punters would surely demand a refund. Imaginary romps with people you know so well they're almost family, and with whom, in your waking life, you would rather die than have sex? Routinely waking up like a teenage boy in a sweaty heap and a tiny puddle? Utterly depraved sessions with Simon Cowell, complete with still-belted high-waisted jeans and open-necked shirt? (For the record: that wasn't only me. A staggering four of my girlfriends routinely shagged Cowell in their pregnancy dreams, and never, ever again.) Prepare for the possibility that your subconscious will embarrass and humiliate you on an almost daily basis for anything up to the full forty weeks. My friend C spent her pregnancy not only battling morning sickness and persistently wonky blood pressure, but also enduring recurring scenes of obscenity with Antony Worrall Thompson. As my own pregnancy hormones soared, my sex dreams were so torrid that I began to think my sleep-depriving hip sciatica was simply my body's way of shielding me from shame. Or preparing me for what lay on the horizon . . .

384

Zero sex drive

Yes, even if throughout pregnancy a woman has been climbing the walls with desire, wanting to shag everything from her spouse to a telegraph pole, it's extremely common to find her libido crashes and burns post-delivery. Breastfeeding, a difficult labour, sleep deprivation, depression or a fretful baby can push sex to the very bottom of the agenda for god knows how long. It's just how it often goes. If the mismatch persists despite proper communication and reassurance (counselling is proven to help), then it seems pretty vital that couples make sure non-sexual intimacy remains part of their relationship. It's much easier to resume a healthy sex life if you've been holding hands and cuddling during the drought, than if you've been sitting awkwardly and guiltily on opposite sides of the flatscreen. One should take comfort in the fact that, like roadworks or air turbulence, it is upsetting, inconvenient and undesirable, but it will end. What may take even longer to work out is . . .

Boobs become a no-go area

Post-baby, many breastfeeding women who would ordinarily find boob-play a big turn-on can suddenly find themselves banning all adult contact with anything located between neck and ribcage. Having a baby jabbing, suckling, pawing and guzzling at your nipples all day, as wonderful as it can be in so many ways, can also leave you desperate for a bit of respite and physical autonomy. Besides, a mere stroke of the nipple, whoever it's from, can easily trigger milk let-down when you'd like to be thinking about almost anything else for five minutes. Non-essential use is simply not a priority, and there's no great hardship in pausing your boobs' other functions until you're back in business. After I finished nursing my two sons (at six months and seventeen months, respectively) I felt an overwhelming need to reclaim my body as my own, treating my tits to a load of sexy new bras (the first time I bought lovely underwear after my second baby was one of the most purely pleasurable moments of my life), allowing myself to enjoy them selfishly again and getting my first-ever tattoo. Whatever you do, it's a joy to enjoy your body again after several possible months of . . .

'Does my fanny look big in this?'

After pregnancy and particularly after vaginal delivery, it is entirely normal to temporarily lose all confidence in the sexual and aesthetic appeal of one's nether regions. Genitalia – rarely beautiful to begin with – can become even less so, but cosmetic appearance aside (tits-deep in nappies and PND, I simply couldn't summon the energy to care that my new fanny bore a passing resemblance to Sir Andrew Lloyd Webber), the vagina's functionality may also seem in jeopardy. After any tear, episiotomy, stitches or even just uncomplicated childbirth, one can become paralysed with fear that sexual intercourse will split your entire body in two (it won't. Your six-week gynae check will assess the healing and give either the green or amber light for sex). Meanwhile, one's partner can feel rejected, frustrated or jealous, putting pressure on you that worsens the anxiety and compounds the problem. The single best piece of advice I've ever heard on this came from Dr Petra Boynton during my own fear-driven sex drought: try without anyone present. A vibrator or other safe, inanimate object has no feelings, ego or emotional investment. Do several trial runs in the safety of solitude. Introduce a human only when you feel completely confident and secure that your fanny will remain painlessly intact.

Incidentally, a final note for the men: that hugely popular and completely hilarious analogy about how watching your wife give birth is

385

like seeing your favourite pub burn down. Please don't make it. It's rude, embarrassing, unfunny and misogynistic. It is endlessly dismaying to me that those who tell it ever manage to get laid again. Most decent spouses, male or female, will feel overwhelmingly proud of what their wife has achieved, and relieved just to be getting some action.

How not to become your partner's social secretary

For some reason, many men who are quite capable of going out, seeing friends and maintaining family contact when single, abrogate responsibility for the lot once in a relationship. Don't allow your partner to:

... surrender his social life

I have witnessed many newly coupled souls – and it is, in my experience, generally the men – failing to maintain their friendships in favour of time spent with their partner. This may be understandable and romantic in the first flush of love but don't let the pattern establish itself. Encourage your partner to make arrangements that don't include you.

... expect to be perennially involved in yours

386

Obviously, Doing Stuff Together is a fundamental joy of being in a relationship, whether with his friends and family, yours, or simply *à deux*. But you each have a right and a responsibility to enjoy your own social life without the other tagging along by default. So while you should of course be proud and happy to take each other to events, coming packaged non-negotiably as a couple is unattractive to others and unhealthy for you. If you break up, it can leave a partner who has abandoned his friendship group lonely, lost and with bridges to awkwardly rebuild.

... make you remember his family's birthdays

His phone's calendar has a 'repeat annually' function for a reason.

Why you really don't have to do date night

It's easy to believe that to keep the magic alive, you and your partner should, as often as possible, recreate whatever felt exciting when you initially got together. Couples in stagnating relationships are often advised, for instance, to make time for date nights, seemingly to relive the honeymoon period and remind each other of whatever it was that drew them together in the first place. But in perfectly contented relationships,

'A staggering four of my girlfriends routinely shagged Cowell in their pregnancy dreams, and never, ever again.'

too, couples can put themselves under pressure to recapture the electricity of courtship, seemingly worried that not doing so would be some kind of admission that the partnership is now effectively a two-person waiting room for death. The thing is, as a relationship matures, so the habits and rituals that mark its progress may gain or lose significance. Dressing to impress your partner possibly lacks the same impact now you're doing it alongside them. You may be sharing taxi costs, but now you might be factoring in babysitting expenses instead. After a hard day's work, the novelty of dragging yourself out for a pricy meal when there was perfectly serviceable quiche in the fridge may quickly pall. So instead of the Evening Dinner Date, consider the Daytime Mooch Date. If your kids are old enough to be left for a couple of hours on a Saturday morning, go out with your partner, having kept getting ready to an acceptable public-facing minimum, and have a local wander without any specific place to be or particular booking to fulfil. Pick up some bits for lunch, stop somewhere for coffee and cake, people-watch, peer into an estate agent's window and play 'fantasy pick a flat'. I much prefer this kind of date because, over a decade into my relationship, a low-key, idle mooch is a much better representation of the contented place we're at, and in turn I paradoxically find it much more romantic than the conscious effort of a sprauntzy dinner date. Fewer things feel more bonding and cosy than nipping out together for essential provisions, bringing them home and shutting out the world. Sometimes all that going out together achieves is making you realise how much you like staying in together.

But if you do want date night

Have sex first, before you go out. If you wait until you've been out for a three-course meal with wine and a side of dough balls, shagging is the very last thing you'll feel like doing. Do it while you're lighter, brighter and sprightlier. You'll be able to relax knowing you won't have to perform later, and enjoy the conspiratorial fun shared by two people who've just had sex. There is nothing lovelier than falling through the front door, tired, full and already sexually satisfied, knowing that what little is left of the evening can be spent watching *Schitt's Creek*.

How to go Dutch

Seriously. I thought the expectation that men always pay the bill on first dates died pre-*Baywatch*, but some women still support it. Lots, in fact – a third of twenty-four to thirty-five-year-old women and a quarter of us overall still think a man should pay the entire bill on a first date. Well over half of us think he should offer. How can any self-respecting person bear to even tick these boxes on an anonymous survey, never mind have the brass neck to make an affronted face at the presumption of equality? A straw poll of the single men in my life confirms that dating, for them, is an expensive business and, unsurprisingly, they resent it.

Why would anyone but Mrs Beeton endorse such a terrifically unfair dynamic? It's a question of manners, chivalry and tradition, apparently. But good manners means holding open a door, chewing with your mouth closed, being respectful and considerate. It's not 'good manners' for a man to feel obliged to pay more than his fair share – it's bad manners for anyone to expect a free ride purely by virtue of being born with ovaries. It's also a clear declaration from the very beginning of a relationship that its two participants are not equal in power or status. He is the provider, she should be provided for, regardless of whether she's a hospital porter, headteacher or hedge fund manager and he's counting pennies from a jam jar. As for tradition, that also prohibited us from inheriting money, owning property and opening a bank account, but we've happily confined those to the distant past. The tradition of women not paying their way stems necessarily from women having no means to pay, and being awarded only pin money for essentials. Tolerating a sexist, anachronistic ritual only when it leaves you up on the deal is a bad look and lets the remaining three-quarters of us right down.

One doesn't want to piss on the proverbial bonfire of anyone kind enough to want to pick up the tab, of course. There's nothing wrong with accepting dinner from a willing and solvent man or woman (provided he's not aggressively insistent and won't accept 'no, thanks' for an answer – if he is, then dinner is the least of your future worries), but it's a fine line between accepting generosity and expecting it as your god-given right. You wouldn't go to the pub with friends, order a drink, then duck out of your round, nor would you expect a total stranger to buy you a sandwich. So why expect a new man to buy your supper and your approval? If he suggests some wildly expensive restaurant you can't possibly stretch to,

389

'Tolerating a sexist,
anachronistic ritual
only when it leaves
you up on the deal is
a bad look.'

then do as you would with mates: say you'd prefer somewhere cheaper and see if he'd rather subsidise than miss out.

Which certainly isn't to say that paying for dinner is done only in reluctance. The joy in treating someone to a lovely evening can be equal to that experienced on the receiving end. But even if a man seemingly wants to pay and you're happy for him to, it's morally dubious to accept if you have absolutely no intention of ever seeing him again. It's certainly not about owing him anything in return for a steak supper, but about wanting to at least imagine a time when you might be able to repay the favour by treating him back. This is surely the nature of all relationships, romantic and otherwise. When I treat a friend to lunch, it's based on the tacit consensus that our friendship is ongoing, that we occasionally spoil one another, that our relationship is a comforting, perpetual exchange.

Besides, food is way too important to be conditional. To order extravagantly on someone else's dollar is even ruder, but order modestly out of politeness and you're cutting off your nose to spite your face. If I'm paying my way, I can order what I like and hang the consequences, whether that means ordering double measures and three extra sides, or guiltlessly shooing away his hand as it reaches towards my plate. Share the bill, never the chips.

Should one ever have break-up sex?

I know that, for many, this is as important a part of breaking up as the avoidance of your favourite coupley pub, and the pruning of romantic photos from your Instagram grid. And god knows, we should do what we need to do to push through the heartbreak. But personally, I don't do curtain calls and haven't for most of my romantic life. Mainly because, for me, what prompts me to accept that it's time to end things is the total loss of sexual intimacy, but also, because after the initial, mutual excitement over the transgressive nature of a passionate final fling, break-up sex always seems to make at least one person feel like shit. Usually, that person is the one who either initiated, or responded to, sexual advances in the hope that their exiting partner might rediscover such a deep connection that they decide to rethink the whole split. In reality, this practically never happens, and even when it does, one heightened sexual exchange is hardly a solid foundation on which to repair something that, just thirty minutes ago, seemed irreparably fractured.

It's normal and right to feel sad when a relationship ends – that doesn't mean the decision is wrong. Break-up sex halts the progress of acceptance, hinders recovery and can easily send someone who was just about coping crashing back into feeling rejected and confused – and understandably so. At best, one party will feel fine post-coitus and even that is dependent on their own ability to disregard the other's feelings (which may, of course, be the source of the whole sorry problem). Beyond a forbidden, furtive shag, what possible good can come of it all?

How to leave a bad first date

I still get shivers thinking about the episode of Channel 4's *First Dates* in which one participant brutally departed during the lunch, having concluded that the poor sap sitting opposite was so unsuitable as not even to be worthy of a polite, post-date 'thanks-but-no-thanks'. He may have regarded his bluntness as a kindness, but even without factoring in the added humiliation of being dumped mid-starter under the unblinking eye of a fixed-rig camera, there is a more humane way to extract yourself from the kind of date where you quickly realise 'first' is also going to be 'only'.

392

An excuse made up on the spot to explain a hurried departure may get you the hell out of Dodge, but frankly, only the least perceptive of dates won't realise you've concocted it for the purpose. Moreover, you'll know they know and you'll leave with a pinch of guilt and awkwardness. Much better to get your excuse in at kick-off. On arrival, apologise and explain that you may have to leave early because of a Previously Unforeseen Thing. At an apposite moment (apparently), check a text during a loo visit and, on your return, if you need an escape, mournfully explain that the PUT has come to pass and you need to go. This will carry a much greater air of legitimacy than some kind of spontaneous nursery flood or granny fire that's conveniently occurred just as conversation's run dry. Conversely, if the date's going well, you can return to the table with the great news that the PUT has blessedly gone away and you're free to continue your evening together. And if it's going really well, you might even confess that the whole thing was just a ruse.

Why bad boys are an absolute waste of your time

Why do so many women still describe their ideal type as 'a bad boy'? My single male friends tell me they're still told this frequently on dates, and I'm surprised to hear it. I suppose that having been in long-term relationships with two emotionally unavailable, sexually messed-up, power-game-playing, commitment-phobic narcissists in my distant youth, I had rather optimistically assumed that the appeal of the bad boy had died the moment I finally came to my senses. A little research and I find to my horror that the appeal of these men isn't just prevalent – it appears also to be scientific fact. A study at Durham University into the bad-boy phenomenon showed that female undergraduates (I suspect age is a big factor here) were more likely to be sexually attracted to men possessing 'the dark triad' of narcissism, psychopathy and Machiavellianism. Common traits of this type include 'a desire for attention, admiration, favours and prestige; the manipulation, exploitation, deceit and flattery of others; a lack of remorse, morality concerns and sensitivity, and cynicism'.

As baffling as this seems, I know these traits all too well, and also how, within a relationship, they can gradually trick you into a skewed sense of what's normal. Bad boy makes it sound much jollier than it is, as though these men are iconoclastic teen-idol types like James Dean. The reality of life with a bad boy, however, is a drip-fed diet of gentle criticism and push-pull affection designed to keep you exactly at clutch biting point. This may involve being routinely chucked out of bed post-coitus because 'I'm not ready for a girlfriend', or being dumped on your birthday, only to be wooed back a week later when he's bored and lonely. It can mean not receiving a Christmas present despite investing several years of your time in someone, because it's all 'just conformist crap', or enduring a cavalier attitude to monogamy because he would rather not be confined to the dreary societal norms you've swallowed unquestioningly (reader, all these things actually happened to me). All this is justified by beat writer clichés and dreary sob stories about how his dad didn't love him. It's not always this dramatic, of course. The tiny, insidious stuff has even greater effect. Missed dates and put-downs, days without so much as a text, last-minute no-shows because something better has come up, the constant reminders that one shouldn't get ideas above one's station.

Ask a bad-boy chaser why she persists in courting these dreadful men and she will often say, 'Nice guys are dull; I want someone who's

393

not a pushover', as though men can't possibly be expected to stand up for themselves unless they have a cruel streak (try telling a nice cardigan-wearing nerd that his awful trainers need binning and see weapons-grade stubbornness in action). Nice people are dull insofar as they're reliable. Reliable is wonderful. Reliability is knowing that someone would never stay out all night without calling to let you know they're not getting laid or murdered. Reliability is someone who doesn't equate your request for a lift from the station after dark with a desire to be married and impregnated with triplets. It's frying you some eggs, ensuring his phone is switched on, not leering at your embarrassed friends, and neither noticing nor caring that you've gained five pounds in Christmas brie. It's a returned text, a sincere expression of emotion without an ulterior motive; it's deciding he really likes someone and making the uncomplicated decision to see lots of them. Reliability is being told you're lovely and not being too terrified to say it back.

Unhelpfully, our culture buys into poor behaviour as a romantic idea. The internet is awash with 'fun' features about how we all love a bad boy, many of them dispensing advice on how to conduct oneself around someone who already doesn't deserve us. This is absolutely infuriating because it encourages women to join in the game of emotional dysfunction. Don't sleep with him on the first date! Don't return his calls! Don't say, 'I love you'! Wait at least one hour before replying to a text! But despite the gazillion Google hits suggesting the contrary, here's the crucial thing one learns: you will never change him. Not because he's some untamable free spirit, but because he's an arsehole with arrested development, who has learned over time that you will put up with behaviour that erodes your identity and sense of self-worth. He either doesn't like you enough, doesn't like himself enough, or both. He might, deep down, be capable of good, but it's too late for you to be on its receiving end.

The way one actually deals with bad boys is far more organic. One becomes hopelessly, irredeemably bored. The occasional laughs and memories of great sex get lost in a tedious and lonely existence of tongue-biting, second guessing and constant, low-level ennui. One becomes too embarrassed to discuss his behaviour with friends, too fatigued by this parallel universe of headfucks, outside of which, other people are just hanging out and watching telly with their loved ones, feeling annoyed about enviably tangible stuff like unemptied dishwashers and disappointing takeaways. Ordinary, unexciting, emotionally healthy

'If your lady boner is activated by someone treating you as unworthy of love, attention or care, then some stereotypical bad boy is the least of your worries.'

lives become almost pornographic in their appeal, until one day: enough. Off you pop. Then you look at yourself and ask how you ended up with someone who treats you like a nobody, and whether you've been unconsciously trying to prove to yourself that they're right. Are you persistently pursuing men who reinforce your own ambivalent feelings about yourself? If your lady boner is activated by someone treating you as unworthy of love, attention or care, then some stereotypical bad boy is the least of your worries. He's just a sideshow and a distraction from the essential work that you're going to need to do on yourself.

Should you change your name?

Keep yours, adopt your partner's, hyphenate both? Prefix any of the above with 'Ms'? The simple answer is, thankfully, that you should do whatever you like. I never considered changing my name. Equality is a factor – if my partner isn't expected to change his name, then why should I? Why should I even declare my marital status when engaging in everyday life admin such as booking an eye test or renewing a railcard? Beyond that, I'm not sure political opinions aren't a bit of a red herring. It seems to me that the trend for maintaining one's own legal identity is less about advertising my feminism than enjoying the self-worth and maintaining the individual freedoms that hard-fought feminism has given me. I didn't keep my name (both times) to make a point. I kept it because it's my name. It's who I am. Not someone's wife, nor someone's mother. But myself. That said, I'm hardly going to lose it if the odd piece of junk mail arrives wrongly addressed to 'Mrs Maier'.

Other women tell me they wanted to change their names so they could share a name with their children. I understand and respect this rationale entirely, but it was one of the many reasons I didn't want to change mine. I adore my children, but I felt an unequivocal desire to hang on to a part of the old me, albeit a symbolic one. I wanted to retain a piece of myself that had nothing to do with my role as a mother, but represented the fully formed person that had existed before them. I was very happy for them to take their father's name, because I had no desire to cause upset and, crucially, it would be my sons' only name from birth. It's the switch later in life that seems so alien to me.

I'm told some women simply have no emotional attachment to their old names. But how, I always wonder? Hughes is the name that was called out in class registration, sandwiched between the same two pupils for years on end. It was the name on my first pay cheque for forty pounds, and the one on the fake ID I used to blow it all on. It was the name on the pass certificate handed to me in the driving test centre car park, on the passport that took me on my first, vodka-soaked, menthol-smoked, Teletext-booked, £170 girls' holiday to Mallorca. It was the name I first saw in a magazine, under a hundred-word review of a forgettable film called *Drop Dead Fred*, which told me now I'd really made it. It's the name I've seen spelled 'Sally Huges' at least a thousand times and the one that's compelled me to take on any idiot who's accused my legitimate Welsh name as some media affectation. Sali Hughes is the person who worked through more difficult times, who shouldn't have to skulk away and let Sali Maier reap the benefits. How can there be no emotional attachment to it? It's my name. It's who I've been since birth. A lovely man with a lovely name will never change that.

And ironically, the man who gave his wife that name, and ultimately gave me the same, is the person who knew that I'd never give it up. On my first wedding day, my father – not an outwardly emotional man – made a speech that, in about seven minutes flat, told me he knew me better than anyone. 'Even if Sali was marrying a man called Hughes, I know she'd bloody refuse to change her name,' he said. And he was right. So I am, as a married woman, Ms Sali Hughes. Choose whichever combination you want. It's no one's business but yours, and convention should be the least of your considerations.

Questions to ask before getting hitched *(marriage or civil partnership)*

I think just these nine specific questions, asked seriously and frankly before you put a ring on it, should pay dividends and keep you out of the courts.

1. How much money do you have?
   Hear me out. This is not about being minted. It's about whether you measure your answer according to the black balance on your current account, or by the limit figure on your credit card. This is the fundamental divider of people (well, that and 'cheese or chocolate', 'Madonna or Kylie'. The former in both cases, obviously).

If you are debt-averse while your partner is a buy-now, pay-later type, or vice versa, then you have a potentially big source of future conflict on your hands. Couples argue about money more than anything else, and however eye-rollingly quirky, inconsequential and even romantic your partner's excessive spending habits seem in the beginning, I guarantee that when the scales fall away, they will make you feel nervous, financially insecure and resentful.

2. What are your energy levels?

There's a great deal to be said for one of you having the impetus and motivation to wrench you both off the sofa and into the weekend, but a dramatic mismatch, in which he needs a packed schedule of activities and you need to alternate *Queer Eye* and *Drag Race* with a Toblerone balanced on your boobs, will cause rot to set in unless you're both happy to spend lots of your free time apart.

3. What does paradise look like?

You need someone you can travel with, and the honeymoon is too late to discover you can't. Holiday compatibility is extremely important (be suspicious of any man who forces you to ski, is my advice), because there are few things more annoying than someone pestering you to visit monuments, memorials and water parks when your ideal state is burning through a Jacqueline Susann, half-cut on rum. Tiresome for you, frustrating for any partner shelling out for the privilege of twiddling their thumbs over a precious fortnight off work. The same goes for destinations. If someone likes alpine hiking while another likes frying on a beach, then you're either going to have to make huge compromises (alternate years with good grace) or holiday separately with friends.

4. How much sex is enough?

The legendary scene in *Annie Hall* where a couple sits in separate analysts' offices, on a split screen, discussing how often they have sex, best sums up the corrosive issue of mismatched libido. 'Hardly ever – maybe three times a week,' he complains. 'Constantly. I'd say three times a week,' she groans. At the risk of damning myself publicly, three times a week is neither typical nor realistic in the long term. Sex ebbs and flows. In all likelihood, there will be the joy of an unexplained purple patch where sex happens daily for a few weeks, drought periods where one or both partners are too knackered, stressed or physically inhibited to initiate it, bookended by long spells of 'we can't live without it so really must make time for it' relative harmony. But if one person's default is banging while another's is a boxset, then that gap is likely to widen over time, and that's not fair on either party. Choosing someone with a libido in the same ballpark as yours is setting yourself up for success.

5. What time is bedtime?

Are you up and showered when clubbers are finally falling into their pits? Or are you watching films until all hours and sleeping it off the next day? Whether you're a morning or night person, choosing a diametrically opposed partner can be problematic. If you're content to share a bed for only a few hours a night, then great. But if you'll be intolerant of him barely staying awake through *EastEnders*, or furiously opening curtains at 10 a.m. like the mother of a teenager, then ask yourself if your body clocks are actually a ticking timebomb.

6. Does 'family' mean you or everyone?

A great deal of importance is placed on agreeing plans for future children before committing to marriage (and it's certainly vital), but people rarely stop to think about the wider family, and whether people want to marry them, too. One man I know comes home most days from work to find his very nice mother-in-law's car parked in the drive, and her seated at the kitchen table, drinking his tea and chatting to his wife. This drives him almost as mad as it would me, but she's never known anything else. Trust me, these things can become huge. Ditto holidaying with your in-laws, visiting for every Sunday lunch, handing over front door keys to extended family, having them proffer an opinion on everything from where you should bank to what you should call your first-born. What's normal, happy and healthy for one person can be an intolerable invasion of privacy for another. There's no right or wrong, no legislating for background and family. But it can be very hard to undo, even unfair to try to tinker with, an intensely close relationship between someone and their parents. Make it crystal clear what you can and can't handle before marrying into the mob.

7. What are their interests?

People who believe your interests must be the same are plain greedy – it's hard enough finding a good mate without making their acceptance conditional on a love of Ian Rankin and salsa. All that really matters is whether you're okay with how important those

399

interests are to your partner. If football means he's gone every Saturday for a match and every Sunday for training, and he has no intention of scaling back, then that's hardly a straight swap for your thrice-yearly attendance at comedy gigs. On the other hand, their occasional weekend spent walking in the country while you batch-cook a freezer full of curry is a gift from the relationship gods.

8. What are their ambitions?

It takes, if not a village to build a career, then at least a couple. It is completely manageable, occasionally even preferable, if one partner is way more ambitious than the other. Someone invariably needs to be able to take their foot off the gas and put on a whites wash while the other is focused on world domination. But, the critical question is: are you okay with your partner's level of aspiration? If their ambition results in success, will you be proud, or might you be jealous? Will you resent the time they spend on their career when you'd like to clock off at 5 p.m. and talk about the state of your basil plant? Or do you have bigger ambitions for your partner than they have for themselves, and will you be embarrassed and frustrated if they're content with a middling career and a nice sit-down? These questions are pivotal to the success of both your marriage and your respective careers. Don't just wait to see how it goes.

9. How noisy are they?

I am convinced someone's relationship with silence can be a success or failure indicator in their relationship with you. If you feel sitting in silence signals a problem that needs to be talked through, or suggests that a human connection is faulty, then finding someone who feels similarly can save everyone's time and feelings. Likewise, if sitting in companionable silence is a state of grace for you, then you'd do well to choose someone who doesn't need the affirmation of constant human contact and conversation. That said, for much of my non-working life I am essentially mute, while my husband is the noisiest person I've ever met – singing, relentlessly talking to himself, the dog, the radio and me – but the crucial point here is that he doesn't mind in the slightest that I simply ignore him for at least 90 per cent of the time. If he took it personally or I didn't tolerate it, we'd have a big problem. The key question, as ever, is not 'are we the same?' but 'can I spend the rest of my life contractually bound to our differences?'

Why you should only marry someone you can drive with

A simpatico approach to long car journeys is a real relationship plus, not least in how it can affect whatever's happening at the end of the trip. A weekend away will get a lovely kick-start if you've had a laugh on the drive there. Likewise, the veil of melancholy that can drift over a long trip home from a lovely holiday or event can often be ameliorated by an agreeable post-mortem or cheerful mutual distraction on the way back. Conversely, a tense and irritable voyage can only psychologically eat into time away or compound the misery of your return.

If you're both chatterboxes, then good conversation will speed the journey. But crucially, companionable travelling often means making a friend of silence. If one traveller prefers quiet on the road, defer to them, especially if they're the driver. Have some distractions planned – if you or your partner generally struggle to concentrate on podcasts, a moving tin box on a featureless road might prove the ideal environment to share one. Make your own fun with a cheap service-station compilation CD and play Beat the Intro (we do this on every long journey). Save the driver from boredom by googling quizzes to read them on the motorway. Stop for snacks – there's a conspiratorial pleasure in loading up on and sharing bags of the kind of sweets, crisps and chocolate you'd never normally look at twice.

401

How to have maintenance sex

According to studies, we are having less sex than we used to. This drop in sexual intercourse is attributed to a variety of external factors, both extremely positive – such as the increased empowerment and autonomy of young adults over their sex lives – and worrying – an overall increase in working hours and in digital distractions such as social media and home entertainment streaming. It would seem that 'Netflix and chill' is often far from a euphemism for sexual contact, but a displacement activity to avoid it. It stands to reason that the less we have to do, the more we make our own fun (and babies – more are conceived in the cold, dark, tedious months than in autumn, spring or summer), and conversely, when we have too much to do, sex becomes less of a priority. Quite simply, we may be too busy tweeting and watching *The Crown* to have sex with our partners.

This is of particular interest to me, since I've known several women who complain about not having enough sex, and the myriad stories legitimise my often scoffed-at belief that their partners should regularly

'The crude reality is that it's hard to be furious about an empty rinse aid dispenser or a damp towel on the floor when you've recently been given head.'

make time for it – whether or not both parties completely fancy it at the moment the opportunity presents itself. It's not a question of stoically 'lying back and thinking of England' and certainly never about doing anything against one's will. But in a busy, demanding life, sex is like going to the gym or putting out the bins – we may not always feel motivated to do it, but we should look at the wider, long-term benefits and at least consider cracking on.

This is a deeply unpopular view, I do realise. By today's standards, sex should be wonderful, romantic, sexy, adventurous, athletic, mutually climactic. Both parties should be wholly focused, thoroughly warmed up and equally turned on. I worry our expectations of Hollywood-style 'good sex' have become so idealised that we've forgotten the importance of a good old-fashioned maintenance shag. The sexual equivalent of making a slice of toast rather than cooking a full English, this sort of straightforward seeing-to has few bells and whistles but can be just as satisfying and necessary. It's this sort of convenient, timely sex, not the soft-lit, sensual marathon (which, let's face it, happens only on high days and holidays), that oils the cogs of the relationship machine. We neglect it at our peril.

For most of us, sex is important not just because we need it, but because it represents a unique connection between two people that has nothing to do with our friends, kids or colleagues. As importantly, it makes us more forgiving of myriad infuriating things that would, without shared physical intimacy, make us want to hack up our partner's jumpers with a breadknife. The crude reality is that it's hard to be furious about an empty rinse aid dispenser or a damp towel on the floor when you've recently been given head. For the sake of continued or renewed harmony, it's invariably worth turning off the telly or putting down the iPad to get naked for a bit (my friend S says sex with her husband of fifteen years is like going to the cinema: 'Every time I do it, I thoroughly enjoy it and wonder why we don't go more often'). One may not instinctively be in the mood, but within the confines of a loving, mutually respectful relationship, one rarely regrets having sex, only avoids getting started. When it's all over, one is usually delighted and relieved to have gone for it, even if it hasn't begun as enthusiastically for one or both of you.

Naturally, some relationships simply don't need sex to survive or even thrive. Amiable companionship, kissing, hugging and shared interests are enough to sustain many marriages, no doubt. Often, one

403

partner's difficult labour, breastfeeding or menopause, or either party's physical or mental health, forces sex out of the relationship, either temporarily or permanently, and people make the best of a bad situation, as they vowed to if they are married. But when there are no mitigating factors, merely laziness, disinterest or the distraction of everyday life, the success of a sexless relationship depends on the serendipitous likelihood of both partners feeling exactly the same way. How often are two people so completely in sync as to want very little or no sex? Much more likely is that one half of the relationship is tolerating the other and would very much like it in their lives (I most often hear of men not putting out, but your mileage and social group may, of course, vary), or worse, is feeling wounded, rejected and dissatisfied.

Some ebb and flow in sexual appetite is normal, but I know from experience that too much ebb can be terminal. A month becomes three and before you know it, over a year may have passed. It's not fair to withdraw sex from someone's life without consultation and consent. It's a bit like coming home from the office and announcing that you've decided you'll never again go on holiday, or eat in a restaurant, or travel anywhere by car. And yet it happens frequently. Instead of simply compromising to bridge the perfectly manageable gap between two libidos, people just stop having sex altogether.

I don't believe many of us want that. But kids, work and extracurricular activities can easily aid our avoidance. Flopping on the sofa to watch a boxset can seem a more relaxing way to spend rare downtime. It's easier to lie in bed waiting for an available wireless network than to reconnect with your partner. But it's also unrealistic to expect the mood to always strike both of you at the same moment, and at a time when sex is practical. What is realistic is to mentally flip through your household's calendar, think 'this may be the last chance we have this week' and squeeze in a swift one before the kids get home from LaserZone. There's something bonding and actually pretty funny about saying 'we can't be arsed to have sex, but we really need to' and mucking in for the good of the relationship, even if it's with an eye on the clock and an ear to the front door. If you hold out for Occasion Sex, you may find it becomes fatally occasional. Don't underestimate the relationship-nourishing power of the routine rooting.

Should you cohabit?

I've lived with four boyfriends and each relationship has benefited hugely from the opportunity to try before I buy. For me, two-home courtship has a definite shelf life. Cabbing across town to shag urgently on the staircase may seem sexy, but what's in no way hot is pulling on yesterday's tights to wear to work the next morning. The Holly Golightly fantasy fades fast when you're permanently lugging an overnight bag, or realising that once again you've been caught short and your hairdryer, charger or Tampax are miles away, while you sit in an XL Inspiral Carpets T-shirt and face cream that smells of turps. Even if you manage to secure a drawer at his, one of you is always out of their own space, searching for the right frying pan or tutting at the dispensing direction of the toilet roll (over, for god's sake, over). It's at this point that it's wise to consider how long you can stand the status quo, and whether it might be worth pooling resources and moving in together.

How to divvy up chores

Chores are not the place to get political. May the best cook cook. Often that will be the woman, often not, but I guarantee you will no longer give a damn about gender stereotypes when he's insisted on making you his 'killer spag bol' and you've had to swallow down sick. Living together is about knowing who's good at what and allocating jobs accordingly (and evenly). I'm a good cook and launderer, but I am useless at hoovering and assembling flatpack, as well as wholly unwilling to iron. My skill set (and mood) benefits heavily from the presence of a partner who can grout, rewire and catch mice. I'll happily do spiders and clean the loo. Which reminds me . . .

405

To lock the bathroom or not?

Around 90 per cent of living together is bathroom. Whether you're a door locker or not, you are going to have to accept that you will now know too much about one another's toilet habits. One boyfriend always sat down to pee. I knew quickly we had no future. My friend rightly got rid of hers when he wandered in on her treaty bubble bath, pulled down his jeans and sat down to poo. You will need to decide early on whether you will pee openly, lock doors, both fart, or spend your weekends in constipated agony, sending him on pointless errands just so you can relieve yourself in peace. On the bright side, you may one day dangerously overstretch your borrowing capability in order to get two loos with his and hers washbasins (truly, I am finally living the dream).

How to respect the privacy of loved ones

We can all understand the impulse. There are many reasons why one might be inclined to snoop, even feel justified in doing so. One acquaintance was so worried her teenage daughter was covering up her boyfriend's coercive control that she read her diary, and she was right. Another was concerned that her fifteen-year-old was smoking weed, and so checked his texts for potential drug deals and perhaps some nonsensical wittering about King Crimson and Crunchy Nut cornflakes. There were none, only a load more probably innocent exchanges that sparked ten entirely new neuroses. I myself monitored my children's Instagram activity and routinely vetted their follower requests because that's just being net smart. Even now, I am pretty sure I'd read anything private if I was truly worried about either of my kids. It's my job to protect them until they're old enough to do it themselves.

406

Adults are surely a different matter. We're autonomous; big enough to look after ourselves. No one is entitled to know every innermost thought of another human and no relationship, however close, should be without a basic data protection policy. We most of us lock the bathroom door when we nip to the loo, so why should we accept our partners having access-all-areas to our brains? Besides, without context, almost any narrative is unreliable. We impose onto our partner's typed thoughts and statements our own bias, perceptions and insecurities. A woman texting 'lovely to see you earlier' probably bumped into your partner unexpectedly and is just being nice because real life tends to be undramatic and nuanced, but our imaginations are more exciting and dogmatic. Snooping on a partner yields only two possible results: a guilty or innocent verdict.

One of the even bigger problems with snooping is that it usually arms the spy with information while compromising their opportunity to act on it. You might throw caution to the wind and confess if your discovery is so awful that your snooping pales by comparison (one acquaintance discovered via Facebook Messenger that his wife had been having an affair for three years, and felt her actions more than justified

'If you hold out for Occasion Sex, you may find it becomes fatally occasional.'

his means), but more often than not, you're likely to come away with little more than a few normal everyday criticisms of your life together, and inadmissible evidence of an idle flirtation with someone inconsequential. Then what? You like them less for only being human, and you daren't discuss it because you've broken your partner's trust.

To hack into someone's private world represents the crossing of a Rubicon that I believe can never end well. Those who disagree have clearly never been spied on themselves. Because to be the victim of relationship hacking is to know a unique sense of violation. Every word typed or thought expressed is reinterpreted and skewed, every action is logged or met with suspicion. One can fall almost instantly out of love. Nowadays, many years after my one relationship with a compulsive snooper, I still don't like people picking up my phone – even my kids. There's nothing sinister on it – no clandestine meeting plans, no dubious browser history, no nude selfies (I'm grateful to come from a generation for whom this was never really A Thing) – just thousands of pictures of kids, daft dogs and skin creams, and a load of unread five-year-old messages warning me of unclaimed PPI. But I desperately need some privacy. And however tempting it is to snoop, I believe very strongly that you deserve yours.

'To be the victim of
relationship hacking
is to know a unique
sense of violation.'

Index